Laboratory Manual

FOR EXERCISE PHYSIOLOGY, EXERCISE TESTING, AND PHYSICAL FITNESS

Terry J. Housh
UNIVERSITY OF NEBRASKA–LINCOLN

Joel T. Cramer
UNIVERSITY OF NEBRASKA–LINCOLN

Joseph P. Weir
UNIVERSITY OF KANSAS

Travis W. Beck
UNIVERSITY OF OKLAHOMA

Glen O. Johnson
UNIVERSITY OF NEBRASKA–LINCOLN

Holcomb Hathaway, Publishers
Scottsdale, Arizona
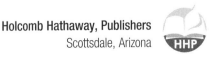

Library of Congress Cataloging-in-Publication Data

Names: Housh, Terry J., author.
Title: Laboratory manual for exercise physiology, exercise testing, and physical fitness /
Terry J. Housh, University of Nebraska-Lincoln [and five others].
Description: Scottsdale, Arizona : Holcomb Hathaway, Publishers, Inc., [2016]
  | Includes index.
Identifiers: LCCN 2015039040 | ISBN 9781621590460 (print) | ISBN 9781621590477
  (ebook)
Subjects: LCSH: Exercise—Psychological aspects—Laboratory manuals. |
  Exercise tests—Laboratory manuals. | Physical
  fitness—Testing—Laboratory manuals.
Classification: LCC QP301 .H76 2016 | DDC 612/.044078—dc23 LC record available at
http://lccn.loc.gov/2015039040

Photo Credits: *Front cover:* Maxim Petrichuk/123RF. *Back cover,* magiceyes/123RF. *Page 1,*
Cathy Yeulet/123RF; *page 45,* Tono Balaguer/123RF; *page 101,* Patrick Chai/123RF; *page 169,*
Hongqi Zhang/ 123RF; *page 201,* Aleksandar Mijatovic/123RF; *page 211,* Scott Griessel/
123RF; *page 247,* ifong/123RF; *page 309,* Wavebreak Media Ltd/123RF.

Please note: The authors and publisher have made every effort to provide current website
addresses in this book. However, because web addresses change constantly, it is inevitable
that some of the URLs listed here will change following publication of this book.

Holcomb Hathaway, Publishers, Inc.
8700 E. Via de Ventura Blvd., Suite 265
Scottsdale, Arizona 85258
480-991-7881
www.hh-pub.com

10   9   8   7   6   5   4   3   2   1

Print ISBN: 978-1-62159-046-0
Ebook ISBN: 978-1-62159-047-7

Printed in the United States of America.

Contents

UNIT 5
MUSCULAR ENDURANCE   201

UNIT 6
MUSCULAR POWER   211

UNIT 7
BODY COMPOSITION AND BODY BUILD   247

Preface

Over the past several decades, we have seen a dramatic increase in interest in physical fitness as it relates to health and sports performance. As a result, the number of academic programs that train professionals in the various scientific aspects of exercise and sport science, as well as healthy lifestyles, has also increased. These programs often are designed to prepare students for careers in physical activity settings such as health clubs, the Y, and corporate fitness centers, as well as public and private schools, venues in which a health and fitness orientation is becoming commonplace. Typically, college and university courses in exercise and sport sciences departments include not only classroom work, but also laboratory and active learning experiences. *Laboratory Manual for Exercise Physiology, Exercise Testing, and Physical Fitness* is a comprehensive text to address the needs of institutions with sophisticated laboratories and equipment as well as those that do not have the equipment, facilities, and/or budget to provide students with high-tech lab experiences.

This text is designed for exercise physiology, exercise testing, physical fitness, and wellness courses, among others. It covers seven major components of physical fitness and sport performance: aerobic fitness, fatigue thresholds, muscular strength, muscular endurance, muscular power, body composition and body build, and flexibility. In addition, an introductory section includes labs for Participation Health Screening, Medical Clearance and Informed Consent, Measuring Heart Rate, Measuring Blood Pressure, Resting and Exercise Electrocardiogram, and Pulmonary Function. The laboratories include norms and classification tables, allowing students to determine how their results, and those of their subjects, compare to non-athletes of the same age and gender as well as, in some cases, athletes in various sports. Laboratories include the following sections:

Background: Provides students with the information they'll need to understand what will be measured/assessed in the laboratory.

Terms and Abbreviations: Familiarize students with the vocabulary and symbols used throughout the lab.

Procedures: Offer step-by-step directions that are clear and logical with photographic examples to provide a visual guide to students for the various lab procedures.

Equations and Sample Calculations: Allow students the opportunity to apply basic mathematics, statistical analyses, and computer applications to discussions of how the systems of the body work. Many of the laboratories in this text involve the application of mathematical modeling to physiological systems.

Lab Worksheets: Enable students to perform the given lab using either themselves or classmates as subjects and to record their results.

Extension Activities and Questions: Provide students with additional opportunities to practice the lab procedures and explore issues of validity, reliability, and accuracy related to the lab.

ABOUT THE AUTHORS

The authors of this text have a common association through the University of Nebraska–Lincoln. Over the years, these associations have grown into close friendships, making the opportunity to coauthor this text a true personal and professional pleasure. Glen O. Johnson (along with William G. Thorland) began the Ph.D. program in Exercise Physiology at UNL in the late 1970s. Johnson served as a mentor to the other coauthors of this manual, and Terry J. Housh was the first Ph.D. graduate in 1984. Joseph P. Weir, Joel T. Cramer, and Travis W. Beck received Ph.D. degrees in 1993, 2003, and 2007, respectively. Currently, Johnson, Housh, and Cramer are professors in the Department of Nutrition and Health Sciences at UNL and continue to advise Exercise Physiology doctoral students. Weir is a professor and Chair of the Department of Health, Sport, and Exercise Sciences at the University of Kansas. Beck is an associate professor in the Department of Health and Exercise Science at the University of Oklahoma, where he mentors Exercise Physiology Ph.D. students. In addition to this manual, the authors worked together on *Physical Fitness Laboratories on a Budget* and on the text *Introduction to Exercise Science* (both published by Holcomb Hathaway) with Terry Housh and Glen Johnson as authors and editors. Joel Cramer and Travis Beck were chapter contributors. Terry Housh is also coauthor of *Applied Exercise and Sport Physiology*, Fourth Edition (Holcomb Hathaway, 2016).

Unit 1

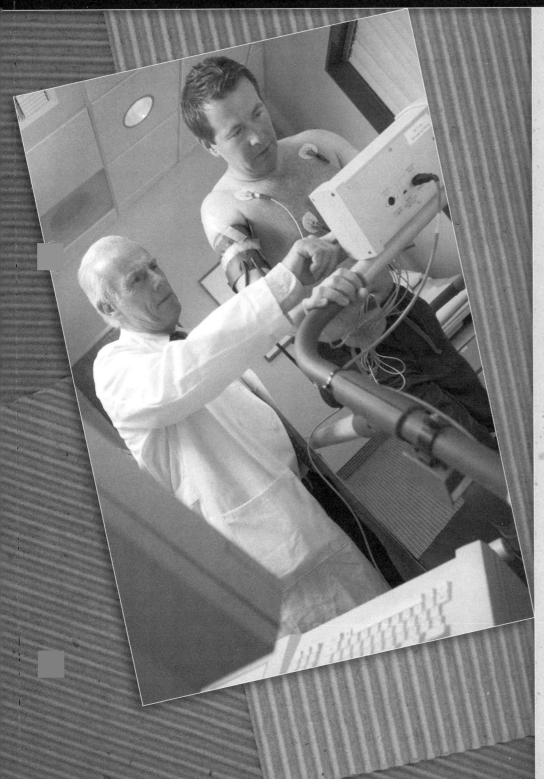

BACKGROUND

The American College of Sports Medicine (ACSM) recommends that medical supervision is not necessary during exercise for healthy individuals (children, adolescents, men <45 years of age, and women <55 years of age) who have no symptoms or known presence of heart disease or major coronary risk factors.[1] Therefore, the primary purpose of preparticipation health screening is to identify those individuals who should be excluded from exercise due to medical contraindications.

The ACSM has provided recommendations for preparticipation health screening procedures for various populations.[1] Specifically, the ACSM defines preparticipation health screening as a three-step process that involves: (a) risk stratification and medical clearance, (b) additional preparticipation assessment, and (c) exercise test considerations. Of these three steps, risk stratification and medical clearance are the most important for performing exercise testing with healthy individuals. Additional preparticipation assessment and exercise test considerations are necessary when evaluating the elderly and individuals with disease conditions that could limit their ability to perform physical activity.

In addition, it may be important to have potential participants complete an informed consent document. The primary purpose of the informed consent document is to provide potential participants with clear and exact information about what they will be required to do during the exercise test. When participants fully understand what they must do, they will be instructed to sign the informed consent document, after which they will be allowed to do the exercise test. Page 4 shows an example of an informed consent document for a maximum one-repetition bench press (1-RM strength test).

With the exception of clinical exercise physiology laboratories and cardiac rehabilitation centers, most exercise science laboratories examine normal, healthy individuals. However, some individuals may not be aware of their risk stratification, so it is essential that careful screening procedures be completed. If the results of a preparticipation health screening questionnaire indicate that an individual may be at a health risk for exercise, the individual should be encouraged to obtain medical clearance before participation. Determination of whether an individual is actually at risk for exercise can, however, be vague. Thus, the purpose of this laboratory is to describe the procedures used to perform preparticipation health screening.

KNOW THESE TERMS & ABBREVIATIONS

- ACSM = American College of Sports Medicine
- 1-RM = one-repetition maximum
- PAR-Q = Physical Activity Readiness Questionnaire
- risk stratification = categorization of the likelihood of untoward events based on the screening and evaluation of patient health characteristics

PROCEDURES

(See photo 1.1.) An individual's risk during exercise can be assessed with a medical screening instrument such as the Physical Activity Readiness Questionnaire (PAR-Q; see page 5) or a Pre-exercise Testing Health Status Questionnaire (see pages 6–7). The PAR-Q is a common medical screening instrument used by many exercise physiology laboratories. The procedures used to determine risk stratification from both the PAR-Q and Pre-exercise Testing Health Status Questionnaire are described below.

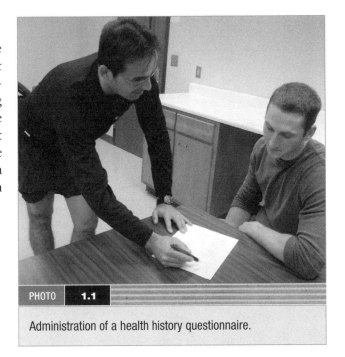

PHOTO **1.1**

Administration of a health history questionnaire.

PAR-Q

1. Begin administering the PAR-Q by instructing the individual to complete the first seven questions.

2. If the individual answers "yes" to one or more of the first seven questions, instruct him or her to contact a physician before performing any exercise. Inform the individual that he or she should tell the physician which questions had "yes" answers on the PAR-Q. The individual should also ask the physician what exercise tests should or should not be performed.

3. If the individual answers "no" to all of the first seven questions, he or she should be allowed to perform the exercise test.

Pre-exercise Testing Health Status Questionnaire

1. Begin the Pre-exercise Testing Health Status Questionnaire by instructing the individual to complete the general information at the top of the questionnaire and sections A through G.

2. Examine the completed questionnaire and determine whether the individual can safely perform the exercise test that you are asking him or her to do. If you feel that the individual may be at a health risk during the exercise test, instruct him or her to contact a physician and receive medical clearance before performing the test.

REFERENCE

1. American College of Sports Medicine. *ACSM's Guidelines for Exercise Testing and Prescription*, 9th edition. Baltimore: Wolters Kluwer/Lippincott Williams & Wilkins, 2014.

INFORMED CONSENT FOR A BENCH PRESS 1-RM TEST

1. Purpose and Explanation of the Test

You will perform a one-repetition maximum (1-RM) bench press strength test using an Olympic barbell, weight plates, and a standard free weight bench. To begin the test, you will perform a warm-up with just the barbell. For each warm-up repetition, you will be required to lower the weight to your chest and then press it upward until your forearms are fully extended. Following the warm-up repetitions, additional weight will be added to the bar, and you will be asked to perform one repetition. If you can successfully complete the repetition, you will be allowed to rest for two minutes while additional weights are added to the bar. You will then be asked to perform one repetition with the new weight. Weights will be continually added to the bar until you are no longer able to complete the movement throughout the full range of motion. The heaviest weight that you were able to lift once will be your bench press 1-RM.

2. Attendant Risks and Discomforts

There is a slight possibility of straining or tearing a muscle during the bench press 1-RM test. Elevations in blood pressure and lightheadedness immediately after the strength test may occur. You may experience muscle soreness for a few days after the test. Every effort will be made to minimize potential risks by allowing for a thorough warm-up prior to the 1-RM test.

3. Responsibilities of the Participant

Information you present about your health status and previous experiences of muscle or joint injuries (e.g., muscle strains, tears, joint dislocations) may affect the safety of your strength test. Your prompt reporting of these conditions is very important to ensure that you are not injured during the 1-RM test. In addition, you will be asked several times during the strength test if you feel any joint or muscle pain.

4. Benefits to Be Expected

The results obtained from your test will provide information regarding your upper-body strength. This information may be helpful for you in the design of future training programs.

5. Inquiries

You are encouraged to ask any questions about the procedures used in the exercise test or the results of your test. If you have any concerns or questions, please ask us for further explanations.

6. Use of Medical Records

The information that is obtained during exercise testing will be treated as privileged and confidential as described in the Health Insurance Portability and Accountability Act of 1996. It is not to be released or revealed to any person except your referring physician without your written consent. However, the information obtained may be used for statistical analysis or scientific purposes with your right to privacy retained.

7. Freedom of Consent

I hereby consent to engage voluntarily in an exercise test to determine my upper-body strength. My permission to perform this test is given voluntarily. I understand that I am free to stop the test at any point if I so desire.

I have read this form, and I understand the test procedures that I will perform and the attendant risks and discomforts. Knowing these risks and discomforts, and having had an opportunity to ask questions that have been answered to my satisfaction, I consent to participate in this test.

Date _____ _Signature of Participant_ _____

Date _____ _Signature of Witness_ _____

Date _____ _Signature of Person Conducting the Test_ _____

Physical Activity Readiness
Questionnaire - PAR-Q
(revised 2002)

PAR-Q & YOU

(A Questionnaire for People Aged 15 to 69)

Regular physical activity is fun and healthy, and increasingly more people are starting to become more active every day. Being more active is very safe for most people. However, some people should check with their doctor before they start becoming much more physically active.

If you are planning to become much more physically active than you are now, start by answering the seven questions in the box below. If you are between the ages of 15 and 69, the PAR-Q will tell you if you should check with your doctor before you start. If you are over 69 years of age, and you are not used to being very active, check with your doctor.

Common sense is your best guide when you answer these questions. Please read the questions carefully and answer each one honestly: check YES or NO.

YES	NO		
☐	☐	1.	**Has your doctor ever said that you have a heart condition <u>and</u> that you should only do physical activity recommended by a doctor?**
☐	☐	2.	**Do you feel pain in your chest when you do physical activity?**
☐	☐	3.	**In the past month, have you had chest pain when you were not doing physical activity?**
☐	☐	4.	**Do you lose your balance because of dizziness or do you ever lose consciousness?**
☐	☐	5.	**Do you have a bone or joint problem (for example, back, knee or hip) that could be made worse by a change in your physical activity?**
☐	☐	6.	**Is your doctor currently prescribing drugs (for example, water pills) for your blood pressure or heart condition?**
☐	☐	7.	**Do you know of <u>any other reason</u> why you should not do physical activity?**

If

you

answered

YES to one or more questions

Talk with your doctor by phone or in person BEFORE you start becoming much more physically active or BEFORE you have a fitness appraisal. Tell your doctor about the PAR-Q and which questions you answered YES.

- You may be able to do any activity you want — as long as you start slowly and build up gradually. Or, you may need to restrict your activities to those which are safe for you. Talk with your doctor about the kinds of activities you wish to participate in and follow his/her advice.
- Find out which community programs are safe and helpful for you.

NO to all questions

If you answered NO honestly to <u>all</u> PAR-Q questions, you can be reasonably sure that you can:

- start becoming much more physically active — begin slowly and build up gradually. This is the safest and easiest way to go.
- take part in a fitness appraisal — this is an excellent way to determine your basic fitness so that you can plan the best way for you to live actively. It is also highly recommended that you have your blood pressure evaluated. If your reading is over 144/94, talk with your doctor before you start becoming much more physically active.

DELAY BECOMING MUCH MORE ACTIVE:

- if you are not feeling well because of a temporary illness such as a cold or a fever – wait until you feel better; or
- if you are or may be pregnant – talk to your doctor before you start becoming more active.

PLEASE NOTE: If your health changes so that you then answer YES to any of the above questions, tell your fitness or health professional. Ask whether you should change your physical activity plan.

<u>Informed Use of the PAR-Q</u>: The Canadian Society for Exercise Physiology, Health Canada, and their agents assume no liability for persons who undertake physical activity, and if in doubt after completing this questionnaire, consult your doctor prior to physical activity.

No changes permitted. You are encouraged to photocopy the PAR-Q but only if you use the entire form.

NOTE: If the PAR-Q is being given to a person before he or she participates in a physical activity program or a fitness appraisal, this section may be used for legal or administrative purposes.

"I have read, understood and completed this questionnaire. Any questions I had were answered to my full satisfaction."

NAME _____

SIGNATURE _____ DATE_____

SIGNATURE OF PARENT _____ WITNESS _____
or GUARDIAN (for participants under the age of majority)

Note: This physical activity clearance is valid for a maximum of 12 months from the date it is completed and becomes invalid if your condition changes so that you would answer YES to any of the seven questions.

© Canadian Society for Exercise Physiology   Supported by: [Canada flag] Health   Santé
                                                                 Canada   Canada

continued on other side...

PRE-EXERCISE TESTING HEALTH STATUS QUESTIONNAIRE

Name _____ Date _____

ID# _____ Birthdate (mm/dd/yy) _____

Home Address _____

Work Phone _____ Home Phone _____

E-mail Address _____

Person to contact in case of emergency _____

Emergency Contact Phone _____

Personal Physician _____ Physician's Phone _____

Gender _____ Age (yrs) _____

Height (ft) (in) _____ Weight (lbs) _____

Does the above weight indicate: ○ *a gain*   ○ *a loss*   ○ *no change*   in the past year?
If a change, how many pounds? _____ (lbs)

A. JOINT-MUSCLE STATUS (✔ *Check areas where you currently have problems.*)

JOINT AREAS

○ Wrists	○ Hips		
○ Elbows	○ Knees		
○ Shoulders	○ Ankles		
○ Upper spine & neck	○ Feet		
○ Lower spine	○ Other		

MUSCLE AREAS

○ Arms	○ Lower back
○ Shoulders	○ Buttocks
○ Chest	○ Thighs
○ Upper back & neck	○ Lower leg
○ Abdominal regions	○ Feet

B. HEALTH STATUS (✔ *Check if you previously had or currently have any of the following conditions.*)

○ High blood pressure

○ Heart disease or dysfunction

○ Peripheral circulatory disorder

○ Lung disease or dysfunction

○ Arthritis or gout

○ Edema

○ Epilepsy

○ Multiple sclerosis

○ High blood cholesterol or triglyceride levels

○ Loss of consciousness

○ Other conditions that you feel we should know about

_____

_____

_____

○ Pregnant

○ Acute infection

○ Diabetes or blood sugar level abnormality

○ Anemia

○ Hernias

○ Thyroid dysfunction

○ Pancreas dysfunction

○ Liver dysfunction

○ Kidney dysfunction

○ Phenylketonuria (PKU)

○ Allergic reactions to medication
Please describe:

_____

_____

_____

○ Allergic reactions to any other substance
Please describe:

_____

QUESTIONNAIRE, page 2

C. PHYSICAL EXAMINATION HISTORY

Approximate date of your last physical examination _____

Physical problems noted at that time _____

_____

Has a physician ever made any recommendations relative to limiting your level of physical exertion?   YES   NO

If YES, what limitations were recommended? _____

_____

Have you ever had an abnormal resting electrocardiogram (ECG)?   YES   NO

D. CURRENT MEDICATION USAGE *(List the drug name and the condition being managed.)*

MEDICATION   CONDITION

_____

_____

E. PHYSICAL PERCEPTIONS *(Indicate any unusual sensations or perceptions. ✔ Check if you have recently experienced any of the following during or soon after physical activity (PA) or during sedentary periods (SED).)*

PA	SED		PA	SED	
○	○	Chest pain	○	○	Nausea
○	○	Heart palpitations (fast irregular heartbeats)	○	○	Lightheadedness
○	○	Unusually rapid breathing	○	○	Loss of consciousness
○	○	Overheating	○	○	Loss of balance
○	○	Muscle cramping	○	○	Loss of coordination
○	○	Muscle pain	○	○	Extreme weakness
○	○	Joint pain	○	○	Numbness
○	○	Other	○	○	Mental confusion

F. FAMILY HISTORY *(✔ Check if any of your blood relatives—parents, brothers, sisters, aunts, uncles, and/or grandparents—have or had any of the following.)*

○ Heart disease   ○ High blood pressure

○ Heart attacks or strokes (prior to age 50)   ○ Diabetes

○ Elevated blood cholesterol or triglyceride levels   ○ Sudden death (other than accidental)

G. CURRENT HABITS *(✔ Check any of the following if they are characteristic of your current habits.)*

○ Smoking. If so, how many per day? _____   ○ Regularly participates in a weight training exercise program.

○ Regularly does manual gardening or yardwork.   ○ Engages in a sports program more than once per week.

○ Regularly goes for long walks.   If so, what does the program consist of?

○ Frequently rides a bicycle.   _____

○ Frequently runs/jogs for exercise.   _____

Worksheet 1.1 | EXTENSION ACTIVITIES

Name _____ Date _____

1. Administer the PAR-Q and Pre-exercise Testing Health Status Questionnaire to someone in your class. Based on the results from the questionnaires, could the individual safely perform the following exercise tests? Circle the appropriate answer next to each exercise test.

   YES   NO   Bench Press One-Repetition Maximum (1-RM) Strength Test

   YES   NO   Leg Extension One-Repetition Maximum (1-RM) Strength Test

   YES   NO   Submaximal Cycle Ergometer Test

   YES   NO   Maximal Cycle Ergometer Test

   YES   NO   Maximal Treadmill Test

   YES   NO   Flexibility Test

   YES   NO   Test for Anaerobic Power

2. Complete the PAR-Q and Pre-Exercise Testing Health Status Questionnaire for yourself. Based on the results, determine whether you would be able to perform most exercise tests safely.

BACKGROUND

Several different physical fitness assessments may involve the measurement of a basic vital sign: heart rate (HR). Sometimes the measurement is performed at rest, which can help determine the pre-exercise health status of the individual or the return to resting conditions after exercise. During exercise, monitoring HR can be an effective method to estimate the intensity of exercise, especially during aerobic exercise. Heart rate is directly related to exercise intensity, and this relationship is most predictable between 50% and 90% of the maximum HR.[1] In addition, for exercise at the same absolute work rate, the HR of an aerobically trained individual will be lower than that of an untrained or unfit person. Thus, for someone who is less physically fit, the HR will generally be higher after completing a fitness test. For example, the Queens College Step Test (see Lab 9) is based on the assumption that less fit individuals will have a higher HR after the 3-minute step test than subjects who are more physically fit. Therefore, measuring HR before, during, and after exercise is an important aspect of physical fitness testing.

On average, most people have resting HR values between 60 and 80 beats per minute (bpm).[4] However, the average resting HR for women tends to be 7–10 bpm higher than for men.[4] Table 2.1 provides specific normative values for resting HR. There are three common clinical classifications of resting HR:

1. Bradycardia, defined as a slow HR of less than 60 bpm

2. Tachycardia, a fast HR of greater than 100 bpm

3. Normal rhythm, a resting HR of 60–100 bpm

Norms for resting heart rate in men and women (age = 18–65+ years). | TABLE | 2.1

Classification	Resting heart rate (bpm)	
	MEN	WOMEN
Low	35–56	39–58
Moderately low	57–61	59–63
< Average	62–65	64–67
Average	66–71	68–72
> Average	72–75	73–77
Moderately high	76–81	78–83
High	82–103	84–104

Data from Golding, L. A. (2000). *YMCA fitness testing and assessment manual,* 4th ed. Champaign, IL: Human Kinetics.

Two primary methods are used for assessing resting HR: (a) palpation and (b) a heart rate monitor. The most common and cost-effective method for measuring HR is palpation. A more expensive but convenient method that has become increasingly popular is a digital-display HR monitor (photo 2.2). Procedures for both methods are described below.

KNOW THESE TERMS & ABBREVIATIONS

- HR = heart rate, measured in beats per minute (bpm)
- HR monitor = equipment used to measure and monitor heart rate; includes a chest strap (identifies the heartbeats and transmits the signal telemetrically photo 2.2a) and a digital display (displays the signal as a real-time HR value photo 2.2b)
- palpation = the act of examining by touch (photos 2.3 and 2.4)

PROCEDURES

Palpation[7]

1. To palpate the HR (or pulse), use the tips of the index and middle fingers. Avoid using the thumb, since small arteries running through the thumb can be confused with the actual palpable HR.

2. Palpate one of the following anatomical landmarks to find the pulse:

    a. The radial artery, which is located on the anterior-lateral surface of the wrist, in line with the base of the thumb.[4] The best location is usually just medial to the styloid process of the radius. The tips of the index and middle fingers should be placed gently on the skin over this area (photo 2.3).

    b. The carotid artery can be found on the anterior surface of the neck, just lateral to the larynx (photo 2.4).[4] Care should be taken when palpating the pulse of the carotid artery, because applying too much

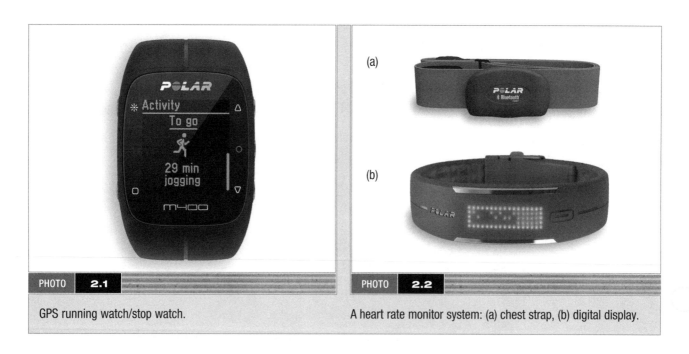

PHOTO	2.1

GPS running watch/stop watch.

PHOTO	2.2

A heart rate monitor system: (a) chest strap, (b) digital display.

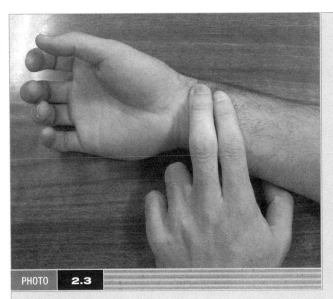

PHOTO **2.3**

Palpation of the radial artery pulse.

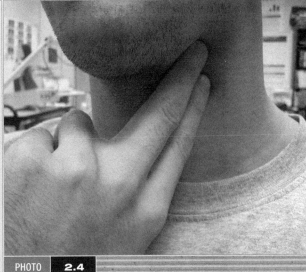

PHOTO **2.4**

Palpation of the carotid artery pulse.

pressure may artificially lower the resultant HR value.[5,9] This may be due to negative feedback from the baroreceptors, which sense pressure, in the aortic arch. There is some debate in the literature whether carotid artery palpation elicits enough pressure to trigger the baroreceptors.[2,6,8]

3. Once the pulse is located, use a stopwatch to keep the time while counting the beats. If the stopwatch is started at the moment the counting begins, count the first beat as "0." If the stopwatch has been running, count the first beat as "1."

4. The HR should be counted for a set period of time, such as 10, 15, 30, or 60 seconds. Use one of the following calculations to determine the HR in bpm:

   a. Counting for 10 seconds: Take the number of beats counted and multiply by 6.

   b. Counting for 15 seconds: Take the number of beats counted and multiply by 4.

   c. Counting for 30 seconds: Take the number of beats counted and multiply by 2.

5. Generally, the shorter-duration HR counts (10 and 15 seconds) are used during and after exercise, when it is important to attain a momentary HR. Since HR can increase with exercise intensity and decrease during recovery, it is sometimes necessary to count the beats during short time periods to obtain an accurate representation of HR at a specific moment during exercise or recovery. In contrast, resting HR measurements are often counted for 30 or 60 seconds to reduce the risk of miscounts and error.

Heart Rate Monitor

Generally, a HR monitor consists of a chest strap and a digital display (photo 2.5). The chest strap contains sensors that identify the heartbeats, and the resultant signal is transmitted telemetrically to the digital display as a real-time HR value in bpm. As with all equipment, different HR monitors may function slightly differently, and the manufacturer's directions should be read and followed. However, most HR monitors work in a similar fashion, and the procedure is as follows:

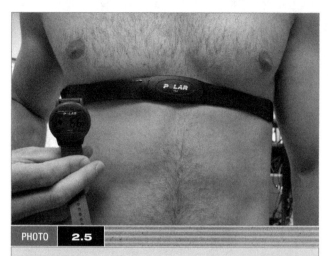

PHOTO **2.5**

Placement of the heart rate monitor strap and the digital display of resting heart rate.

1. Most chest straps require a little moisture (water) applied with a damp cloth over the sensor areas to improve their ability to sense heartbeats.

2. Once the chest strap has been wetted, place the strap just distal to the pectoralis major muscles by adjusting the elastic band (see photo 2.5). The strap should be firm, but not tight enough to indent the skin. For both men and women, the chest strap should be placed in direct contact with the skin.

3. When properly placed, the digital display should provide HR values that update regularly (within seconds).

Sample Calculations

Gender: *Female*

Age: *24 years*

Resting heart rate count (radial pulse) for 30 seconds: *38 beats*

Step 1: Calculate the resting heart rate in beats per minute (bpm).

38 beats x 2 = 76 bpm

Step 2: Compare the resting heart rate (bpm) to the norms in table 2.1.

A score of 76 bpm would be classified as > Average for a woman, according to table 2.1.

REFERENCES

1. Beam, W. C. and Adams, G. M. *Exercise Physiology Laboratory Manual,* 7th edition. New York: McGraw-Hill, 2014.
2. Couldry, W. C., Corbin, C. B., and Wilcox, A. Carotid vs. radial pulse counts. *Phys. Sportsmed.* 10(12): 67–72, 1982.
3. Cramer, J. T., and Coburn, J. W. Fitness testing protocols and norms. In *NSCA's Essentials of Personal Training*, eds. R. W. Earle and T. R. Baechle. Champaign, IL: Human Kinetics, 2005, pp. 218–263.
4. Heyward, V. H. *Advanced Fitness Assessment and Exercise Prescription,* 7th edition. Champaign, IL: Human Kinetics, 2014.
5. McArdle, W. D., Katch, F. I., and Katch, V. L. *Exercise Physiology: Energy, Nutrition, and Human Performance,* 6th edition. Philadelphia: Lippincott Williams & Wilkins, 2007.
6. Oldridge, N. B., Haskell, W. L., and Single, P. Carotid palpation, coronary heart disease and exercise rehabilitation. *Med. Sci. Sports Exerc.* 13(1):6–8, 1981.
7. Ryan, E. D., and Cramer, J. T. Fitness testing protocols and norms. In *NSCA's Essentials of Personal Training*, eds. R. W. Earle and T. R. Baechle, 2nd edition. Champaign, IL: Human Kinetics, 2012, pp. 201–250.
8. Sedlock, D. A., Knowlton, R. G., Fitzgerald, P. I., Tahamont, M. V., and Schneider, D. A. Accuracy of subject-palpated carotid pulse after exercise. *Phys. Sportsmed.* 11(4): 106–116, 1983.
9. White, J. R. EKG changes using carotid artery for heart rate monitoring. *Med. Sci. Sports Exerc.* 9: 88, 1977.

RESTING HEART RATE FORM

Name _____ *Date* _____

Gender: _____

Age: _____

30-second radial pulse count: _____

1. Resting heart rate (bpm) = _____

2. Resting heart rate classification = _____ (see table 2.1)

EXTENSION ACTIVITIES

Name _____ *Date* _____

Use the following data with table 2.1 to answer the questions below.

Gender: _Female_

Age: _32 years_

30-second radial pulse count: _41 beats_

1. Calculate the subject's resting heart rate.

   Resting heart rate (bpm) = _____

2. Classify the subject's resting heart rate based on table 2.1.

   Resting heart rate classification = _____

BACKGROUND

In addition to measuring heart rate, physical fitness assessments may involve the measurement of another basic vital sign: blood pressure (BP). Blood pressure is commonly defined as a measurement of the force of the blood acting against the vessel walls during and between heartbeats.[2] The pressure exerted against the vessels during a heartbeat (systole) is called the *systolic blood pressure,* while the pressure recorded between heartbeats (diastole) is called the *diastolic blood pressure.* The BP measurement is a combination of both the systolic and diastolic pressure and is usually written as "systolic / diastolic" (e.g., 120 / 80). BP is usually measured in units of millimeters of mercury (mmHg). A common and normal BP measurement would be written as 120 / 80 mmHg.

Sounds are emitted as a result of the pressure exerted against the vessel walls, and these sounds are called Korotkoff sounds. The detection and disappearance of Korotkoff sounds when external pressure is applied provides the basis of traditional BP assessments. Sphygmomanometry is the most common and clinically acceptable technique to measure BP.[3] The American Heart Association regards the mercury sphygmomanometer (photo 3.1) as the gold standard measurement device for clinical BP assessment.[3] However, other techniques, such as aneroid (pressure gauge) and automated (photo 3.2) sphygmomanometers, are increasingly common, but these may be more prone to errors than mercury sphygmomanometers.[3] Nevertheless, with either

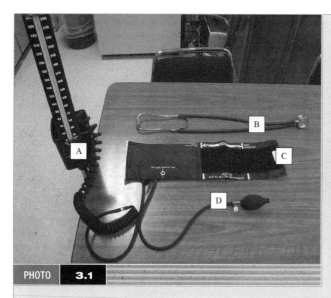

PHOTO **3.1**

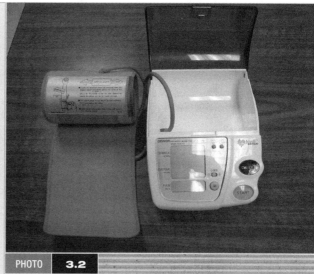

PHOTO **3.2**

A mercury sphygmomanometer. (A) Mercury column with pressure gradients listed from 0 to 300 mmHg, (B) stethoscope, (C) cuff, (D) air bulb and pressure release valve for inflating the cuff.

An automated sphygmomanometer.

| | Classification of hypertension (JNC*-7). | TABLE | 3.1 |

Blood pressure classification	Systolic blood pressure (mmHg)	Diastolic blood pressure (mmHg)
Normal	< 120	< 80
Prehypertensive	120–139	80–89
Stage 1 hypertension	140–159	90–99
Stage 2 hypertension	≥ 160	≥ 100

*Joint National Committee on Prevention, Detection, Evaluation, and Treatment of High Blood Pressure

Source: JNC 7: A. V. Chobanian, G. L. Bakris, H. R. Black, et al. Seventh Report of the Joint National Committee on prevention, detection, evaluation, and treatment of high blood pressure. *Hypertension* 42: 1206–1252, 2003

mercury or aneroid sphygmomanometry, auscultation with a stethoscope placed over the brachial artery is necessary to hear the Korotkoff sounds. Therefore, sphygmomanometry is commonly called the "cuff," "auscultation," or "Korotkoff" technique.[3]

The premise of sphygmomanometry with auscultation is that the brachial artery is occluded with an air-inflated cuff placed around the arm (just distal to the shoulder). The amount of pressure used to inflate the cuff to occlude brachial artery blood flow should be greater than the individual's systolic BP.[3] As the cuff is deflated slowly, blood will eventually squeeze past the occlusion point (cuff) at a pressure that is equal to the systolic BP. A stethoscope is placed over the brachial artery distal to the cuff to auscultate the sounds made by the blood (i.e., Korotkoff sounds). The cuff pressure at which the first audible Korotkoff sounds occur while the cuff is deflating is denoted as the systolic BP, and the cuff pressure of the last audible Korotkoff sounds is recorded as the diastolic BP.

BP assessments are important for detecting hypertension (table 3.1) and monitoring the antihypertensive effects of an exercise program or dietary changes.[4] BP measurements are most often performed at rest (before exercise). BP can be assessed during and after exercise; however, these techniques require advanced skills for measurement and interpretation and will not be covered in this context.[1] The BP measurement technique described in this laboratory focuses on resting BP to evaluate the presence of hypertension and, consequently, the readiness of individuals to undergo other physical fitness tests. For example, if successive BP measurements indicate the possibility of hypertension (table 3.1) for an individual, then physical fitness testing may have to be postponed until medical clearance is granted by a physician. For more information on pre-exercise health status evaluations, see Lab 1.

KNOW THESE TERMS & ABBREVIATIONS

- auscultation = listening to sounds arising from organs to aid in diagnosis and treatment

○ BP = blood pressure, measured in millimeters of mercury (mmHg). BP is defined as a measurement of the force of the blood acting against the vessel walls during and between heartbeats.

○ systolic blood pressure = the pressure exerted against the vessels during a heartbeat (systole)

○ diastolic blood pressure = the pressure recorded between heartbeats (diastole)

○ Korotkoff sounds = the sounds emitted as a result of the pressure exerted against the vessel walls; these sounds provide the basis of traditional BP assessments

○ sphygmomanometer = the instrument used to measure blood pressure in an artery, consisting of a pressure gauge and a cuff, used with a stethoscope. Mercury and aneroid sphygmomanometers are available.

○ hypertension = an abnormally high BP reading (≥ 140 / 90)

PROCEDURES

Mercury Sphygmomanometry (Auscultation Technique)[3,4]

1. To prepare for a resting BP assessment, the subject should be relaxed and comfortably seated upright with the legs uncrossed and the back and arms supported (photo 3.4). All clothing that covers the location of the cuff should be removed. The room temperature should be comfortable (not hot or cold), the environment should be free from distracting background noises, the subject's bladder should be relieved prior to the test, and no talking should be allowed by the subject or the tester during the test. Resting BP should always be taken prior to exercise, and caffeine, alcohol, and nicotine should be avoided for at least 30 minutes prior to any BP measurement.

2. Since various cuff sizes are available, the appropriate cuff size should be determined by measuring the arm circumference with a tape measure (photo 3.3) at 50% of the distance from the shoulder to the elbow. Once the arm circumference has been recorded, determine the appropriate BP cuff size with table 3.2.[3]

3. Place the cuff around the left or right arm so that the cuff is level with the heart. To do this, it is important to position the subject so that the arm is resting in the same horizontal plane as the heart. BP measurements taken with the arm hanging below or raised above the heart level will be inaccurate.[3] In addition, most cuffs have an identification line that is to be placed over the brachial artery. This feature allows the air bladder within the cuff to be positioned directly over the brachial artery. This is important for the occlusion of the artery during cuff inflation. Position the cuff so that the bottom edge of the cuff is approximately 1 inch (2.5 cm) above the antecubital space (elbow crease).

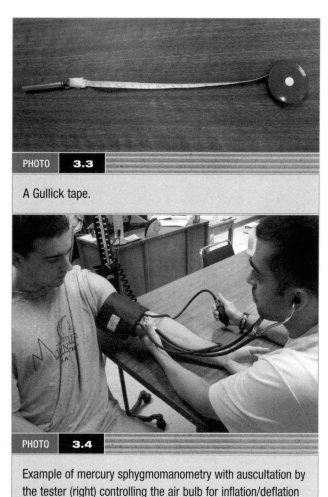

PHOTO 3.3

A Gullick tape.

PHOTO 3.4

Example of mercury sphygmomanometry with auscultation by the tester (right) controlling the air bulb for inflation/deflation of the cuff while monitoring the mercury column (upper left).

Determining cuff dimension using arm circumference. **TABLE 3.2**

Size	Measured cuff dimensions	Measured arm circumference
Small adult	12 x 22 cm	22–26 cm
Adult	16 x 30 cm	27–34 cm
Large adult	16 x 36 cm	35–44 cm

4. Once seated and relaxed, allow the subject to rest for at least 5 minutes prior to the first BP measurement.

5. With the subject's palm facing up, place the stethoscope head in the antecubital space firmly but not hard enough to indent the skin. It is recommended that the tester use his or her dominant hand to control the air bulb and the inflation/deflation of the cuff, while the nondominant hand should be used to hold the stethoscope (see photo 3.4; the tester is right-handed).

6. Assure that the mercury column (or aneroid pressure gauge) is easily readable by the tester. In photo 3.4, the mercury column is visible and at eye level for the tester. For aneroid pressure gauges, it is recommended to place the gauge in the tester's lap or clip it to the cuff to enable a quick and accurate pressure reading.

7. It is important to avoid contacting the stethoscope head with the air tubes connected to the mercury sphygmomanometer. If the air tubes contact the stethoscope head, the sound may be mistaken for a Korotkoff sound and may result in erroneous BP measurements. Therefore, position the air tubes away from the stethoscope head as much as possible.

8. Once the cuff, stethoscope, and sphygmomanometer have been properly placed, make sure the air release valve is closed on the air bulb and then quickly inflate the cuff either to 160 mmHg or to 20 mmHg above the anticipated systolic BP.

9. Upon reaching the maximum inflation pressure, carefully turn the air release valve counterclockwise to release the cuff pressure. The rate of pressure release should be approximately 2 to 3 mmHg per second.

10. While the cuff is deflating, listen carefully for the Korotkoff sounds. Record the systolic BP as an even number to the nearest 2 mmHg where the first Korotkoff sound is heard. Record the diastolic BP as an even number to the nearest 2 mmHg where the last Korotkoff sound is heard. Usually, Korotkoff sounds are described as sharp tapping noises that are similar to tapping the stethoscope head (bell) gently with a finger. After the Korotkoff sounds have disappeared, observe the mercury column for another 10 to 20 mmHg of deflation to confirm the absence of sounds.

11. When it is confirmed that no more Korotkoff sounds are audible, rapidly deflate and remove the cuff.

12. After a minimum of 2 minutes of rest, measure BP again using the same technique described above. If the two consecutive measurements of

either systolic BP or diastolic BP differ by more than 5 mmHg, take a third BP measurement. After either two or three consecutive BP measurements, calculate the average systolic and diastolic BP. The average systolic and diastolic BP values should be used as the final scores.

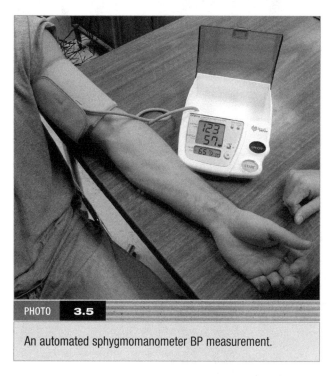

PHOTO 3.5

An automated sphygmomanometer BP measurement.

Automated Sphygmomanometry

The American Heart Association recommends that any BP measurement technique other than mercury sphygmomanometry (including automated systems) should be validated prior to being used in practice.[3] Substantial errors in BP measurements and erroneous values may occur in both validated and unvalidated devices, but the probability of errors is reduced with validation.[3]

Most automated sphygmomanometers operate very similarly to the regular auscultation technique described above, except that a stethoscope is not required. Subject positioning and cuff placement are usually the same. Therefore, steps 1–4 and step 12 (above) may be applied. Because individual manufacturers may have different procedures, the manufacturer's directions should be carefully followed for any automated BP assessments. Photo 3.5 shows an automated sphygmomanometer BP assessment.

Sample Calculations

Gender: _Male_

Age: _19 years_

BLOOD PRESSURE	TRIAL 1	TRIAL 2	TRIAL 3
systolic (mmHg) =	124	118	118
diastolic (mmHg) =	72	66	70

Step 1: Calculate the average systolic and diastolic blood pressure values.

systolic: $(124 + 118 + 118) \div 3 = 120$

diastolic: $(72 + 66 + 70) \div 3 = 69.3$

final blood pressure = 120 / 69.3 mmHg

Step 2: Classify the final blood pressure measurement using table 3.1.

A score of 120 / 69.3 mmHg would be classified as normal in table 3.1.

BLOOD PRESSURE FORM	Worksheet **3.1**

Name _____   Date _____

Gender: _____

Age: _____

BLOOD PRESSURE:	TRIAL 1	TRIAL 2	TRIAL 3
Systolic (mmHg)	_____	_____	_____
Diastolic (mmHg)	_____	_____	_____

1. Final resting blood pressure (mmHg) = _____

2. Resting blood pressure classification = _____ (see table 3.1)

EXTENSION ACTIVITIES	Worksheet **3.2**

Name _____   Date _____

Use the following data with table 3.1 to answer the questions below.

Gender: _Female_

Age: _32 years_

BLOOD PRESSURE:	TRIAL 1	TRIAL 2	TRIAL 3
Systolic (mmHg)	136	130	132
Diastolic (mmHg)	78	84	82

1. Calculate the subject's blood pressure.

   Final resting blood pressure (mmHg) = _____

2. Classify the subject's blood pressure based on table 3.1.

   Resting blood pressure classification = _____ (see table 3.1)

REFERENCES

1. American College of Sports Medicine. *ACSM's Guidelines for Exercise Testing and Prescription,* 9th edition. Baltimore: Wolters Kluwer/Lippincott Williams & Wilkins, 2014.

2. Beam, W. C. and Adams, G. M. *Exercise Physiology Laboratory Manual,* 7th edition. New York: McGraw-Hill, 2014.

3. Pickering, T. G., Hall, J. E., Appel, L. J., Falkner, B. E., Graves, J., Hill, M. N., Jones, D. W., Kurtz, T., Sheps, S. G., and Roccella, E. J. Recommendations for blood pressure measurement in humans and experimental animals. Part 1: Blood pressure measurement in humans: A statement for professionals from the subcommittee of professional and public education of the American Heart Association Council on high blood pressure research. *Circulation* 111: 697–716, 2005.

4. Ryan, E. D., and Cramer, J. T., Fitness testing protocols and norms. In *NSCA's Essentials of Personal Training,* eds. R. W. Earle and T. R. Baechle, 2nd edition. Champaign, IL: Human Kinetics, 2012, pp. 201–250.

BACKGROUND

The electrocardiogram (EKG or ECG) is a graphical recording of the electrical activity of the heart muscle (myocardium). Typically, the EKG is recorded from 10 electrodes placed in specific locations on the chest, arms, and legs.[2] These 10 electrodes combine to form 12 separate leads that provide different views of the heart (figure 4.1; table 4.1).[2,3] At rest and during exercise, the EKG tracing is used to determine the heart's rate and rhythm. Deviations in the EKG tracing are used to diagnose conduction disturbances, heart disease, and damage to the myocardium.[3,4]

The EKG records the movement of an electrical impulse as it travels through the heart's conduction system, stimulating the myocardium to contract and pump the blood throughout the body. The electrical impulse is initiated at the sinoatrial (SA) node within the right atrium, which contains specialized cells that are capable of self-excitation (autorhythmicity) at a regular interval of 60 to 100 beats per minute (bpm).[2] As the electrical impulse moves through the heart, it produces a specific pattern that is recorded on the EKG strip (figure 4.2).[2]

Three basic components of the EKG tracing (figure 4.3) are used to examine cardiac function: the P wave, the QRS complex, and the T wave. The first upward deflection on the EKG tracing is the P wave, which represents the atrial depolarization as the electrical impulse moves from the SA node through the atria to the AV node, located between the atria and the ventricles. After the P wave there is a brief flat baseline called the PR segment. The PR segment

Mason-Likar 10 electrode placement. **FIGURE** **4.1**

Right arm (RA): upper right arm–chest region just below the mid-point of the clavicle

Left arm (LA): upper left arm–chest region just below the mid-point of the clavicle

Right leg (RL): lower right abdominal region, at the midclavicular line, at the level of the last rib

Left leg (LL): lower left abdominal region, at the midclavicular line, at the level of the last rib

V$_1$: right sternal border, 4th intercostal space

V$_2$: left sternal border, 4th intercostal space

V$_3$: midway between V$_2$ and V$_4$

V$_4$: fifth intercostal space, midclavicular line

V$_5$: anterior axillary line, level with V$_4$

V$_6$: midaxillary line, level with V$_5$

Note: The leg electrodes may also be placed at the level of the navel. This placement, however, may result in motion artifact. The placement of the leg electrodes on the last rib at the midclavicular line (as indicated above) tends to result in less motion artifact and has no effect on the EKG tracing.

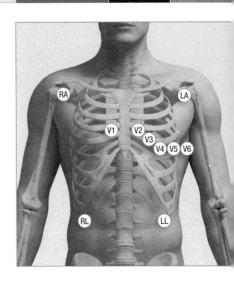

TABLE	4.1	Electrocardiogram leads.

*LIMB AND AUGMENTED LEADS			CHEST LEADS		
Lead	**Electrode Placement**	**Heart Surface Viewed**	**Lead**	**Electrode Placement**	**Heart Surface Viewed**
Lead I	Left arm (+), right arm (−)	Lateral	V$_1$	4th intercostal space, right sternal border	Septum
Lead II	Left leg (+), right arm (−)	Inferior	V$_2$	4th intercostal space, left sternal border	Septum
Lead III	Left leg (+), left arm (−)	Inferior	V$_3$	midway between V$_2$ and V$_4$	Anterior
aVR	Right arm (+)	None	V$_4$	midclavicular line, 5th intercostal space	Anterior
aVL	Left arm (+)	Lateral	V$_5$	anterior axillary line, level with V$_4$	Lateral
aVF	Left leg (+)	Inferior	V$_6$	midaxillary line, level with V$_5$	Lateral

*The limb leads can be positioned on the left and right arm–chest regions just below the mid-point of the clavicle and the left and right lower abdominal regions, at the midclavicular line, at the level of the last rib.

Source: Pescatello, L. S. American College of Sports Medicine. *ACSM's guidelines for exercise testing and prescription,* 9th edition. Philadelphia: Lippincott Williams & Wilkins, 2014, Appendix C, pp. 413.

FIGURE	4.2	EKG tracing.

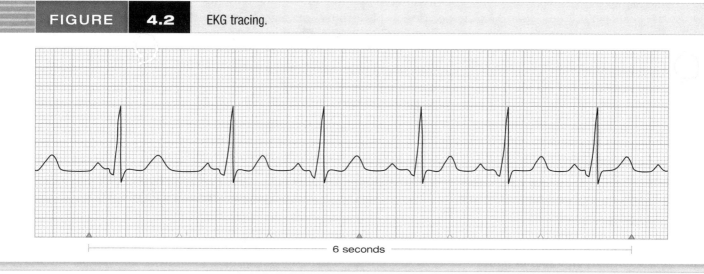

6 seconds

reflects the slight delay of the electrical impulse as it moves through the AV node and junctional tissue. The first downward deflection after this baseline is the Q wave, which is followed by an upward R wave and a downward S wave to form the QRS complex. The QRS complex reflects ventricular depolarization as the impulse continues to the AV bundle (bundle of His), down the left and right bundle branches, and finally to the Purkinje fibers (cardiomyocytes that conduct an electrical impulse). Following the QRS complex is a short, flat baseline called the ST segment that precedes the T wave. The T wave reflects the recovery period or repolarization of the ventricles. The ST segment should be flat and level with other areas of baseline (PR segment). Changes in the ST segment above and below baseline are evidence of a cardiac pathology (figure 4.4).[3,4] For example, a lack of blood flow to the heart (myocardial ischemia) will result in ST segment depression.[3,4]

A representation of an EKG tracing including the P, Q, R, S, and T waves, the QRS complex, the PR segment, and the ST segment.

FIGURE 4.3

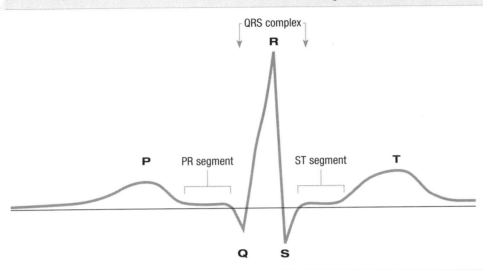

ST segment depression.

FIGURE 4.4

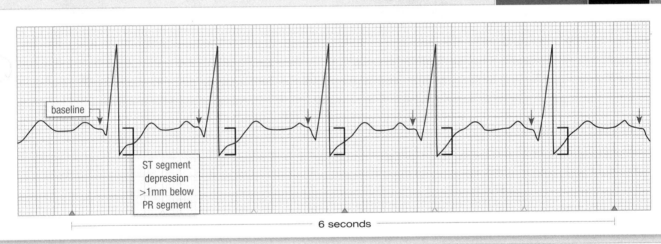

Under some conditions, the normal conduction of the electrical impulse through the heart may be altered and result in an irregular rhythm, or arrhythmia. Sometimes, the impulse frequency of the SA node may be less than 60 bpm, resulting in bradycardia (slow heart rate). A resting heart rate greater than 100 bpm is termed tachycardia (fast heart rate). During sinus bradycardia and tachycardia, the impulse is still generated by the SA node so the sinus rhythm is normal (P wave, QRS complex, and T wave are normal), but the rate is altered. Other arrhythmias may occur that result from an impulse that is generated outside the SA node. A premature ventricular contraction (PVC) is a relatively common arrhythmia that may result in the feeling of a skipped or extra heartbeat. Because a PVC occurs outside the normal conduction system, it depolarizes the cardiac cells of only the ventricles, which causes a wide QRS complex that is not immediately preceded by a P wave (figure 4.5).[1] Isolated PVCs can occur at rest or during exercise and do not necessarily indicate an underlying heart condition.[3,4]

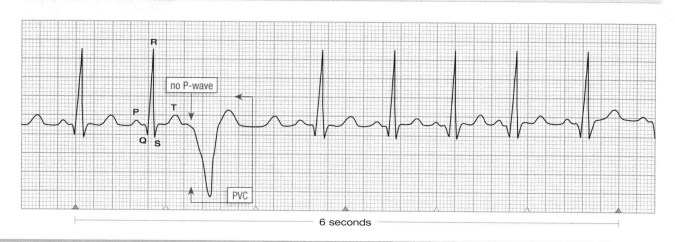

FIGURE 4.5 Premature ventricular contraction (PVC).

The resting EKG can be used to determine the heart rate and rhythm and identify potential pathologies.[1] An EKG performed during exercise has two primary purposes in a laboratory setting: (1) to accurately measure heart rate and (2) to increase the safety of the exercise test by examining the EKG for any abnormal tracings that would warrant stopping the test, such as ST segment depression.[1] A diagnosis of cardiovascular disease, however, can be made only by a physician and is beyond the scope of this laboratory. This laboratory is meant only to provide a basic introduction into the EKG and will describe (1) the measurement of heart rate for an EKG tracing at rest and during exercise, (2) the identification of arrhythmias (bradycardia, tachycardia, and PVCs), and (3) the identification of ST segment depression.

KNOW THESE TERMS & ABBREVIATIONS

- bradycardia = slow resting heart rate (< 60 bpm)
- EKG = electrocardiogram
- PVC = premature ventricular contraction
- PR segment = isoelectric point; flat baseline between the P wave and QRS complex
- Purkinje fibers = large-diameter cardiomyocytes that conduct electrical impulses
- P wave = reflects atrial depolariation
- QRS complex = reflects ventricular depolarization
- ST segment = flat baseline between the QRS complex and T wave
- tachycardia = fast resting heart rate (>100 bpm)
- T wave = repolarization of the ventricles

PROCEDURES

A number of brands of EKG recorders are available, and each brand will have slightly different operating instructions. Therefore, it is recommended that you review the operating instructions for the EKG recorder you will be using for this laboratory activity. The procedures described in this laboratory for a resting and exercise EKG are consistent among various EKG recorders. The exercise EKG will be recorded during an incremental exercise test performed on a Monark cycle ergometer.

Resting EKG

1. The subject's shirt should be removed for the electrode placement preparation and EKG procedures. Women should be instructed prior to the testing day to wear a sport bra or swimsuit top.

2. Record the subject's demographic information on worksheet 4.1.

3. The subject may be seated or in a supine position for the electrode preparation and placement.

4. Identify all 10 of the electrode placement sites (see figure 4.1, p. 21).[2] These 10 electrodes combine to form 12 separate leads (see table 4.1). Although all 10 electrodes will be placed and used during the EKG recording, this lab activity will include the use of one of the most common leads, lead II, for the EKG interpretation. Other leads are often used for a more comprehensive EKG interpretation. A detailed description of EKG interpretation can be found in Appendix C of the ACSM *Guidelines for Exercise Testing and Interpretation.*[3]

5. Any body hair at the electrode site should be removed with a disposable razor. The sites should be cleaned with an alcohol swab or other mild cleaner. Gently rub each site with an abrasive pad to remove the dead skin. This will allow for a clearer EKG signal.

6. Apply the electrodes to each of the 10 sites indicated in figure 4.1. Gently press the edges of the electrode to be sure there is good contact with the skin.

7. Once the electrodes are placed, have the subject lie supine if not already doing so.

8. Attach the wires from the EKG recorder to the electrodes. The wires are labeled according to the electrode to which they should be attached.

9. Instruct the subject to relax all muscles as much as possible. The electrical activity of any skeletal muscle contraction near the electrode sites can be recorded by the EKG and may cause interference, making the EKG difficult to interpret.

10. Turn on the EKG recorder and follow the manufacturer's instructions for patient data entry.

11. Record the 12-lead EKG for 10 to 15 seconds.

12. After the EKG strip is printed, examine the tracing to be sure the signal is clear of interference. (*Note:* If the EKG tracing is not clear, adjust the wires and check with the subject to be sure he or she is completely relaxed, then rerun the test for another 10 to 15 seconds.)

13. If the EKG tracing appears to be clear of interference, remove all of the electrodes and wipe the sites clean of any gel or adhesive. (*Note:* If the subject will complete an exercise test with an EKG recording, the electrodes and wires can be left in place.)

14. Calculate the heart rate using lead II. The EKG is recorded on graph paper, which contains heavy black lines spaced 5 mm apart. Between each heavy black line there are 5 small squares. Each small square is 1 mm. The paper also contains tick marks across the bottom, spaced 75 mm apart (75 small boxes). The EKG paper runs at 25 mm • s^{-1}, so that the time from one tick mark to the next (75 mm) is equal to 3 seconds. To calculate heart rate, we will use a 6-second strip, which will include 150 mm (150 small boxes). Count the number of cardiac cycles (R wave to R wave) that occur in 6 seconds and multiply by 10 to determine the heart rate in bpm (see figure 4.6).

15. Examine the EKG tracing for ST segment depression using lead II. ST segment depression is defined by a decrease greater than or equal to 1 mm (1 small box) from baseline (baseline is at the same level of the PR segment)[3] (figure 4.4).

16. Examine the EKG tracing for any PVCs using lead II. A PVC appears as a wide QRS complex that is not immediately proceeded by a P wave (figure 4.5).

Exercise EKG

1. A resting EKG should be performed prior to the exercise EKG. The preparation, electrode placement, and recording of the resting EKG are described in the previous section. Record the subject's demographic information on worksheet 4.2.

2. After the resting EKG is completed, help the subject move to the cycle ergometer without removing the electrodes or wires.

3. Adjust the seat height of the cycle ergometer to allow for near full extension of the subject's legs while pedaling.

4. Record an EKG tracing for 10 to 15 seconds with the subject seated on the bike, but not pedaling.

5. *Incremental test:* The incremental test will be performed at a cadence of 70 rev • min^{-1}. Prior to the start of the test, the subject should pedal at 70 rev • min^{-1} without any resistance for 1 to 2 minutes to become accustomed

FIGURE 4.6 Example of the heart rate calculation from an EKG tracing.

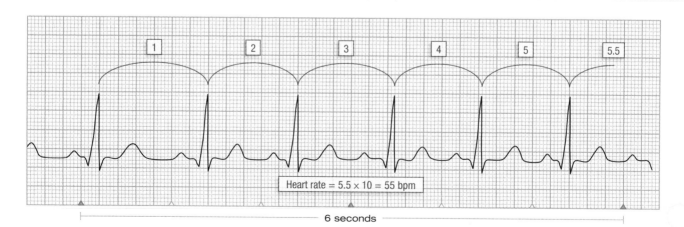

Heart rate = 5.5 × 10 = 55 bpm

6 seconds

to the cadence. When the subject is comfortable with the cadence, begin the test by applying 1 kg of resistance to the cycle ergometer. The resistance should be increased by 0.5 kg every 2 minutes until the subject voluntarily exhausts or the cadence falls below 65 rpm for greater than 10 seconds. Record an EKG tracing during the final 15 seconds of each 2-minute stage, before the resistance is increased.

6. Use lead II of the EKG tracing to calculate heart rate using table 4.3, for each stage.

7. Examine the tracing for ST segment depression and PVCs (see steps 14–16 on p. 26).

Sample Calculations

Sample Resting EKG (see figure 4.7)

Gender: Female   Age: 21   Height (cm): 168 cm   Weight (kg): 60 kg

Resting EKG, tracing sample calculation..   **FIGURE**   **4.7**

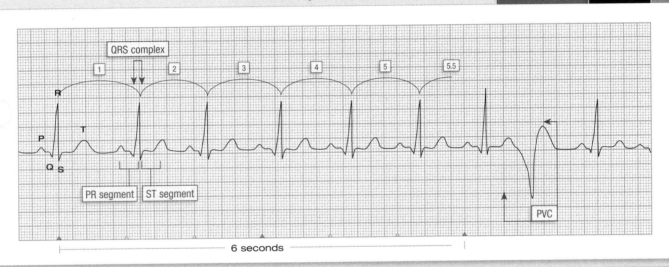

1. Note a P, Q, R, S, and T wave.

2. Note a QRS complex.

3. Note a PR segment and ST segment.

4. Calculate heart rate: number of cardiac cycles (R wave to R wave) in 6 seconds x 10 = heart rate

   5.5 cardiac cycles in 6 seconds x 10 = 55 bpm

   Is there bradycardia (resting HR < 60 bpm)? ___Yes___

   Is there tachycardia (resting HR > 100 bpm)? ___No___

5. Are there any PVCs (look for a wide QRS that is not preceded by a P wave)? ___Yes___

6. Is there ST segment depression (greater than 1 small box below the baseline [PR segment])? ___No___

Sample Exercise EKG (see figure 4.8)

7. Calculate power output:

kgm • min⁻¹ = kg of resistance x 6 m (this is a constant associated with the flywheel for the Monark cycle ergometer) x 70 rev • min⁻¹ (pedal cadence)

8. *Use lead II to calculate heart rate for stage 3 using table 4.2:* number of cardiac cycles (R wave to R wave) in 6 seconds x 10 = heart rate

15 x 10 = 150 bpm

| FIGURE | 4.8 | Sample calculations, exercise EKG, lead II (stage 3). |

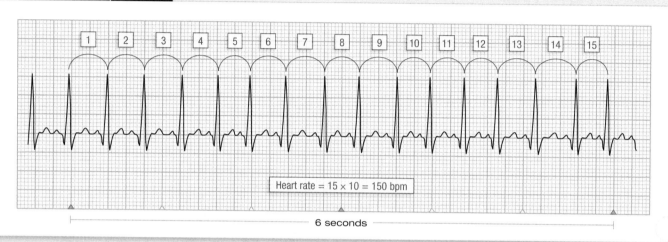

Heart rate = 15 × 10 = 150 bpm

6 seconds

| TABLE | 4.2 | Incremental cycle ergometer test protocol. |

Note: The heart rate was recorded and calculated for each stage using the EKG tracing (see example calculation for stage 3 in #8 above).

Stage	Min	Resistance	Constant		rev·min⁻¹		kgm·min⁻¹	Heart rate
0	0:00	0.0	x	6	x	0	=	0	55
1	2:00	1.0	x	6	x	70	=	420	125
2	4:00	1.5	x	6	x	70	=	630	142
3	6:00	2.0	x	6	x	70	=	840	150
4	8:00	2.5	x	6	x	70	=	1050	172
5	10:00	3.0	x	6	x	70	=	1260	185
6	12:00	3.5	x	6	x	70	=	1470	193

RESTING EKG

Name _____   Date _____

Gender: _____   Age: _____   Height (cm): _____   Weight (kg): _____

EXERCISE EKG

Name _____   Date _____

Gender: _____   Age: _____   Height (cm): _____   Weight (kg): _____

Incremental cycle ergometer test protocol.   TABLE   **4.3**

Note: The heart rate should be calculated and recorded for each stage of the test using the EKG tracing.

Stage	Min	Resistance	Constant			rev·min⁻¹		kgm·min⁻¹	Heart rate
0	0:00	0.0	x	6	x	0	=	0	
1	2:00	1.0	x	6	x	70	=	420	
2	4:00	1.5	x	6	x	70	=	630	
3	6:00	2.0	x	6	x	70	=	840	
4	8:00	2.5	x	6	x	70	=	1050	
5	10:00	3.0	x	6	x	70	=	1260	
6	12:00	3.5	x	6	x	70	=	1470	

Worksheet 4.3 — EXTENSION ACTIVITIES

1. Ann just underwent an EGK assessment. The EKG tracing was examined by a physician and it showed ST segment depression of 2 mm. What might this indicate?

2. The physician also noticed a PVC. How do you identify a PVC?

3. Define the terms *bradycardia* and *tachycardia*.

The following questions apply to the EKG tracing in figure 4.9.

FIGURE 4.9 — Extension activity: EKG tracing.

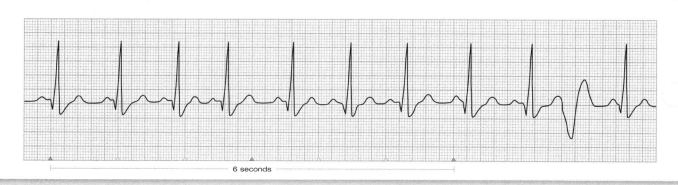

6 seconds

4. Label a P, Q, R, S, and T wave.
5. Label a QRS complex.
6. Label a PR and ST segment.
7. Calculate the heart rate: number of cardiac cycles (R wave to R wave) in 6 seconds x 10 = heart rate

   _____ (number of cardiac cycles in 6 seconds) x 10 = _____ bpm

8. Are there any arrhythmias or ST segment changes? If so, label them on the EKG tracing.

Working with a partner, perform a resting EKG. Use lead II from your resting EKG tracing to answer the following questions.

PASTE YOUR RESTING EKG TRACING HERE

9. Label a P, Q, R, S, and T wave.
10. Label a ST segment.
11. Determine the resting heart rate: number of cardiac cycles (R wave to R wave) in 6 seconds x 10 = heart rate

    _____ (number of cardiac cycles) x 10 = _____ bpm

12. Does the resting heart rate indicate bradycardia? Tachycardia? Explain how you know this.

13. Examine the EKG. Are there any arrhythmias (PVC) or ST segment changes? If so, label them on the EKG tracing.

Working with a partner, perform an exercise EKG. Use stage 3, lead II from your exercise EKG tracings to answer the following questions.

PASTE YOUR EXERCISE EKG TRACING FOR STAGE 3 HERE

14. Label a P, Q, R, S, and T wave.
15. Label a ST segment.
16. Determine the heart rate: number of cardiac cycles (R wave to R wave) in 6 seconds x 10 = heart rate

    _____ (number of cardiac cycles) x 10 = _____ bpm

17. Examine the EKG. Are there any arrhythmias (PVC) or ST segment changes? If so, label them on the EKG tracing.

EXTENSION QUESTIONS

1. What are some common mistakes that may occur in administering this lab?

2. Identify possible sources of error in this lab.

3. Assess the practicality of using this lab in the field.

4. Research the reliability and validity of this lab using online resources, journal articles, and other credible sources.

REFERENCES

1. Beam, W. C. and Adams, G. M. *Exercise Physiology: Laboratory Manual,* 7th edition. New York: McGraw-Hill, 2014.

2. Dubin, D. *Rapid Interpretation of EKG's,* 6th edition. Fort Myers, CO: Cover Publishing, 2000.

3. Pescatello, L. S. American College of Sports Medicine. *ACSM's Guidelines for Exercise Testing and Prescription,* 9th edition. Baltimore: Wolters Kluwer/Lippincott Williams & Wilkins, 2014.

4. Swain, D. P. American College of Sports Medicine. *ACSM's Resource Manual for Guidelines for Exercise Testing and Prescription,* 7th edition. Baltimore: Wolters Kluwer/Lippincott Williams & Wilkins, 2014.

BACKGROUND

The pulmonary system includes the nasal cavity, pharynx, epiglottis, larynx, trachea, bronchus, lungs, and alveoli. The primary functions of the pulmonary system are to participate in the processes of external and internal respiration.[7,13] External respiration refers to the movement of oxygen and other gases from the outside environment into and out of the lungs, while internal respiration refers to the exchange of gases between the alveoli within the lungs and the blood cells.[7,13]

Two types of tests, static and dynamic, can be used to assess pulmonary function. *Static tests* measure variables such as vital capacity (VC), residual volume (RV), and total lung capacity (TLC), which depend on an individual's physical size/stature as well as the anatomical structure of the lungs.[4,7] Vital capacity represents the maximum amount of gas that can be expired after a maximal inspiration and provides an estimate of the size of the lungs.[3] RV is the volume of air that remains in the lungs after a maximal exhalation. Vital capacity and RV are used to determine body composition during underwater weighing (see Lab 33).[14] Total lung capacity is the sum of VC plus RV. Lung volumes tend to be larger in tall individuals than in short individuals, and larger in males than females. In a laboratory setting, static lung volumes are measured using a paper tracing from a mechanical spirometer or with an electronic spirometer that provides a digital tracing and computer calculated volumes.

Dynamic tests include forced vital capacity (FVC) and forced expiratory volumes (FEV) and are used to measure rate of airflow to diagnose respiratory disorders such as asthma or emphysema[2,4,13] (see table 5.1). Forced vital capacity is the volume of air that is exhaled during the entire duration of an FEV test, while FEV represents the volume of air that can be forcefully exhaled in a

| | Classification of spirometric abnormality based on $FEV_{1.0}$. | TABLE 5.1 |

Degree of Severity	$FEV_{1.0}$ % Predicted
Mild	Less than the LLN but $\geq$ 70
Moderate	60–69
Moderately severe	50–59
Severe	35–49
Very severe	<35

$FEV_{1.0}$ forced expiratory volume in one second; LLN, lower limit of normal

Data derived from *ACSM Guidelines*.[2]

FIGURE **5.1** Lung volumes and capacities.

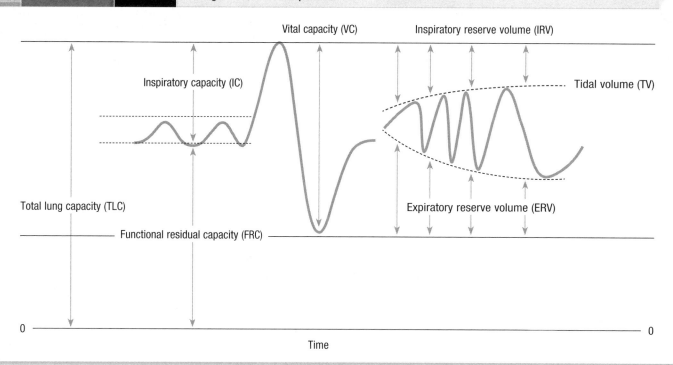

specified period of time. The FEV$_{1.0}$ test calculates a forceful expiration across a 1-second period. Figure 5.1 depicts lung volumes and capacities.[4,13]

The measure of ventilation during exercise can provide important information regarding pulmonary function and exercise tolerance.[13] Dynamic parameters include pulmonary or minute ventilation ($\dot{V}_E$), breathing rate (BR), tidal volume (TV), and ventilatory equivalent ($\dot{V}_E/\dot{V}O_2$).[13] When comparing fit and unfit subjects, a fit subject will produce lower $\dot{V}_E$, BR, and TV values than the unfit subject at any submaximal exercise intensity.[13] In both populations, however, there is a linear relationship between ventilation and exercise intensity (increase in ventilation with an increase in exercise intensity), while a positive, curvilinear relationship exists between BR, TV, and exercise intensity (BR and TV increase in a linear fashion with exercise intensity before leveling out). A depiction of normal ventilatory kinetics can be seen in figure 5.2.[4,13]

In normal populations, pulmonary function is not a significant limiting factor to aerobic performance at or below sea level. In clinical populations with pulmonary disorders (i.e., asthma and chronic obstructive pulmonary disease (COPD)), however, the pulmonary system can limit aerobic performance.[2,13] Laboratory procedures that measure lung volumes and capacities are useful in assessing pulmonary function and diagnosing potentially life-threatening conditions.

KNOW THESE TERMS & ABBREVIATIONS[8,9]

Lung Volumes (table 5.2)

- tidal volume (TV) (approximately 500 mL at rest) = reflects the depth of breathing; it is the volume of gas inspired or expired during each respiratory cycle.

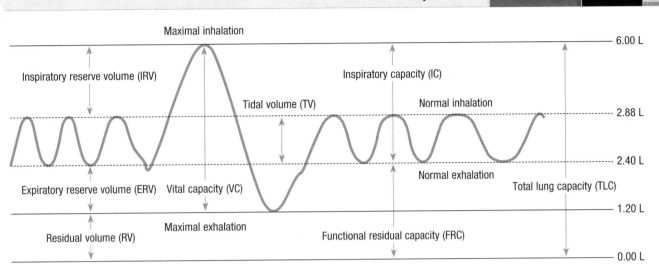

Normal ventilatory kinetics. **FIGURE** **5.2**

- inspiratory reserve volume (IRV) (approximately 1900–3100 mL) = the maximum amount of gas that can be inspired from the end-tidal (the end of a breath) inspiratory level.

- expiratory reserve volume (ERV) (approximately 800–1200 mL) = the maximum volume of gas that can be expired from the end-tidal expiratory level. It is also known as the volume of air present in the resting lungs after a passive exhalation, or resting lung volume (RLV).

- residual volume (RV) (approximately 1000–1200 mL) = the volume of air that remains in the lungs even after a maximal exhalation. After a maximal exhalation, approximately one quarter of total lung capacity (24% for males and 28% for females) will remain as residual volume.

Corrected lung volumes and capacities. **TABLE** **5.2**

Measure	Male (mL)	Female (mL)
Tidal volume (TV)	500	500
Inspiratory reserve volume (IRV)	3300	1900
Expiratory reserve volume (ERV)	1000	700
Residual volume (RV)	1200	1100
Vital capacity (VC)	4800	3100
Inspiratory capacity (IC)	3800	2400
Functional residual capacity (FRC)	2200	1800
Total lung capacity (TLC)	6000	4200

Source: Data derived from Martini.[9]

Lung Capacities[8,9] (table 5.2)

○ inspiratory capacity (IC) (approximately 2400–3600 mL) = the maximum amount of gas that can be inspired from the resting expiratory level. It includes the tidal volume and inspiratory reserve volume.

○ functional residual capacity (FRC) (approximately 1800–2400 mL) = the amount of gas remaining in the lungs at the resting expiratory level. It includes the expiratory reserve volume and residual volume.

○ vital capacity (VC) (approximately 3200–4800 mL) = the maximum amount of gas that can be expired with a forceful effort following a maximal inspiration. It includes the tidal volume, inspiratory reserve volume, and expiratory reserve volume.

○ total lung capacity (TLC) (approximately 4200–6000 mL) = the sum of VC and RV.

Ventilation and Pulmonary Measurements[4,13] (table 5.3)

○ BTPS = body temperature pressure (water vapor) saturated; used to refer to the conditions within the lungs.

○ BTPS correction factor = used to convert flow and volume measured at ambient conditions within the lungs. Ambient conditions are called ATP (ambient temperature, pressure); the conditions within the lungs are called BTPS.

○ minute ventilation ($\dot{V}_E$) = the amount of air expired in 1 minute.

○ breathing rate (BR) = the number of breaths taken each minute.

○ ventilatory equivalent ($\dot{V}_E/\dot{V}O_2$) = the ratio of minute ventilation to oxygen consumption.

○ forced vital capacity (FVC) = the total volume of air that is exhaled during the FEV test.

○ forced expiratory volume (FEV) = the volume of air that is forcefully expired during a maximal exhalation. It is typically measured in a specific increment of time; for example, 0.5 second, 1 second, and so on.

○ forced expiratory volume in 1 second ($FEV_{1.0}$) = the volume of air that can be forcefully exhaled in 1 second.

TABLE 5.3	Corrected pulmonary function measurement.	

Measure	Male (mL)	Female (mL)
Forced vital capacity (FVC)	4930	3530
Forced expiratory volume at 1 second ($FEV_{1.0}$)	4100	3020
$FEV_{1.0}$/FEV	83.0	85.5

Source: Data derived from Hankinson.[6]

PROCEDURES[1,3,4]

This lab will focus on procedures and testing relevant to the mechanical, wet-type spirometer with lung volume and capacity recordings on a paper trace spirogram. If the lab has access only to an electronic type spirometer, however, the same breathing techniques can be used.

Subjects should not smoke, consume a large meal, or consume alcohol within 4 hours of the test. In addition, subjects should wear clothing that will allow full chest and abdominal expansion. Testing should be completed in the seated position unless the subject is unable to fully expand the chest, in which case testing may be conducted while the subject stands. Testers should rehearse the commands and have the subjects practice the breathing maneuvers prior to each test.

Measuring Inspiratory Reserve Volume, Tidal Volume, and Expiratory Reserve Volume[1]

1. Testers should check the drum, spirogram paper, and tracing pen to ensure that all components are in working order (photo 5.1).
2. Testers should record the room air temperature and the temperature of the air in the spirometer.
3. The subject should fit himself or herself with a nose clip and seal his or her lips around the disposable mouthpiece.
4. Turn the power to the drum on, at the slowest rotating speed.
5. Have the subject inhale and exhale normally for several breaths. After two to three resting breaths, have the subject perform a maximal inhalation, hold for 1 second, and then complete a maximal expiration, expelling all the air from the lungs (photo 5.2). Have the subject return to a normal breathing pattern for two to three breaths.
6. IRV, TV, and ERV can now be measured using the spirogram recording (figure 5.2) and BTPS correction factors (table 5.4) (measured volume x BTPS correction factor).[3]

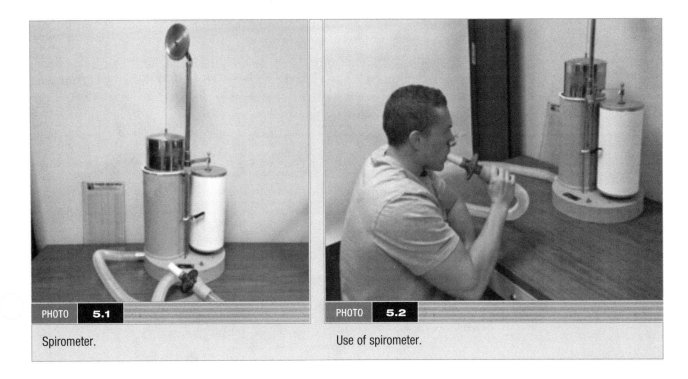

PHOTO 5.1	PHOTO 5.2
Spirometer.	Use of spirometer.

TABLE	5.4	Correction factors (CF) for coverting volume from ATPS to BTPS conditions.

Air Temperature (T_A)	CF	Air Temperature (T_A)	CF
20°	1.102	27	1.063
21	1.096	28	1.057
22	1.091	29	1.051
23	1.085	30	1.045
24	1.080	31	1.039
25	1.075	32	1.032
26	1.068	33	1.026

Measuring Forced Vital Capacity and Forced Expiratory Volume[1,11]

Ensure that the pen indicators are reset to the starting position on the drum. If necessary, replace the spirogram tracing paper. Change the timing knob setting to correspond to the desired FEV duration; for example 1.0 second ($FEV_{1.0}$).

Prior to starting the test, inform the subject(s) that they will be instructed to perform a maximal inhalation and exhalation. Emphasize that when exhaling, they must exhale as fast as possible for the first second and then continue to exhale for as long as they are able to empty their lungs as thoroughly as possible.

1. To begin the test, have the subject secure a nose clip and perform a deep, maximal inhalation of the room air before sealing his or her lips around the disposable mouthpiece attached to the spirometer. Once the lips are sealed, have the subject forcefully exhale all the air from his or her lungs as quickly as possible as noted above.

2. Repeat this procedure three times to get the largest value possible. Ensure that the spirometer is reset at the end of each trial. If the subject continues to produce increasing values (0.15 L above the previous trial), the test can be performed additional times.

3. Record the highest value for FVC and $FEV_{1.0}$ and multiply by the BTPS correction factor.

4. Once testing is complete, flush the air out of the drum by raising and lowering the spirometer bell three to five times.

Measuring RV

A number of methods are available to measure RV, including the nitrogen washout[5] and O_2 dilution;[14] the RV can also be estimated as a percentage of VC or by subtracting the known expiratory reserve volume (ERC) from the functional residual capacity (FRC). This lab will estimate RV as a gender-specific percentage of VC.[14]

1. Measure the subject's vital capacity (see previous section).
2. Determine the BTPS correction factor (table 5.4). Three other factors may need consideration when calculating BTPS: ambient pressure, instrument or bell factor, and the use of graph paper in BTPS units.[12]
3. Multiply the subject's vital capacity by the appropriate BTPS correction factor and then multiply by the gender specific constant (see equation below).

Equations[4,8]

tidal volume (TV) = IC − IRV

residual volume (RV) = FRC − ERV

VC_{BTPS} = VC x BTPS

RV = VC_{BTPS} x 0.24 (males) or VC_{BTPS} x 0.28 (females)

inspiratory capacity (IC) = TV + IRV

inspiratory reserve volume (IRV) = IC − TV

functional residual capacity (FRC) = ER + RV

vital capacity (VC) = IRV +TV + ERV

Sample Calculations

Gender: _Male_

Age: _22_

Body Weight: _82 kg_

Height: _187 cm_

Air Temperature (°C): _24_ P_B (mmHg): _755_

Relative Humidity: _35%_

BTPS correction factor (table 5.4): _1.080_

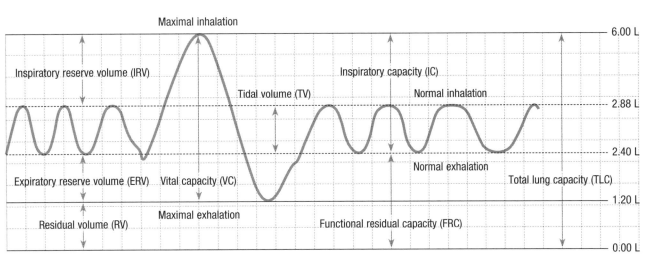

Using the equations above and the spirometer tracing, calculate the following variables:

IRV (L) = _3.12_   TV (L) = _.48 L_   ERV (L) = _1.2_

RV (L) = _4.8_ x 0.24 = _1.2 L_ (Estimation)

	T1	T2	T3	Highest FVC$_{ATPS}$	Actual BTPS (corrected) FVC$_{BTPS}$
FVC (L) =	4.7	4.8	4.8	4.8	5.2

Predicted FVC$_{BTPS}$ (L) =   6.2

table 5.5

	T1	T2	T3	Highest FEV$_{1.0ATPS}$	Actual BTPS (corrected) FEV$_{1.0BTPS}$
FEV$_{1.0}$ (L) =	4.4	4.6	5.0	5.0	5.4

Predicted FEV$_{1.0BTPS}$ (L) =   5.1

table 5.6

Evaluation   Classification Label (table 5.7)

%PFVC	5.2	/	6.2	x 100	83.8	%	Normal
	Actual		Predicted table 5.5				
%PFEV$_{1.0}$	5.4	/	5.1	x 100	105	%	Good
	Actual		Predicted table 5.6				
%FEV$_{1.0}$/FVC	5.4	/	5.2	x 100	104	%	Good
	Act FEV$_{1.0}$		Act FVC				

TABLE 5.5   Predicted forced vital capacity (FVC$_{BTPS}$) based on gender, height (cm), and age (y).

Height (cm)	Males Age (y)				Females Age (y)			
	20–24	25–29	30–34	35–39	20–24	25–29	30–34	35–39
155–159	4.29	4.22	4.15	4.06	3.52	3.52	3.50	3.46
160–164	4.58	4.52	4.44	4.35	3.76	3.76	3.74	3.70
165–169	4.89	4.83	4.75	4.66	4.00	4.00	3.98	3.94
170–174	5.21	5.14	5.07	4.98	4.25	4.25	4.23	4.20
175–179	5.53	5.47	5.39	5.30	4.51	4.51	4.49	4.45
180–184	5.87	5.80	5.73	5.64	4.78	4.78	4.76	4.72
185–189	6.21	6.15	6.07	5.98	5.05	5.05	5.03	4.99
190–194	6.56	6.50	6.42	6.33	5.33	5.33	5.31	5.27

Males: PFVC = $-0.1933 + 0.00064 \times Age - 0.000269 \times Age^2 + 0.00018642 \times Ht^2$

Females: PFVC = $-0.3560 + 0.0187 \times Age - 0.00382 \times Age^2 + 0.00014815 \times Ht^2$

Source: Data derived from Hankinson et al.[7]

| Predicted forced expiratory volume (PFEV$_{1.0BTPS}$) based on gender, height (cm), and age (y). | TABLE | 5.6 |

Height (cm)	Males Age (y)				Females Age (y)			
	20–24	25–29	30–34	35–39	20–24	25–29	30–34	35–39
155–159	3.66	3.55	3.44	3.31	3.09	3.03	2.95	2.87
160–164	3.88	3.78	3.66	3.54	3.28	3.21	3.14	3.05
165–169	4.12	4.01	3.89	3.77	3.47	3.40	3.33	3.24
170–174	4.35	4.25	4.13	4.01	3.66	3.60	3.52	3.44
175–179	4.60	4.49	4.38	4.25	3.86	3.80	3.72	3.64
180–184	4.85	4.75	4.63	4.51	4.08	4.00	3.93	3.84
185–189	5.11	5.01	4.89	4.77	4.28	4.21	4.14	4.05
190–194	5.38	5.27	5.16	5.03	4.50	4.43	4.36	4.27

Males: PFEV$_{1.0}$ = 0.5536 − 0.01303 x Age − 0.000172 x Age^2 + 0.00014098 x Ht^2

Females: PFEV$_{1.0}$ = 0.4333 − 0.00361 x Age − 0.000194 x Age^2 + 0.00011496 x Ht^2

Source: Data derived from Hankinson et al.[7]

| Category of lung function including degrees of lung restriction or obstruction. | TABLE | 5.7 |

Classification	% Predicted
High lung function	≥ 120%
Good lung function	100–119%
Normal lung function	80–99%
Mild restriction (FVC) or obstruction (FEV)	65–79%
Moderate restriction (FVC) or obstruction (FEV)	50–64%
Severe restriction (FVC) or obstruction (FEV)	35–49%
Very severe restriction (FVC) or obstruction (FEV)	< 35%

FVC = forced vital capacity

FEV = forced expiratory volume

Source: Data derived from Morris.[10]

Worksheet 5.1 — DETERMINATION OF LUNG VOLUMES AND CAPACITIES

Name _____ Date _____

Body Weight (kg): _____

Age: _____

Height (cm): _____

Air Temperature (°C): _____ P_B (mmHg): _____ Relative Humidity: _____

BTPS correction factor (table 5.4): _____

Using the lung capacity and volume equations as well as your spirometer tracing, calculate the following variables:

IRV (L) = _____ TV (L) = _____ ERV (L) = _____ RV (L) = (VC_{BTPS} = _____ x gender specific correction

factor = _____) = _____ (Estimation)

	T1	T2	T3	Highest FVC_{ATPS}	Actual BTPS (corrected) FVC_{BTPS}
FVC (L) =	_____	_____	_____	_____	_____

Predicted FVC_{BTPS} (L) = table 5.5 _____

	T1	T2	T3	Highest $FEV_{1.0\,ATPS}$	Actual BTPS (corrected) $FVC_{1.0\,BTPS}$
$FEV_{1.0}$ (L) =	_____	_____	_____	_____	_____

Predicted $FEV_{1.0\,BTPS}$ (L) = table 5.6 _____

Evaluation _____ Classification Label (table 5.7) _____

%PFVC _____ / _____ x 100 = _____ % _____
       Actual   Predicted

%PFEV$_{1.0}$ _____ / _____ x 100 = _____ % _____
       Actual   Predicted

%FEV$_{1.0}$/FVC _____ / _____ x 100 = _____ % _____
       Act FEV$_{1.0}$ Act FVC

EXTENSION ACTIVITIES

Name _____   *Date* _____

1. Graph the relationship between HT and VC for both males and females.
2. Graph the relationship between the condition of restrictive lung disease and forced vital capacity.

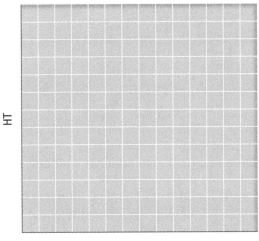

Vital capacity

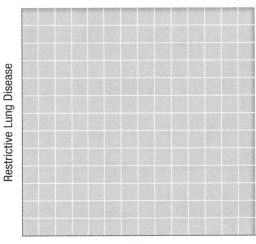

FVC

3. Paula Profusion (165 cm; 30 yrs) performed a pulmonary function test using a bell spirometer, and her results are below. Use her lung volume and capacity values to complete the following calculations:

Air temperature: 26°C, BTPS correction factor (table 5.4) = _____

IRV: 2067 mL   TV: 318 mL
IC: 2450 mL   ERV: 795 mL
FRC: 1750 mL   FVC: 3450 mL
TLC: 4200 mL FEV_1: 2980 mL

VC: _____ mL

RV: _____ mL

FVC_{BTPS}: _____ mL   Predicted FVC_{BTPS}: _____ mL

$FEV_{1.0BTPS}$: _____ mL   Predicted $FEV_{1.0BTPS}$: _____ mL

$\%FEV_{1.0}/FVC$: _____ mL

Lung function category (table 5.7): _____

REFERENCES

1. American College of Chest Physicians. Clinical spirometry: recommendations of the section on pulmonary function testing committee on pulmonary physiology. *Dis. Chest* 4:214; 1963.

2. American College of Sports Medicine. *ACSM's Guidelines for Exercise Testing and Prescription*, 9th edition. Baltimore: Wolters Kluwer/Lippincott Williams & Wilkins, 2014.

3. American Thoracic Society. Lung function testing: selection of reference values and interpretative strategies. *Am. Rev. Respir. Dis.* 144:1202–1218, 1991.

4. Beam, W., and Adams, G. *Exercise Physiology Laboratory Manual*, 7th edition. New York: McGraw-Hill, 2014.

5. DuBois, A. B., Botelho, S. Y., Bedell, G. N., Marshall, R., and Comroe Jr., J. H. A rapid plethysmographic method for measuring thoracic gas volume: a comparison with a nitrogen washout method for measuring functional residual capacity in normal subjects. *J. Clin. Invest.* 35(3):322, 1956.

6. Hankinson, J. L., Crapo, R. O., and Jensen R. L. Spirometric reference values for the 6-s FVC maneuver. *Chest* 124: 1805–1811, 2003.

7. Hankinson, J. L., Odencrantz, J. R., and Fedan, K. B. Spirometric reference values from a sample of the general U.S. population. *Am. J. Respir. Crit. Care Med.* 159: 179–187, 1999.

8. Housh, T. J., Housh, D. J., and DeVries, H. A. *Applied Exercise and Sport Physiology*, 4th edition. Scottsdale, AZ: Holcomb Hathaway, 2016.

9. Martini, F. H., Ober, W. C., Garrison, C. W., Welch, K., and Hutchings, R. T. Respiratory physiology. In *Fundamentals of Anatomy and Physiology*, 3rd edition. Englewood Cliffs, NJ: Prentice-Hall, 1995, pp. 846–858.

10. Morris, J. F. Spirometry in the evaluation of pulmonary function. *West. J. Med.* 125:110–118, 1976.

11. Universities Occupational Safety and Health Educational Resource Center. *NIOSH Spirometry Training Guide.* Morgantown, WV, December 2003.

12. Wasserman, K., Hansen, J. E., Sue, D. Y., Stringer, W. W., Sietsema, K. E., Sun, X., and Whipp, B. J. *Principles of Exercise Testing and Interpretation: Including Pathophysiology and Clinical Applications.* Philadelphia: Lippincott Williams & Wilkins, 2011.

13. Wilmore, J. H. A simplified method for determining residual volume. *J. Appl. Physiol.* 27:96–100, 1968.

14. Wilmore, J. H., Vodak, P. A., Parr, R. B., Girandola, R. N., and Billing, J. E. Further simplification of a method for determination of residual volume. *Med. Sci. Sports Exerc.* 12(3):216–218, 1979.

Unit 2

AEROBIC FITNESS

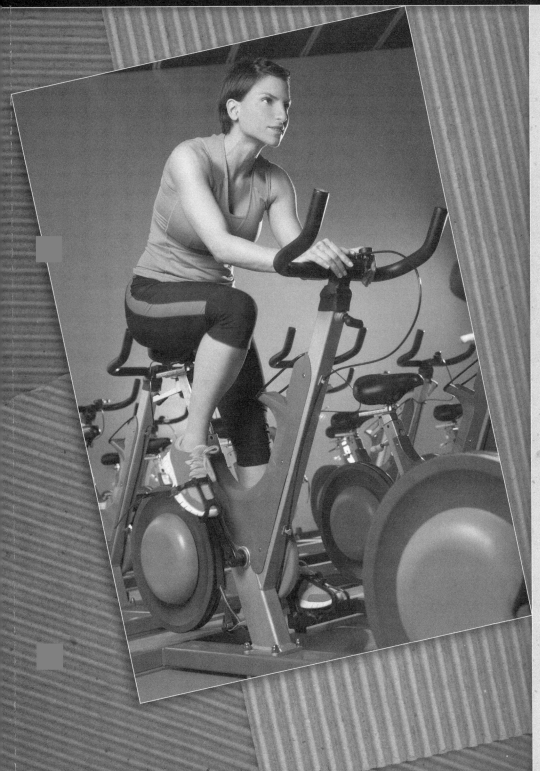

45

Lab 6

Direct Measurement of Oxygen Consumption Rate, Respiratory Exchange Ratio, and Caloric Expenditure Rate from Open-Circuit, Indirect Calorimetry

BACKGROUND

Oxygen consumption rate ($\dot{V}O_2$ = volume of oxygen consumed per minute) is an indirect measure of aerobic ATP production and is reflective of cardiorespiratory function. In addition, maximal oxygen consumption rate ($\dot{V}O_2$ max) is one of the best predictors of endurance performance.

In most exercise physiology laboratories, $\dot{V}O_2$ is determined from gas exchange parameters measured using a metabolic cart and an open-circuit technique (photo 6.1). Typically, this means that, while exercising on a treadmill or cycle ergometer, the subject breathes room air through one side of a mouthpiece, and the expired samples are directed to the oxygen (O_2) and carbon dioxide (CO_2) gas analyzers in the metabolic cart through the other side of the mouthpiece (photo 6.2). In addition to $\dot{V}O_2$, other information can be obtained from these tests, such as the respiratory exchange ratio (R value) and caloric expenditure rate (CER).

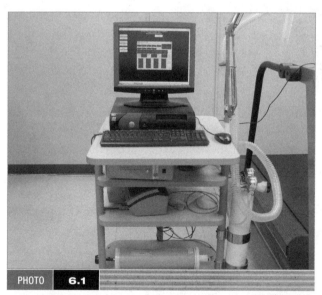

PHOTO **6.1**

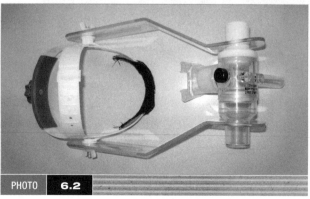

PHOTO **6.2**

R Value

The R value is defined as the ratio of CO_2 produced to O_2 consumed ($\dot{V}CO_2/\dot{V}O_2$) and reflects the foodstuffs (carbohydrates or fats) that are being used to produce ATP. [*Note:* The technique described in this laboratory ignores the small contribution of protein to ATP production during exercise, and technically, the R value is therefore more accurately termed the non-protein R value.] Theoretically, the R value ranges from 0.70 to 1.00 (although it is common to have R values during high-intensity exercise that are greater than 1.00). An R value of 0.70 indicates that fats are being used to fuel the exercise, while an R value of 1.00 indicates that carbohydrates are being used. R values between 0.70 and 1.00 indicate that a combination of fats and carbohydrates is being metabolized to produce ATP. During low-intensity exercise, fats are the primary fuel source for ATP production, and the R value tends to be about 0.70 to 0.80. As the intensity of exercise is increased (for example, shifting from a walking to a running pace), the R value increases, and ATP is then produced from a combination of fat and carbohydrate sources. With maximal-intensity exercise, the R value is 1.00 (or greater), and carbohydrates are used exclusively for ATP production.

Fats R = 0.70	Fats and Carbohydrates R = 0.85	Carbohydrates R = 1.00
Low-intensity exercise	Moderate-intensity exercise	Maximal-intensity exercise

Caloric Expenditure Rate

Caloric expenditure rate (CER) during exercise can be calculated from the $\dot{V}O_2$ and the R value. The number of calories expended during exercise is, in part, dependent on the foodstuffs (fats and carbohydrates) that are being used to produce ATP. If we know the R value, we can use table 6.1 to determine the kilocalories expended per liter of oxygen consumed. To calculate CER, we simply multiply the value from table 6.1 by the $\dot{V}O_2$ value measured during exercise.

KNOW THESE TERMS & ABBREVIATIONS

- $\dot{V}O_2$ L • min^{-1} = volume of O_2 consumed
- $\dot{V}CO_2$ L • min^{-1} = volume of CO_2 produced
- $\dot{V}CO_{2I}$ L • min^{-1} = volume of CO_2 inspired
- $\dot{V}CO_{2E}$ L • min^{-1} = volume of CO_2 expired
- $\dot{V}O_{2I}$ L • min^{-1} = volume of O_2 inspired
- $\dot{V}O_{2E}$ L • min^{-1} = volume of O_2 expired
- $\dot{V}_I$ L • min^{-1} = volume of inspired gas (room air)
- $\dot{V}_E$ L • min^{-1} = volume of expired gas
- R value = respiratory exchange ratio ($\dot{V}CO_2$ / $\dot{V}O_2$)

Kilocalories expended per liter of O_2 consumed at a given R value.   **TABLE 6.1**

R	Kilocalories per liter of O$_2$ consumed ($\dot{V}O_2$)	Percentage of kilocalories derived from Carbo-hydrates	Fats	R	Kilocalories per liter of O$_2$ consumed ($\dot{V}O_2$)	Percentage of kilocalories derived from Carbo-hydrates	Fats	R	Kilocalories per liter of O$_2$ consumed ($\dot{V}O_2$)	Percentage of kilocalories derived from Carbo-hydrates	Fats
0.70	4.686	0	100	0.80	4.801	33	67	0.90	4.924	68	32
0.71	4.690	1	99	0.81	4.813	37	63	0.91	4.936	71	29
0.72	4.702	5	95	0.82	4.825	40	60	0.92	4.948	74	26
0.73	4.714	8	92	0.83	4.838	44	56	0.93	4.961	77	23
0.74	4.727	12	88	0.84	4.850	47	53	0.94	4.973	81	19
0.75	4.739	16	84	0.85	4.862	51	49	0.95	4.985	84	16
0.76	4.751	19	81	0.86	4.875	54	46	0.96	4.998	87	13
0.77	4.764	23	77	0.87	4.887	58	42	0.97	5.010	90	10
0.78	4.776	26	74	0.88	4.899	61	39	0.98	5.022	94	6
0.79	4.788	30	70	0.89	4.911	64	36	0.99	5.035	97	3
								1.00	5.047	100	0

- ⊙ CER = caloric expenditure rate ($\dot{V}O_2$ × kilocalories expended per liter of O_2 consumed)

- ⊙ STPD = standard temperature pressure dry correction factor

- ⊙ $\dot{V}O_2$ max = maximal oxygen consumption rate

PROCEDURES (see photos 6.3–6.4)

There are many treadmill and cycle ergometer protocols used in laboratory and clinical settings. Table 6.2 provides a list of commonly used protocols in clinical and laboratory settings for diagnostic purposes and/or to determine $\dot{V}O_2$ max, gas exchange threshold, ventilatory threshold, and respiratory compensation point (see Lab 14). The choice of which one to use depends on the goals of the test (diagnostic or functional), the variables to be measured ($\dot{V}O_2$ max, ventilatory threshold, etc.), the exercise capacity of the subjects being tested (patients or athletes, etc.), and the age of the subjects (children, adults, or elderly). The procedures outlined in this laboratory are designed only to provide information about the effects of three different exercise intensities on the measurement of $\dot{V}O_2$, R value, and CER. Thus, this specific protocol should not be considered a recommendation for testing any particular population of subjects. Typically, during treadmill tests, exercise intensity can be increased by changing the velocity and/or grade (incline). Each stage should be 3 minutes in duration (although other durations are commonly used) so that a steady state $\dot{V}O_2$ value can be obtained.

1. Calibrate the metabolic cart according to the manufacturer's procedures.

2. Place and adjust the breathing valve while the subject straddles the treadmill (photo 6.3).

3. Attach the hose from the expiratory end of the breathing valve to the metabolic cart.

4. Set the treadmill velocity at a walking pace of 3.0 mph (4.8 km • hr⁻¹) and 0% grade (photo 6.4). Have the subject step onto the treadmill, using the handrails for stabilization, and walk at this speed and grade for 3 minutes. Collect and analyze expired gas samples for the final 30 seconds of the 3-minute stage.

5. At the end of the first 3-minute stage of exercise at 3.0 mph and 0% grade, increase the treadmill velocity to a jogging pace of 6.0 mph (9.7 km • hr⁻¹) and 0% grade. Again, collect and analyze expired gas samples for the final 30 seconds of the 3-minute stage.

6. At the end of the second 3-minute stage of exercise at 6.0 mph, raise the treadmill incline to a grade of 2%. Thus, the subject will be jogging at 6.0 mph and 2% grade. Collect and analyze expired gas samples for the final 30 seconds of the 3-minute stage.

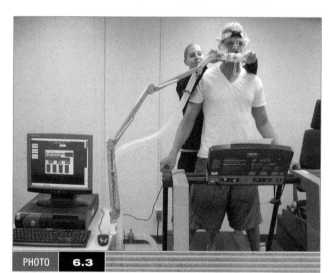

PHOTO 6.3

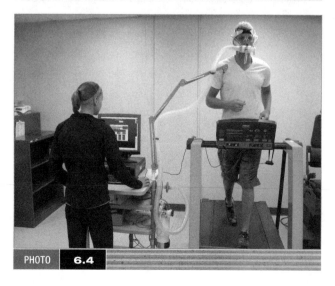

PHOTO 6.4

At the end of the three stages, data can be calculated (or will be available directly from the metabolic cart) for three separate exercise intensities: 3.0 mph, 0% grade; 6.0 mph, 0% grade; and 6.0 mph, 2% grade (worksheet 6.1). The $\dot{V}O_2$, R value, and CER value should demonstrate progressive increases with each increase in exercise intensity.

Commonly used treadmill and cycle ergometer protocols in clinical and laboratory settings for diagnostic purposes and/or to determine $\dot{V}O_2$ max.	TABLE	6.2

Treadmill Protocols

BRUCE PROTOCOL

Application: Clinical testing, cardiac stress testing, physically active individuals

Stage	Duration (min)	Velocity (mph)	Grade (%)
1	3	1.7	10
2	3	2.5	12
3	3	3.4	14
4	3	4.2	16
5	3	5.0	18
6	3	5.5	20
7	3	6.0	22

BRUCE RAMP PROTOCOL

Application: Clinical testing, cardiac stress testing, physically active individuals

Stage	Duration (min)	Velocity (mph)	Grade (%)
1	1	1.0	0
2	1	1.3	5
3	1	1.7	10
4	1	2.1	10
5	1	2.3	11
6	1	2.5	12
7	1	2.8	12
8	1	3.1	13
9	1	3.4	14
10	1	3.8	14
11	1	4.1	15
12	1	4.2	16
13	1	4.5	16
14	1	4.8	17
15	1	5.0	18
16	1	5.3	18
17	1	5.6	19
18	1	5.8	20

(continued)

TABLE 6.2 Continued.

MODIFIED BALKE PROTOCOL

Application: Clinical testing, deconditioned individuals, patients

Stage	Duration (min)	Velocity (mph)	Grade (%)
1	2	2.0	0
2	2	3.0	0
3	2	3.0	2.5
4	2	3.0	5.0
5	2	3.0	7.5
6	2	3.0	10.0
7	2	3.0	12.5
8	2	3.0	15.0
9	2	3.0	17.5
10	2	3.0	20.0
11	2	3.0	22.5
12	2	3.0	25.0

BERGSTROM-COCHRANE PROTOCOL

Application: Athletes, conditioned individuals; determination of $\dot{V}O_2$ max, gas exchange, ventilatory threshold, and respiratory compensation point

Stage	Duration (min)	Velocity (mph)	Grade (%)
1	2	4.0	0
2	2	5.0	0
3	2	6.0	0
4	2	7.0	0
5	2	8.0	0
6	2	9.0	0
7	2	9.0	2
8	2	9.0	4

Note: Continue test at 9 mph and increase grade by 2.0% every 2 minutes until voluntary exhaustion.

Cycle Ergometer Protocols

INCREMENTAL PROTOCOL

Application: Unconditioned to athletic individuals; determination of $\dot{V}O_2$ max, gas exchange threshold, ventilatory threshold, and respiratory compensation point

Stage	Duration (min)	Power Output (W)	Pedal Rate (rpm)
1	2	30	70
2	2	60	70
3	2	90	70
4	2	120	70

Note: Continue test by increasing the power output by 30 W every 2 minutes until voluntary exhaustion. This protocol begins at a power output of 30 W and a standard pedal rate of 70 rpm. These parameters, however, can be modified based on the fitness level and cycling experience of the individual. Low to moderately fit individuals and inexperienced cyclists can begin the protocol at 20 W and often prefer a pedal rate of 50–70 rpm. Highly trained individuals and experienced cyclists can begin the protocol at 80 or 110 W and often prefer a pedal rate of 80–90 rpm.

Continued. TABLE **6.2**

RAMP PROTOCOL

Application: Unconditioned to athletic individuals; determination of $\dot{V}O_2$ max, gas exchange threshold, ventilatory threshold, and respiratory compensation point

Stage	Duration (min)	Power Output (W)	Pedal Rate (rpm)
1	1 W every 4 seconds = 15 W • min⁻¹	30	70

Note: Continue test by increasing the power output by 1 W every 4 seconds until voluntary exhaustion. This protocol begins at a power output of 30 W and a standard pedal rate of 70 rpm. These parameters, however, can be modified based on the fitness level and cycling experience of the individual. Low to moderately fit individuals and inexperienced cyclists can begin the protocol at a pedal rate of 50–70 rpm. Highly trained individuals and experienced cyclists can begin the protocol at 90 or 120 W and often prefer a pedal rate of 80–90 rpm.

SAMPLE CALCULATIONS

Calculation of $\dot{V}O_2$ (Expressed in L • min⁻¹)

The determination of $\dot{V}O_2$ during exercise requires the measurement of the following values:

1. The volume of inspired gas ($\dot{V}_I$).
2. The concentration of O_2 in expired gas (%O_2 expired or %O_{2E}).
3. The concentration of CO_2 in expired gas (%CO_2 expired or %CO_{2E}).
4. Gas temperature and pressure.

The amount of O_2 consumed per minute ($\dot{V}O_2$) during exercise is equal to the difference between the amount of O_2 inspired ($\dot{V}O_{2I}$) and the amount of O_2 expired ($\dot{V}O_{2E}$).

Equation 1: $\dot{V}O_2 = \dot{V}O_{2I} - \dot{V}O_{2E}$

For example, assume the following data were collected on a subject:

$\dot{V}_I = 100 \text{ L} \bullet \text{min}^{-1}$

$\%O_{2E} = 16.9\%$

$\%CO_{2E} = 3.5\%$

To determine $\dot{V}O_2$ from Equation 1, we must first calculate $\dot{V}O_{2I}$ and $\dot{V}O_{2E}$.

Equation 2: $\dot{V}O_{2I} = \dot{V}_I \times$ STPD correction factor $\times$ (%O_2 in inspired gas/100)

Equation 3: $\dot{V}O_{2E} = \dot{V}_E \times$ STPD correction factor $\times$ (%O_2 in expired gas/100)

Note: Inspired and expired gas volumes are standardized to account for the effects of varying atmospheric temperatures and pressures. This standardization is accomplished by simply multiplying the measured gas volume by an STPD (standard temperature pressure dry) correction factor. The STPD correction factors are available in standard tables, but for this laboratory experience a correction factor will be provided for you.

Assume an STPD correction factor of 0.885.

Typically, during exercise, $\dot{V}_I$ does not equal $\dot{V}_E$ because the volume of O_2 consumed rarely equals the volume of CO_2 produced. If $\dot{V}_I$ is measured, $\dot{V}_E$ can be calculated using the following equation:

Equation 4: $\dot{V}_E$ STPD = $\dot{V}_I \times$ STPD correction factor $\times \dfrac{79.04}{100 - (\%O_{2E} + \%CO_{2E})}$

Thus, for the current example:

$\dot{V}_I$ STPD = 100 L $\cdot$ min^{-1} $\times$ 0.885 = 88.5 L $\cdot$ min^{-1}

$\dot{V}_E$ STPD = 100 L $\cdot$ min^{-1} $\times$ 0.885 $\times \dfrac{79.04}{100 - (16.9 + 3.5)}$

$\dot{V}_E$ STPD = 87.877 L $\cdot$ min^{-1}

Once $\dot{V}_I$ STPD and $\dot{V}_E$ STPD are determined, Equations 2 and 3 can be used to determine $\dot{V}O_{2I}$ and $\dot{V}O_{2E}$.

$\dot{V}O_{2I} = \dot{V}_I$ STPD $\times$ **(20.93/100)**

$\dot{V}O_{2I} = 88.5 \times 0.2093$

$\dot{V}O_{2I} = 18.523$ L $\cdot$ min^{-1}

Note: **The percent of O_2 in inspired gas (room air) is a constant 20.93 percent.**

$\dot{V}O_{2E} = \dot{V}_E$ STPD $\times$ (16.9/100)

$\dot{V}O_{2E} = 87.877 \times 0.1690$

$\dot{V}O_{2E} = 14.851$ L $\cdot$ min^{-1}

Once $\dot{V}O_{2I}$ and $\dot{V}O_{2E}$ are determined, Equation 1 can be used to determine $\dot{V}O_2$.

$\dot{V}O_2 = \dot{V}O_{2I} - \dot{V}O_{2E}$

$\dot{V}O_2 = 18.523$ L $\cdot$ min^{-1} $- 14.851$ L $\cdot$ min^{-1}

$\dot{V}O_2 = 3.672$ L $\cdot$ min^{-1}

The volume of CO_2 produced ($\dot{V}CO_2$) can be calculated in a similar manner. Please notice that the volume of CO_2 in expired gas is greater than in inspired gas. This is because we consume O_2, but we produce CO_2.

Equation 5: $\dot{V}CO_2 = \dot{V}CO_{2E} - \dot{V}CO_{2I}$

$\dot{V}CO_{2E} = \dot{V}_E$ STPD $\times$ (3.5/100)

$\dot{V}CO_{2E} = 87.877 \times 0.035$

$\dot{V}CO_{2E} = 3.076$ L $\cdot$ min^{-1}

$\dot{V}CO_{2I} = \dot{V}_I$ STPD $\times$ **(0.03/100)**

$\dot{V}CO_{2I} = 88.5 \times 0.0003$

$\dot{V}CO_{2I} = 0.027$ L $\cdot$ min^{-1}

Note: **The percent of CO_2 in inspired gas (room air) is a constant 0.03 percent.**

Substituting $\dot{V}CO_{2E}$ and $\dot{V}CO_{2I}$ into Equation 5 results in:

$$\dot{V}CO_2 = \dot{V}CO_{2E} - \dot{V}CO_{2I}$$
$$\dot{V}CO_2 = 3.076 \text{ L} \cdot \text{min}^{-1} - 0.027 \text{ L} \cdot \text{min}^{-1}$$
$$\dot{V}CO_2 = 3.049 \text{ L} \cdot \text{min}^{-1}$$

Calculation of R Value

Once $\dot{V}O_2$ and $\dot{V}CO_2$ are determined, the R value can be calculated using Equation 6.

Equation 6: $R = \dot{V}CO_2 / \dot{V}O_2$

$$R = 3.049 \text{ L} \cdot \text{min}^{-1} / 3.672 \text{ L} \cdot \text{min}^{-1}$$

$$R = 0.83$$

In this example, the R value of 0.83 indicates that approximately 56% of the ATP is produced from fats and 44% from carbohydrate sources (table 6.1).

Calculation of Caloric Expenditure Rate (CER)

Once $\dot{V}O_2$ and the R value are known, the CER can be calculated. Based on the R value, the caloric cost (kilocalories) of the exercise per liter of O_2 consumed ($\dot{V}O_2$) can be determined from table 6.1.

$$CER = \dot{V}O_2 \times \text{kilocalories per liter of } O_2 \text{ consumed}$$

In the current example:

$$CER = 3.672 \times 4.838 \text{ (from table 6.1 with an R value of 0.83)}$$

$$CER = 17.77 \text{ kilocalories expended per minute of exercise}$$

Below are two additional examples of calculations for $\dot{V}O_2$, R value, and CER. As exercise intensity increases, $\dot{V}O_2$, R value, and CER also increase.

Low-Intensity Exercise

$$\dot{V}_I = 35.0 \text{ L} \cdot \text{min}^{-1}$$
$$\%O_{2E} = 17.0\%$$
$$\%CO_{2E} = 3.2\%$$
$$\text{STPD correction factor} = 0.885$$

Calculation of $\dot{V}O_2$

Equation 1: $\dot{V}O_2 = \dot{V}O_{2I} - \dot{V}O_{2E}$

Equation 2: $\dot{V}O_{2I} = 35.0 \text{ L} \cdot \text{min}^{-1} \times 0.885 \times 0.2093$

$$\dot{V}O_{2I} = 6.483 \text{ L} \cdot \text{min}^{-1}$$

Equation 3: $\dot{V}O_{2E} = \dot{V}_E \times 0.885 \times 0.170$

Equation 4: $\dot{V}_E \text{ STPD} = 35.0 \text{ L} \cdot \text{min}^{-1} \times 0.885 \times \dfrac{79.04}{100 - (17.0 + 3.2)}$

$$\dot{V}_E \text{ STPD} = 30.68 \text{ L} \cdot \text{min}^{-1}$$

$$\dot{V}O_{2E} = 30.68 \times 0.170$$
$$\dot{V}O_{2E} = 5.216 \text{ L} \cdot \text{min}^{-1}$$

Equation 1: $\dot{V}O_2 = 6.483 \text{ L} \cdot \text{min}^{-1} - 5.216 \text{ L} \cdot \text{min}^{-1}$
$$\dot{V}O_2 = 1.267 \text{ L} \cdot \text{min}^{-1}$$

Calculation of $\dot{V}CO_2$

Equation 5: $\dot{V}CO_2 = \dot{V}CO_{2E} - \dot{V}CO_{2I}$
$$\dot{V}CO_{2E} = \dot{V}_E \text{ STPD} \times (3.2/100)$$
$$\dot{V}CO_{2E} = 30.68 \text{ L} \cdot \text{min}^{-1} \times 0.032$$
$$\dot{V}CO_{2E} = 0.982 \text{ L} \cdot \text{min}^{-1}$$
$$\dot{V}CO_{2I} = \dot{V}_I \text{ STPD} \times (0.03/100)$$
$$\dot{V}CO_{2I} = 30.975 \text{ L} \cdot \text{min}^{-1} \times 0.0003$$
$$\dot{V}CO_{2I} = 0.0093 \text{ L} \cdot \text{min}^{-1}$$

Thus, from Equation 5: $\dot{V}CO_2 = 0.982 \text{ L} \cdot \text{min}^{-1} - 0.0093 \text{ L} \cdot \text{min}^{-1}$
$$\dot{V}CO_2 = 0.973 \text{ L} \cdot \text{min}^{-1}$$

Calculation of R value

$$R = \dot{V}CO_2 / \dot{V}O_2$$
$$R = 0.973 / 1.267$$
$$R = 0.77$$

Calculation of CER

$$\text{CER} = \dot{V}O_2 \times \text{kilocalories per liter of } O_2 \text{ consumed}$$
$$(\text{kcal} \cdot \text{L}^{-1}) \text{ (from table 6.1)}$$
$$\text{CER} = 1.267 \text{ L} \cdot \text{min}^{-1} \times 4.764 \text{ (kcal} \cdot \text{L}^{-1})$$
$$\text{CER} = 6.04 \text{ kcal} \cdot \text{min}^{-1}$$

High-Intensity Exercise

$$\dot{V}_I = 135.0 \text{ L} \cdot \text{min}^{-1}$$
$$\%O_{2E} = 17.6\%$$
$$\%CO_{2E} = 3.2\%$$
$$\text{STPD correction factor} = 0.885$$

Calculation of $\dot{V}O_2$

Equation 1: $\dot{V}O_2 = \dot{V}O_{2I} - \dot{V}O_{2E}$

Equation 2: $\dot{V}O_{2I} = 135.0 \text{ L} \cdot \text{min}^{-1} \times 0.885 \times 0.2093$
$$\dot{V}O_{2I} = 25.01 \text{ L} \cdot \text{min}^{-1}$$

Equation 3: $\dot{V}O_{2E} = \dot{V}_E \times 0.885 \times 0.176$

Equation 4: $\dot{V}_E \text{ STPD} = 135.0 \text{ L} \cdot \text{min}^{-1} \times 0.885 \times \dfrac{79.04}{100 - (17.6 + 3.2)}$

$$\dot{V}_E \text{ STPD} = 119.24 \text{ L} \cdot \text{min}^{-1}$$

$$\dot{V}O_{2E} = 119.24 \times 0.176$$

$$\dot{V}O_{2E} = 20.986 \text{ L} \cdot \text{min}^{-1}$$

Equation 1: $\dot{V}O_2 = 25.01 \text{ L} \cdot \text{min}^{-1} - 20.986 \text{ L} \cdot \text{min}^{-1}$

$$\dot{V}O_2 = 4.024 \text{ L} \cdot \text{min}^{-1}$$

Calculation of $\dot{V}CO_2$

Equation 5: $\dot{V}CO_2 = \dot{V}CO_{2E} - \dot{V}CO_{2I}$

$$\dot{V}CO_{2E} = \dot{V}_E \text{ STPD} \times (3.2/100)$$

$$\dot{V}CO_{2E} = 119.24 \text{ L} \cdot \text{min}^{-1} \times 0.032$$

$$\dot{V}CO_{2E} = 3.816 \text{ L} \cdot \text{min}^{-1}$$

$$\dot{V}CO_{2I} = \dot{V}_I \text{ STPD} \times (0.03/100)$$

$$\dot{V}CO_{2I} = 119.475 \text{ L} \cdot \text{min}^{-1} \times 0.0003$$

$$\dot{V}CO_{2I} = 0.036 \text{ L} \cdot \text{min}^{-1}$$

Thus, from Equation 5: $\dot{V}CO_2 = 3.816 \text{ L} \cdot \text{min}^{-1} - 0.036 \text{ L} \cdot \text{min}^{-1}$

$$\dot{V}CO_2 = 3.78 \text{ L} \cdot \text{min}^{-1}$$

Calculation of R value

$$R = \dot{V}CO_2 / \dot{V}O_2$$

$$R = 3.78 / 4.024$$

$$R = 0.94$$

Calculation of CER

$$CER = \dot{V}O_2 \times \text{kilocalories per liter of } O_2 \text{ consumed}$$
$$(\text{kcal} \cdot \text{L}^{-1}) \text{ (from table 6.1)}$$

$$CER = 4.024 \times 4.973 \text{ (kcal} \cdot \text{L}^{-1})$$

$$CER = 20.01 \text{ kcal} \cdot \text{min}^{-1}$$

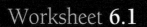

Worksheet 6.1 | DIRECT MEASUREMENT OF $\dot{V}O_2$, R VALUE, AND CER

Name _____ *Date* _____

Stage 1: 3 mph and 0% grade

$\dot{V}_I$ = _____ L • min^{-1} *Calculate:* $\dot{V}O_2$ = _____ L • min^{-1}

$\%O_{2E}$ = _____ % $\dot{V}CO_2$ = _____ L • min^{-1}

$\%CO_{2E}$ = _____ %   R value = _____

STPD = _____   CER = _____ kcal • min^{-1}

Stage 2: 6 mph and 0% grade

$\dot{V}_I$ = _____ L • min^{-1} *Calculate:* $\dot{V}O_2$ = _____ L • min^{-1}

$\%O_{2E}$ = _____ % $\dot{V}CO_2$ = _____ L • min^{-1}

$\%CO_{2E}$ = _____ %   R value = _____

STPD = _____   CER = _____ kcal • min^{-1}

Stage 3: 6 mph and 2% grade

$\dot{V}_I$ = _____ L • min^{-1} *Calculate:* $\dot{V}O_2$ = _____ L • min^{-1}

$\%O_{2E}$ = _____ % $\dot{V}CO_2$ = _____ L • min^{-1}

$\%CO_{2E}$ = _____ %   R value = _____

STPD = _____   CER = _____ kcal • min^{-1}

Worksheet 6.2

Name   *Date*

1. Listed below are gas exchange data collected using an open-circuit procedure during a treadmill test. For each stage of the test calculate:

   a. $\dot{V}O_2$ (L • min^{-1})

   b. $\dot{V}CO_2$ (L • min^{-1})

   c. R value

   d. CER (kcal • min^{-1})

   e. Indicate what type of foodstuff (fats, carbohydrates, or combination) is being used to produce ATP.

Stage	$\dot{V}_I$	$\%O_{2E}$	$\%CO_{2E}$
1	60.3 L • min^{-1}	16.25%	4.02%
2	71.95 L • min^{-1}	15.48%	5.03%
3	103.79 L • min^{-1}	15.74%	5.16%

Note: Assume an STPD correction factor of 0.885.

BACKGROUND

The determination of maximal oxygen consumption rate ($\dot{V}O_2$ max) provides information related to an individual's level of cardiorespiratory fitness and is a valuable predictor of endurance exercise and sports performance. In Lab 8, the Astrand–Rhyming submaximal cycle ergometer test utilizes the relationship between heart rate and power output to estimate $\dot{V}O_2$ max. In this laboratory, regression equations for males and females are used to estimate $\dot{V}O_2$ max without the need for subjects to exercise. The equations in this laboratory employ demographic variables such as age, height, and body weight as well as descriptive variables related to exercise habits, including the duration of exercise, intensity of exercise, and years of training. Typically, the errors associated with these equations (± 10 to 15%) are approximately the same as those for exercise-based estimates of $\dot{V}O_2$ max.[1,2,3] The accuracy of the equations, however, is influenced by the level of fitness of the subject and, therefore, in this laboratory equations are provided that can be used for both untrained and aerobically trained individuals.

KNOW THESE TERMS & ABBREVIATIONS

- R = multiple correlation coefficient; a numerical measure of how well a dependent variable can be predicted from a combination of independent variables (a number between –1 and 1)

- regression equations = statistical methods that are developed and used to relate two or more variables

- SEE = standard error of estimate; a measure of the accuracy of the predictions made using a regression equation

- $\dot{V}O_2$ max = maximal oxygen consumption rate

PROCEDURES

Record the following information on worksheet 7.1.

1. Your height in cm, body weight in kg, and age in years.

2. Refer to the Borg Rating of Perceived Exertion Scale (see Lab 21, p. 160) to estimate the typical intensity of training using the following statement:[2,3] "Indicate, in general, the intensity at which you perform your exercise regimen."

3. Indicate the duration of training using the following question:[2,3] "How many hours per week do you exercise?"

4. Record the years of training using the following question:[2,3] "How long have you consistently (no more than one month without exercise) been exercising?"

5. Determine the natural log of years of training. That is, enter the client's years of training and then hit "LN," or natural log function, on a hand-held calculator. You may also search online for "What is the natural log of _____?" In the blank insert the years of training.

6. Determine $\dot{V}O_2$ max in L • min^{-1} or mL • min^{-1}

7. Calculate $\dot{V}O_2$ max in mL • kg^{-1} • min^{-1} using the relevant equation below.

8. Identify fitness category from table 7.1 on p. 60.

Equations

Untrained Males[1]

$\dot{V}O_2$ max (L • min^{-1}) = (0.046 x height in cm) – (0.021 x age in years) – 4.31

R (multiple correlation coefficient) = 0.87

SEE = 0.458 L • min^{-1}

Untrained Females[1]

$\dot{V}O_2$ max (L • min^{-1}) = (0.046 x height in cm) – (0.021 x age in years) – 4.93

R = 0.87

SEE = 0.458 L • min^{-1}

*Aerobically Trained Males[3]

$\dot{V}O_2$ max (mL • min^{-1}) = (27.387 x body weight in kg) + (26.634 x height in cm) – (27.572 x age in years) + (26.161 x duration of training in hours per week) + (114.904 x intensity of training using the Borg Scale) + (506.752 x natural log of years of training) – 4609.791

R = 0.82

SEE = 378 mL • min^{-1}

*Aerobically Trained Females[2]

$\dot{V}O_2$ max (mL • min^{-1}) = (18.528 x body weight in kg) + (11.993 x height in cm) – (17.197 x age in years) + (23.522 x duration of training in hours per week) + (62.118 x intensity of training using the Borg Scale) + (278.262 x natural log of years of training) – 1375.878

R = 0.83

SEE = 247 mL • min^{-1}

* "Aerobically trained" is defined as having participated in continuous aerobic exercise three or more sessions per week for a minimum of 1 hour per session, for at least the past 18 months.[2,3]

Sample Calculations

AEROBICALLY TRAINED MALE[3]

Height: _180 cm_

Body weight: _80 kg_

Age: _25 years_

Intensity of training: _15_

Duration of training: _6 h • wk^{-1}_

Years of training: _____8_____ : natural log of 8 = 2.08

Equation: $27.387 \times 80 = 2190.96$

plus $26.634 \times 180 = 6985.08$

minus $27.572 \times 25 = 6295.78$

plus $26.161 \times 6 = 6452.75$

plus $114.904 \times 15 = 8176.31$

plus $506.752 \times 2.08 = 9230.35$

minus $4609.791 = \dot{V}O_2 \max (mL \cdot min^{-1}) = 4620.56 \ mL \cdot min^{-1}$

$\dot{V}O_2 \max (mL \cdot kg^{-1} \cdot min^{-1}) = 4620.56/80 = 57.76 \ mL \cdot kg^{-1} \cdot min^{-1}$

Fitness category from table 7.1 = Superior

UNTRAINED FEMALE[1]

Height: _166 cm_

Body weight: _59 kg_

Age: _22 years_

Equation: $0.046 \times 166 = 7.64$

minus $0.021 \times 22 = 7.18$

minus $4.93 = \dot{V}O_2 \max (L \cdot min^{-1}) = 2.25 \ L \cdot min^{-1}$

$\dot{V}O_2 \max (mL \cdot min^{-1}) = 2.25 \times 1000 = 2250 \ mL \cdot min^{-1}$

$\dot{V}O_2 \max (mL \cdot kg^{-1} \cdot min^{-1}) = 2250 / 59 = 38.14 \ mL \cdot kg^{-1} \cdot min^{-1}$

Fitness category from table 7.1 = Excellent

TABLE 7.1 Men's and women's aerobic fitness classifications.

Men		Age (years)					
CATEGORY	MEASURE	13–19	20–29	30–39	40–49	50–59	60+
I. Very Poor	$\dot{V}O_2 \max (mL \cdot kg^{-1} \cdot min^{-1})$	<35.0	<33.0	<31.5	<30.2	<26.1	<20.5
II. Poor	$\dot{V}O_2 \max (mL \cdot kg^{-1} \cdot min^{-1})$	35.0–38.3	33.0–36.4	31.5–35.4	30.2–33.5	26.1–30.9	20.5–26.0
III. Fair	$\dot{V}O_2 \max (mL \cdot kg^{-1} \cdot min^{-1})$	38.4–45.1	36.5–42.4	35.5–40.9	33.6–38.9	31.0–35.7	26.1–32.2
IV. Good	$\dot{V}O_2 \max (mL \cdot kg^{-1} \cdot min^{-1})$	45.2–50.9	42.5–46.4	41.0–44.9	39.0–43.7	35.8–40.9	32.3–36.4
V. Excellent	$\dot{V}O_2 \max (mL \cdot kg^{-1} \cdot min^{-1})$	51.0–55.9	46.5–52.4	45.0–49.4	43.8–48.0	41.0–45.3	36.5–44.2
VI. Superior	$\dot{V}O_2 \max (mL \cdot kg^{-1} \cdot min^{-1})$	>56.0	>52.5	>49.5	>48.1	>45.4	>44.3

Women		Age (years)					
CATEGORY	MEASURE	13–19	20–29	30–39	40–49	50–59	60+
I. Very Poor	$\dot{V}O_2 \max (mL \cdot kg^{-1} \cdot min^{-1})$	<25.0	<23.6	<22.8	<21.0	<20.2	<17.5
II. Poor	$\dot{V}O_2 \max (mL \cdot kg^{-1} \cdot min^{-1})$	25.0–30.9	23.6–28.9	22.8–26.9	21.0–24.4	20.2–22.7	17.5–20.1
III. Fair	$\dot{V}O_2 \max (mL \cdot kg^{-1} \cdot min^{-1})$	31.0–34.9	29.0–32.9	27.0–31.4	24.5–28.9	22.8–26.9	20.2–24.4
IV. Good	$\dot{V}O_2 \max (mL \cdot kg^{-1} \cdot min^{-1})$	35.0–38.9	33.0–36.9	31.5–35.6	29.0–32.8	27.0–31.4	24.5–30.2
V. Excellent	$\dot{V}O_2 \max (mL \cdot kg^{-1} \cdot min^{-1})$	39.0–41.9	37.0–40.9	35.7–40.0	32.9–36.9	31.5–35.7	30.3–31.4
VI. Superior	$\dot{V}O_2 \max (mL \cdot kg^{-1} \cdot min^{-1})$	>42.0	>41.0	>40.1	>37.0	>35.8	>31.5

Source: Cooper, Kenneth H. *The Aerobics Way.* Toronto: Bantam Books, 1977, pp. 280–281. Printed with permission of Kenneth H. Cooper, MD, MPH, www.cooperaerobics.com, and J.B. Lipponcott via Copyright Clearance Center.

NON-EXERCISE-BASED ESTIMATION OF $\dot{V}O_2$ MAX

Worksheet 7.1

Name _____   Date _____

height = _____ cm   intensity of training (from Borg scale) = _____   years of training = _____

body weight = _____ kg   duration of training = _____ hr • wk^{-1} natural log of years of training = _____

age = _____ yr

Equations

Untrained Male

          0.046 × height = _____

minus   0.021 × age = _____

minus   4.31 = $\dot{V}O_2$ max (L • min^{-1}) = _____ L • min^{-1}

$\dot{V}O_2$ max (mL • min^{-1}) = _____ × 1000 = _____ mL • min^{-1}

$\dot{V}O_2$ max mL • kg^{-1} • min^{-1} = _____ / body weight = _____ mL • kg^{-1} • min^{-1}

Fitness category (table 7.1, page 60) = _____

Untrained Female

          0.046 × height = _____

minus   0.021 × age = _____

minus   4.93 = $\dot{V}O_2$ max (L • min^{-1}) = _____ L • min^{-1}

$\dot{V}O_2$ max (mL • min^{-1}) = _____ × 1000 = _____ mL • min^{-1}

$\dot{V}O_2$ max (mL • kg^{-1} • min^{-1}) = _____ / body weight = _____ mL • kg^{-1} • min^{-1}

Fitness category (table 7.1) = _____

Aerobically Trained Male

          27.387 × body weight = _____

plus   26.634 × height = _____

minus   27.572 × age = _____

plus   26.161 × duration of training = _____

plus   114.904 × intensity of training = _____

plus   506.752 × natural log of years of training = _____

minus   4609.791 = $\dot{V}O_2$ max (mL • min^{-1}) = _____ mL • min^{-1}

$\dot{V}O_2$ max (mL • kg^{-1} • min^{-1}) = _____ / body weight = _____ mL • kg^{-1} • min^{-1}

Fitness category (table 7.1) = _____

Aerobically Trained Female

          18.528 × body weight = _____

plus   11.993 × height = _____

minus   17.197 × age = _____

plus   23.522 × duration of training = _____

plus   62.118 × intensity of training = _____

plus   278.262 × natural log of years of training = _____

minus   1375.878 = $\dot{V}O_2$ max (mL • min^{-1}) = _____ mL • min^{-1}

$\dot{V}O_2$ max (mL • kg^{-1} • min^{-1}) = _____ /body weight = _____ mL • kg^{-1} • min^{-1}

Fitness category (table 7.1) = _____

Worksheet 7.2 | EXTENSION ACTIVITIES

Name _____   Date _____

1. Given the following data: (a) calculate $\dot{V}O_2$ max in $L \cdot min^{-1}$, $mL \cdot min^{-1}$, and $mL \cdot kg^{-1} \cdot min^{-1}$, and (b) determine the individual's fitness category from table 7.1 (page 60).

   UNTRAINED MALE

   height = 175 cm

   body weight = 78 kg

   age = 30 yr

   $\dot{V}O_2$ max ($L \cdot min^{-1}$) = _____ $L \cdot min^{-1}$

   $\dot{V}O_2$ max ($mL \cdot min^{-1}$) = _____ $mL \cdot min^{-1}$

   $\dot{V}O_2$ max ($mL \cdot kg^{-1} \cdot min^{-1}$) = _____ $mL \cdot kg^{-1} \cdot min^{-1}$

   Fitness category (table 7.1) = _____

2. Given the following data: (a) calculate $\dot{V}O_2$ max in $mL \cdot min^{-1}$ and $mL \cdot kg^{-1} \cdot min^{-1}$, and (b) determine the individual's fitness category from table 7.1.

   AEROBICALLY TRAINED FEMALE

   height = 169 cm

   body weight = 65 kg

   age = 27 yr

   intensity of training = 14

   duration of training = 9 $h \cdot wk^{-1}$

   years of training = 6

   $\dot{V}O_2$ max ($mL \cdot min^{-1}$) = _____ $mL \cdot min^{-1}$

   $\dot{V}O_2$ max ($mL \cdot kg^{-1} \cdot min^{-1}$) = _____ $mL \cdot kg^{-1} \cdot min^{-1}$

   Fitness category (table 7.1) = _____

EXTENSION QUESTIONS

1. What are examples of common mistakes that may occur in administering this lab?

2. Identify possible sources of error in this lab.

3. Assess the practicality of using this lab in the field.

4. Research the reliability and/or validity of this lab using online resources, journal articles, and other credible sources.

REFERENCES

1. Jones, N. L., Makrides, L., Hitchcock, C., Chypchar, T., and McCartney, N. Normal standards for an incremental progressive cycle ergometer test. *Am. Rev. Respir. Dis.* 131: 700–708, 1985.

2. Malek, M. H., Housh, T. J., Berger, D. E., Coburn, J. W., and Beck, T. W. A new non-exercise based $\dot{V}O_2$max equation for aerobically trained females. *Med. Sci. Sports Exerc.* 36: 1804–1810, 2004.

3. Malek, M. H., Housh, T. J., Berger, D. E., Coburn, J. W., and Beck, T. W. A new non-exercise based $\dot{V}O_2$max prediction equation for aerobically trained men. *J. Strength Cond. Res.* 19:559–565, 2005.

BACKGROUND

Endurance capabilities are reflected in one's ability to take in and utilize oxygen. Oxygen is a crucial factor in the operation of the electron transport system, where the production of large quantities of adenosine triphosphate (ATP) occurs as a result of oxidative metabolism. The ability to sustain moderate to high-intensity exercise for appreciable lengths of time is based on the rate at which ATP can be produced by oxidative means. Consequently, this rate will be reflected by the rate at which oxygen is consumed (taken in and utilized): oxygen consumption rate or $\dot{V}O_2$. One means of describing the cardiorespiratory endurance fitness level of an individual is by determining maximal oxygen consumption rate ($\dot{V}O_2$ max).

As one performs heavier power outputs on a cycle ergometer, both oxygen consumption rate and heart rate (HR) increase. Oxygen consumption rate increases because the demands of the work require increased production of energy and increased HR to transport oxygen and fuels to the active muscle tissues and remove their metabolic waste products more rapidly. The relationship of power output to oxygen consumption rate remains fairly constant between individuals, as well as for the same individual at various times. Therefore, when we know the power output, the corresponding oxygen consumption rate can be predicted with reasonable accuracy (± about 10%). However, the proportion to which HR increases in comparison to either power output or oxygen consumption rate will vary between individuals or for a certain individual based on level of fitness (endurance capability).

The ability to predict $\dot{V}O_2$ max is based on the fact that the heart pumps more efficiently and oxygen is more readily utilized for metabolism in individuals with higher maximal oxygen consumption capabilities. We can refer to this as increased cardiovascular efficiency, since the heart doesn't have to work as hard (HR is lower) to meet the metabolic demands of a task. Therefore, if two individuals are performing at the same power output (requiring the same rate of oxygen consumption), the individual with the higher $\dot{V}O_2$ max will tend to have a lower HR. The basis of the Astrand–Rhyming Test (named for the distinguished scientists who developed the test, the husband-and-wife team P. O. Astrand and I. Rhyming) is to make use of this relationship.[2]

In essence, we would expect that if two individuals were to work such that similar HRs result (say 150 bpm), the individual with a higher $\dot{V}O_2$ max will actually be performing more physical work (again, this reflects cardiovascular efficiency). Therefore, the basic procedure of the test is to have an individual work at moderate intensity (HR = 120–170 bpm) and record both the HR and the power output. Using these two pieces of data, we can estimate $\dot{V}O_2$ max (± 10 to 15% error) from previously determined relationships available in tables 8.1 and 8.2. This laboratory experience will help you become familiar with the procedures and supportive principles of this basic mode of fitness testing. In addition, you should be able to interpret the results of such testing in terms of fitness levels.

KNOW THESE TERMS & ABBREVIATIONS

- ○ kgm • min^{-1} = kilogram meters per minute
- ○ HR = heart rate
- ○ $\dot{V}O_2$ = oxygen consumption rate; an indirect measure of aerobic ATP production
- ○ $\dot{V}O_2$ max = maximal oxygen consumption rate

PROCEDURES

1. Set the seat height on the Monark cycle ergometer (see photo 8.1) for near full extension of the subject's legs while pedaling.

2. Have the subject warm up at 50 revolutions per minute (rpm) for 3 to 5 minutes at zero resistance. A metronome or digital pedal cadence recorder should be used to ensure proper rate of pedaling (see photo 8.2).

3. Set the first power output at 600 to 900 kgm • min^{-1} (approximately 100 to 150 watts). Determine this by multiplying the pedal cadence (always 50 for this test) × 6 (distance in meters the flywheel on the Monark cycle ergometer travels in one revolution) × resistance setting (see photo 8.3). Thus, a resistance setting of 2 kg at 50 rpm is equal to 600 kgm • min^{-1} (2 kg × 6 m × 50 rpm).

4. Start the 6-minute test as soon as the correct pedaling cadence and power output are achieved (see photo 8.4).

5. Measure and record the 30-second HR for the last 30 seconds of minutes 2 through 6. Record data on worksheet 8.1.

6. At the end of the third minute, adjust the power output (up or down) if it is not likely that the subject will be in the target HR zone (120–170 bpm) at the end of the 6-minute test.

7. If the subject has not reached a steady state HR by the end of the 6 minutes, extend the test until the difference between consecutive minutes is

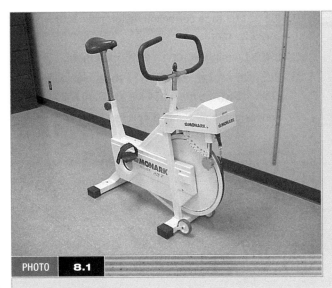

PHOTO **8.1**

Monark cycle ergometer.

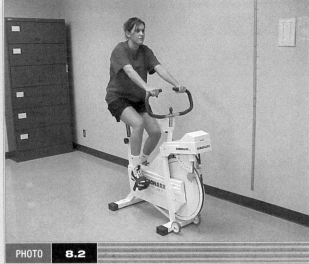

PHOTO **8.2**

Have the subject warm up at 50 rpm for 3 to 5 minutes at zero resistance.

TABLE	8.2	Females' maximal oxygen consumption rate (L • min⁻¹) predicted from cycle ergometer test.[1]

	Power Output (kgm • min⁻¹)					
HR	150	300	450	600	750	900
120	1.8	2.6	3.4	4.1	4.8	
121	1.7	2.5	3.3	4.0	4.8	
122	1.7	2.5	3.2	3.9	4.7	
123	1.7	2.4	3.1	3.9	4.6	
124	1.7	2.4	3.1	3.8	4.5	
125	1.6	2.3	3.0	3.7	4.4	
126	1.6	2.3	3.0	3.6	4.3	
127	1.6	2.2	2.9	3.5	4.2	
128	1.6	2.2	2.8	3.5	4.2	4.8
129	1.6	2.2	2.8	3.4	4.1	4.8
130		2.1	2.7	3.4	4.0	4.7
131		2.1	2.7	3.4	4.0	4.6
132		2.0	2.7	3.3	3.9	4.5
133		2.0	2.6	3.2	3.8	4.4
134		2.0	2.6	3.2	3.8	4.4
135		2.0	2.6	3.1	3.7	4.3
136		1.9	2.5	3.1	3.6	4.2
137		1.9	2.5	3.0	3.6	4.2
138		1.8	2.4	3.0	3.5	4.1
139		1.8	2.4	2.9	3.5	4.0
140		1.8	2.4	2.8	3.4	4.0
141		1.8	2.3	2.8	3.4	3.9
142		1.7	2.3	2.8	3.3	3.9
143		1.7	2.2	2.7	3.3	3.8
144		1.7	2.2	2.7	3.2	3.8
145		1.6	2.2	2.7	3.2	3.7
146		1.6	2.2	2.6	3.2	3.7
147		1.6	2.1	2.6	3.1	3.6
148		1.6	2.1	2.6	3.1	3.6
149			2.1	2.6	3.0	3.5
150			2.0	2.5	3.0	3.5
151			2.0	2.5	3.0	3.4
152			2.0	2.5	2.9	3.4
153			2.0	2.4	2.9	3.3
154			2.0	2.4	2.8	3.3
155			1.9	2.4	2.8	3.2
156			1.9	2.3	2.8	3.2
157			1.9	2.3	2.7	3.2
158			1.8	2.3	2.7	3.1
159			1.8	2.2	2.7	3.1
160			1.8	2.2	2.6	3.0
161			1.8	2.2	2.6	3.0
162			1.8	2.2	2.6	3.0
163			1.7	2.2	2.6	2.9
164			1.7	2.1	2.5	2.9
165			1.7	2.1	2.5	2.9
166			1.7	2.1	2.5	2.8
167			1.6	2.1	2.4	2.8
168			1.6	2.0	2.4	2.8
169			1.6	2.0	2.4	2.8
170			1.6	2.0	2.4	2.7

Note: To convert kgm • min⁻¹ to watts, divide by 6.12.

From P.O. Astrand and K. Rodahl, *Textbook of Work Physiology.* Copyright © 1977 McGraw-Hill Book Company. Used with permission of the author.

Age correction factors for predicting maximal oxygen consumption rate.[1] | TABLE | 8.3

Age (yrs)	Correction Factor
20	1.07
25	1.00
35	0.87
45	0.78
55	0.71
65	0.65

From P. O. Astrand and K. Rodahl, *Textbook of Work Physiology.* Copyright © 1977 McGraw-Hill Book Company. Used with permission.

Men's and women's aerobic fitness classifications. | TABLE | 8.4

Men		Age (years)					
CATEGORY	MEASURE	13–19	20–29	30–39	40–49	50–59	60+
I. Very Poor	$\dot{V}O_2$ max (mL • kg^{-1} • min^{-1})	<35.0	<33.0	<31.5	<30.2	<26.1	<20.5
II. Poor	$\dot{V}O_2$ max (mL • kg^{-1} • min^{-1})	35.0–38.3	33.0–36.4	31.5–35.4	30.2–33.5	26.1–30.9	20.5–26.0
III. Fair	$\dot{V}O_2$ max (mL • kg^{-1} • min^{-1})	38.4–45.1	36.5–42.4	35.5–40.9	33.6–38.9	31.0–35.7	26.1–32.2
IV. Good	$\dot{V}O_2$ max (mL • kg^{-1} • min^{-1})	45.2–50.9	42.5–46.4	41.0–44.9	39.0–43.7	35.8–40.9	32.3–36.4
V. Excellent	$\dot{V}O_2$ max (mL • kg^{-1} • min^{-1})	51.0–55.9	46.5–52.4	45.0–49.4	43.8–48.0	41.0–45.3	36.5–44.2
VI. Superior	$\dot{V}O_2$ max (mL • kg^{-1} • min^{-1})	>56.0	>52.5	>49.5	>48.1	>45.4	>44.3

Women		Age (years)					
CATEGORY	MEASURE	13–19	20–29	30–39	40–49	50–59	60+
I. Very Poor	$\dot{V}O_2$ max (mL • kg^{-1} • min^{-1})	<25.0	<23.6	<22.8	<21.0	<20.2	<17.5
II. Poor	$\dot{V}O_2$ max (mL • kg^{-1} • min^{-1})	25.0–30.9	23.6–28.9	22.8–26.9	21.0–24.4	20.2–22.7	17.5–20.1
III. Fair	$\dot{V}O_2$ max (mL • kg^{-1} • min^{-1})	31.0–34.9	29.0–32.9	27.0–31.4	24.5–28.9	22.8–26.9	20.2–24.4
IV. Good	$\dot{V}O_2$ max (mL • kg^{-1} • min^{-1})	35.0–38.9	33.0–36.9	31.5–35.6	29.0–32.8	27.0–31.4	24.5–30.2
V. Excellent	$\dot{V}O_2$ max (mL • kg^{-1} • min^{-1})	39.0–41.9	37.0–40.9	35.7–40.0	32.9–36.9	31.5–35.7	30.3–31.4
VI. Superior	$\dot{V}O_2$ max (mL • kg^{-1} • min^{-1})	>42.0	>41.0	>40.1	>37.0	>35.8	>31.5

Source: Cooper, Kenneth H. *The Aerobics Way.* Toronto: Bantam Books, 1977, pp. 280–281. Printed with permission of Kenneth H. Cooper, MD, MPH, www.cooperaerobics.com, and J.B. Lipponcott via Copyright Clearance Center.

Worksheet 8.1 | ASTRAND-RHYMING TEST FORM

Name _____ Date _____

Body weight _____ Gender _____

MINUTE	HEART RATE FOR LAST 30 SECONDS OF THE TIME INTERVAL	POWER OUTPUT
1		_____
2	_____	
3	_____	
4	_____	_____
5	_____	
6	_____	

Use if needed

7	_____	
8	_____	

Initial power output _____

Adjusted power output (if applicable) _____

Average HR for last 2 minutes of test _____

A. Preliminary $\dot{V}O_2$ max value from table 8.1 or 8.2 _____ $L \cdot min^{-1}$

B. Multiply preliminary $\dot{V}O_2$ max value by age correction factor (table 8.3) _____ $L \cdot min^{-1}$

C. Multiply $\dot{V}O_2$ max in $L \cdot min^{-1} \times 1000$ = _____ $mL \cdot min^{-1}$

D. Divide the age-corrected $\dot{V}O_2$ max ($mL \cdot min^{-1}$) value by body weight in kg = _____ $mL \cdot kg^{-1} \cdot min^{-1}$

E. Fitness category (table 8.4) _____

Name _____ Date _____

1. A 20-year-old male (175 pounds) performed a submaximal cycle ergometer test. The following power out-puts and heart rates were recorded. Using the blank graph below, predict this individual's maximal oxygen consumption rate ($\dot{V}O_2$ max). Assume a maximal HR of 200 bpm (220 − age = maximal HR) and express your answer relative to body weight (mL • kg^{-1} • min^{-1}). $\dot{V}O_2$ max = _____ mL • kg^{-1} • min^{-1}

Power Output 1 (300 kgm • min^{-1}),
                HR = 100 bpm

Power Output 2 (900 kgm • min^{-1}),
                HR = 150 bpm

Heart Rate (bpm) vs Power Output (kgm • min^{-1})

$\dot{V}O_2$ (L • min^{-1})

2. Activities such as weight training are not commonly used to estimate $\dot{V}O_2$ max. List at least one reason why this type of exercise would not accurately predict aerobic fitness.

3. Use your own data to calculate your estimated $\dot{V}O_2$ max (table 8.1 or 8.2) relative to your body weight (mL • kg^{-1} • min^{-1}) and determine your level of endurance fitness based on the classification from table 8.4.

4. Use the following data to calculate the subject's estimated $\dot{V}O_2$ max relative to body weight (mL • kg^{-1} • min^{-1}) and determine her level of endurance fitness based on the classification from table 8.4.

    a. Gender = female

    b. Age = 35 years

    c. Average HR during the last 2 minutes = 145 bpm

    d. Power output = 600 kgm • min^{-1}

    e. Body weight = 65 kg

$\dot{V}O_2$ max = _____ mL • kg^{-1} • min^{-1}

Classification = _____

EXTENSION QUESTIONS

1. What are some common mistakes that may occur in administering this lab?

2. Identify possible sources of error in this lab.

3. Assess the practicality of using this lab in the field.

4. Research the reliability and/or validity of this lab using online resources, journal articles, and other credible sources.

REFERENCES

1. Astrand, P. O., and Rodahl, K. *Textbook of Work Physiology.* New York: McGraw-Hill, 1977, pp. 350–352.

2. Astrand, P. O., and Rhyming, I. A nomogram for calculation of aerobic capacity (physical fitness) from pulse rate during submaximal work. *J. Appl. Physiol.* 7: 218–221, 1954.

3. Cooper, K. H. *The Aerobics Way.* Toronto: Bantam Books, 1977, pp. 280–281.

BACKGROUND

The Queens College Step Test was designed to provide quick, easy, and accurate predictions of $\dot{V}O_2$ max for college-age men[1] and women.[1,2] This test involves only 3 minutes of stair stepping on a step of 41.3 cm height. Upon completion of the Queens College Step Test, the subject's heart rate is recorded, and this measurement is referred to as the recovery heart rate. In theory, individuals' recovery heart rate will be lower after the Queens College Step Test if they are in better shape (i.e., higher $\dot{V}O_2$ max), and individuals who exhibit poor fitness levels (i.e., lower $\dot{V}O_2$ max) will have a higher recovery heart rate after the step test. A higher recovery heart rate usually reflects a greater amount of exercise-induced stress as a result of the same submaximal stair-stepping task for all participants. Overall, the lower the post-exercise recovery heart rate, the higher the predicted $\dot{V}O_2$ max.

Perhaps the greatest advantages of the Queens College Step Test over other field-based cardiovascular tests (e.g., 12-minute run, 1.5-mile run, or Rockport fitness walking test) are (a) it requires only 3 minutes of submaximal stair stepping and (b) large groups of individuals can be tested in a relatively short time. A common use of the test is to have a group of students organize into pairs. Half of the group performs the Queens College Step Test on a long bench, while the partners monitor and record the recovery heart rate. Upon completion of the first group, the pairs switch tasks so that all students are tested with only two 3-minute step test sessions.

Here are the $\dot{V}O_2$ max prediction equations for the Queens College Step Test:

COLLEGE-AGE MEN[1]
$\dot{V}O_2$ max (mL • kg^{-1} • min^{-1}) = 111.33 − (0.42 × recovery heart rate in beats per minute)

COLLEGE-AGE WOMEN
$\dot{V}O_2$ max (mL • kg^{-1} • min^{-1}) = 65.81 − (0.1847 × recovery heart rate in beats per minute)
r (correlation coefficient) = −0.75
standardized error of prediction = 2.9 mL • kg^{-1} • min^{-1}

KNOW THESE TERMS & ABBREVIATIONS

○ recovery heart rate = the HR taken after the end of exercise (in this lab it is taken 5 seconds after the completion of the Queens College Step Test)

○ regression equations = statistical methods that are developed and used to relate two or more variables

○ $\dot{V}O_2$ max = maximal oxygen consumption rate

PROCEDURES[1,2] (see photos 9.1–9.5)

1. Have the subject (or group of subjects) warm up by walking briskly or jogging for 5 minutes prior to the test.

2. Instruct the subject (or group of subjects) to perform 3 minutes of stepping using a four-step cadence: "up–up–down–down." Ensure that the subjects are stepping with their entire foot on the bench/step and that the contralateral foot makes complete contact with the bench/step at the top (see photos 9.1–9.4). Encourage the participants to alternate legs, such that the consecutive stepping cycles would be performed as: right leg up, left leg up, right leg down, left leg down → right leg up, left leg up, right leg down, left leg down → right leg up, and so forth. One step should be taken with each tick of the metronome, using the following cadences:

   a. Men will maintain a cadence of 24 steps per minute, which is equivalent to 96 beats per minute on a metronome.

   b. Women will complete 22 steps per minute, which is 88 beats per minute on a metronome.

3. Five seconds after the 3-minute Queens College Step Test is complete, measure the subject's recovery heart rate (see photo 9.5) and record it (in beats per minute) on worksheet 9.1.

4. Use one of the regression equations below to predict $\dot{V}O_2$ max.

5. Compare the estimated $\dot{V}O_2$ max score to the norms listed in table 9.1.

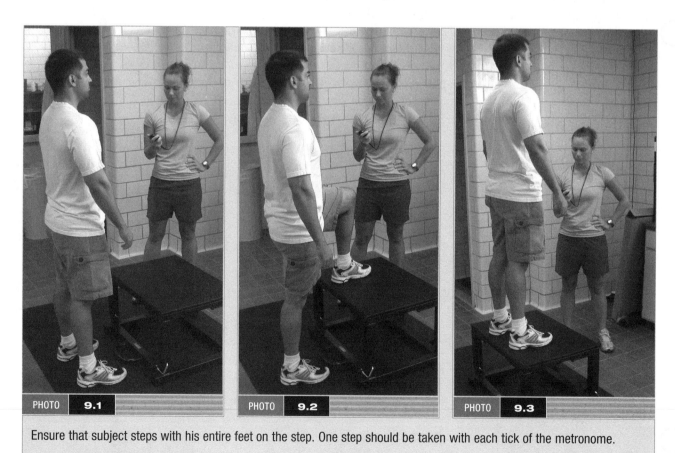

PHOTO 9.1 PHOTO 9.2 PHOTO 9.3

Ensure that subject steps with his entire feet on the step. One step should be taken with each tick of the metronome.

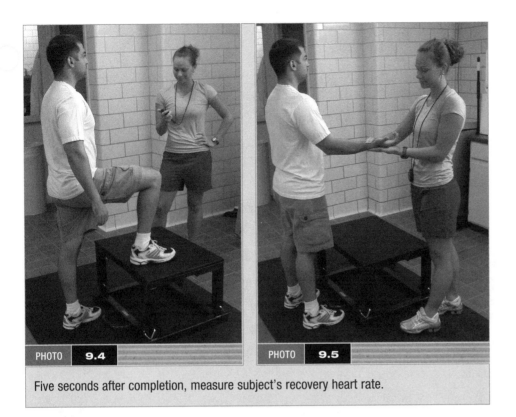

PHOTO **9.4**   PHOTO **9.5**

Five seconds after completion, measure subject's recovery heart rate.

Equations

COLLEGE-AGE MEN[1]

$\dot{V}O_2$ max (mL • kg^{-1} • min^{-1}) = 111.33 – (0.42 × recovery heart rate in beats per minute)

COLLEGE-AGE WOMEN

$\dot{V}O_2$ max (mL • kg^{-1} • min^{-1}) = 65.81 – (0.1847 × recovery heart rate in beats per minute)

Sample Calculations

Gender: ___Male___

Age: ___19 years___

Body weight: ___182 lbs___

Recovery heart rate: ___150 bpm___

Step 1: Calculate the predicted $\dot{V}O_2$ max.

$\dot{V}O_2$ max (mL • kg^{-1} • min^{-1}) = 111.33 – (0.42 × 150 bpm)

= 48.3 mL • kg^{-1} • min^{-1}

Step 2: Compare the predicted $\dot{V}O_2$ max score from the Queens College Step Test to the norms in table 9.1.

A score of 48.3 mL • kg^{-1} • min^{-1} would be classified as Good for a 13- to 19-year-old man, according to table 9.1.

TABLE 9.1 Men's and women's aerobic fitness classifications.

Men				Age (years)				
CATEGORY	MEASURE	13–19	20–29	30–39	40–49	50–59	60+
I. Very Poor	$\dot{V}O_2$ max (mL • kg^{-1} • min^{-1})	<35.0	<33.0	<31.5	<30.2	<26.1	<20.5
II. Poor	$\dot{V}O_2$ max (mL • kg^{-1} • min^{-1})	35.0–38.3	33.0–36.4	31.5–35.4	30.2–33.5	26.1–30.9	20.5–26.0
III. Fair	$\dot{V}O_2$ max (mL • kg^{-1} • min^{-1})	38.4–45.1	36.5–42.4	35.5–40.9	33.6–38.9	31.0–35.7	26.1–32.2
IV. Good	$\dot{V}O_2$ max (mL • kg^{-1} • min^{-1})	45.2–50.9	42.5–46.4	41.0–44.9	39.0–43.7	35.8–40.9	32.3–36.4
V. Excellent	$\dot{V}O_2$ max (mL • kg^{-1} • min^{-1})	51.0–55.9	46.5–52.4	45.0–49.4	43.8–48.0	41.0–45.3	36.5–44.2
VI. Superior	$\dot{V}O_2$ max (mL • kg^{-1} • min^{-1})	>56.0	>52.5	>49.5	>48.1	>45.4	>44.3

Women				Age (years)				
CATEGORY	MEASURE	13–19	20–29	30–39	40–49	50–59	60+
I. Very Poor	$\dot{V}O_2$ max (mL • kg^{-1} • min^{-1})	<25.0	<23.6	<22.8	<21.0	<20.2	<17.5
II. Poor	$\dot{V}O_2$ max (mL • kg^{-1} • min^{-1})	25.0–30.9	23.6–28.9	22.8–26.9	21.0–24.4	20.2–22.7	17.5–20.1
III. Fair	$\dot{V}O_2$ max (mL • kg^{-1} • min^{-1})	31.0–34.9	29.0–32.9	27.0–31.4	24.5–28.9	22.8–26.9	20.2–24.4
IV. Good	$\dot{V}O_2$ max (mL • kg^{-1} • min^{-1})	35.0–38.9	33.0–36.9	31.5–35.6	29.0–32.8	27.0–31.4	24.5–30.2
V. Excellent	$\dot{V}O_2$ max (mL • kg^{-1} • min^{-1})	39.0–41.9	37.0–40.9	35.7–40.0	32.9–36.9	31.5–35.7	30.3–31.4
VI. Superior	$\dot{V}O_2$ max (mL • kg^{-1} • min^{-1})	>42.0	>41.0	>40.1	>37.0	>35.8	>31.5

Source: Cooper, Kenneth H. *The Aerobics Way.* Toronto: Bantam Books, 1977, pp. 280–281. Printed with permission of Kenneth H. Cooper, MD, MPH, www.cooperaerobics.com, and J.B. Lipponcott via Copyright Clearance Center.

QUEENS COLLEGE STEP TEST FORM   Worksheet **9.1**

Name _____   *Date* _____

Gender: _____

Recovery heart rate (bpm):   _____

1. Predicted $\dot{V}O_2$ max (mL $\cdot$ kg^{-1} $\cdot$ min^{-1}) = _____

2. Classification   = _____ (see table 9.1)

EXTENSION ACTIVITIES   Worksheet **9.2**

Name _____   *Date* _____

Use the following data and table 9.1 to answer the questions below.

Gender: ___Female___

Age: ___32 years___

Recovery heart rate: ___187 bpm___

1. Calculate the subject's predicted $\dot{V}O_2$ max from the Queens College Step Test.

    $\dot{V}O_2$ max = _____ mL $\cdot$ kg^{-1} $\cdot$ min^{-1}

2. Classify the subject's predicted $\dot{V}O_2$ max from the Queens College Step Test (see table 9.1).

    Classification = _____

3. On the graph below, draw the expected relationship between recovery heart rate from the Queens College Step Test and $\dot{V}O_2$ max.

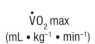 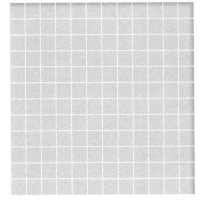

$\dot{V}O_2$ max
(mL $\cdot$ kg^{-1} $\cdot$ min^{-1})

recovery heart rate

EXTENSION QUESTIONS

1. What are some common mistakes that may occur in administering this lab?

2. Identify possible sources of error in this lab.

3. Assess the practicality of using this lab in the field.

4. Research the reliability and/or validity of this lab using online resources, journal articles, and other credible sources.

REFERENCES

1. McArdle, W. D., Katch, F. I., and Katch, V. L. *Exercise Physiology: Energy, Nutrition, and Human Performance*, 6th edition. Philadelphia: Lippincott Williams & Wilkins, 2007.

2. McArdle, W. D., Katch, F. I., Pechar, G. S., Jacobson, L., and Ruck, S. Reliability and interrelationships between maximal oxygen intake, physical work capacity and step-test scores in college women. *Med. Sci. Sports.* 4: 182–186, 1972.

BACKGROUND

The Rockport Fitness Walking Test (RFWT) was developed by Kline et al.[5] as a submaximal field test for predicting maximal oxygen consumption rate ($\dot{V}O_2$ max) using a 1-mile walking protocol. During the RFWT, participants are instructed to walk for 1 mile as fast as possible while maintaining a constant pace. Immediately after the RFWT, heart rate (beats per minute) is assessed, and the time (minutes) to complete the 1-mile walk is recorded. These variables, as well as body weight (lbs) and age (years), are then used in a regression equation to predict $\dot{V}O_2$ max. In theory, a lower post-exercise heart rate and time to complete the 1-mile walk will result in a higher predicted $\dot{V}O_2$ max. Therefore, since the RFWT does not involve running or jogging, as in the 12-minute or 1.5-mile run tests, the RFWT may be appropriate for individuals with lower fitness levels or older adults who may not be able to run.

The original RFWT equations by Kline et al.[5] provided acceptable $\dot{V}O_2$ max predictions for men and women between the ages of 30 and 69 years. Fenstermaker et al.[3] cross-validated the RFWT equations for 65- to 79-year-old women and determined that the RFWT was appropriate for this population as well. However, other studies[2,4] have demonstrated that the original RFWT[5] consistently overpredicted $\dot{V}O_2$ max for college-aged men and women. Therefore, Dolgener et al.[2] modified the original RFWT equations to better predict $\dot{V}O_2$ max for 18- to 29-year-old men and women, and these modified equations have been validated by George et al.[4]

Since the applicable age range is broad (30–79 years) for the original equations by Kline et al.,[5] age is included as a predictor variable. However, the modified equations by Dolgener et al.[2] do not include age as a predictor, because the age range for these equations is narrow (18–29 years).

MEN (30–69 YEARS)[5]

$\dot{V}O_2$ max (mL • kg^{-1} • min^{-1}) = 139.168 − (0.3877 × age in years)
− (0.1692 × body weight in lbs) − (3.2649 × 1.0-mile walk time in min)
− (0.1565 × heart rate in beats per min)
R (multiple correlation coefficient) = 0.83–0.88
SEE (standard error of estimate) = 4.5–5.3 mL • kg^{-1} • min^{-1}

WOMEN (30–79 YEARS)[3,5]

$\dot{V}O_2$ max (mL • kg^{-1} • min^{-1}) = 132.853 − (0.3877 × age in years)
− (0.1692 × body weight in lbs) − (3.2649 × 1.0-mile walk time in min)
− (0.1565 × heart rate in beats per min)
R (multiple correlation coefficient) = 0.59–0.88
SEE (standard error of estimate) = 2.7–5.3 mL • kg^{-1} • min^{-1}

MEN (18–29 YEARS)[2,4]

$\dot{V}O_2$ max (mL • kg^{-1} • min^{-1}) = 97.660 − (0.0957 × body weight in lbs)
− (1.4537 × 1.0-mile walk time in min) − (0.1194 × heart rate in beats per min)

R (multiple correlation coefficient) = 0.50–0.85

SEE (standard error of estimate) = 3.5–5.8 mL • kg^{-1} • min^{-1}

WOMEN (18–29 YEARS)[2,4]

$\dot{V}O_2$ max (mL • kg^{-1} • min^{-1}) = 88.768 – (0.0957 × body weight in lbs)
– (1.4537 × 1.0-mile walk time in min) – (0.1194 × heart rate in beats per min)

R (multiple correlation coefficient) = 0.38–0.85

SEE (standard error of estimate) = 3.0–4.8 mL • kg^{-1} • min^{-1}

KNOW THESE TERMS & ABBREVIATIONS

- RFWT = Rockport Fitness Walking Test
- R = multiple correlation coefficient: a numerical measure of how well a dependent variable can be predicted from a combination of independent variables (a number between –1 and 1)
- regression equations = statistical methods that are developed and used to relate two or more variables
- SEE = standard error of estimate: a measure of the accuracy of the predictions made using a regression equation
- $\dot{V}O_2$ max = maximal oxygen consumption rate
- 1 mile = 1.6 km

PROCEDURES[6]

1. Measure body weight (in lbs) on a scale.

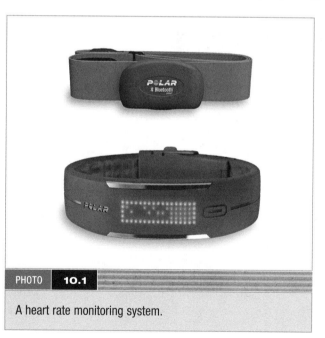

2. Have the subject (or group of subjects) warm up by walking briskly for five minutes prior to the test and put on the heart rate monitor (see photo 10.1).

3. Instruct the subject (or group of subjects) to walk briskly (i.e., as fast as possible) for 1.0 mile (1.6 km) while maintaining a constant pace (see photo 10.2).

4. Immediately after the 1.0-mile walk is complete, measure the subject's heart rate and record it (in beats per minute) on worksheet 10.1.

5. Measure the time it takes to complete the 1.0-mile walk and record it (in minutes) on worksheet 10.1.

6. Use one of the following regression equations to predict $\dot{V}O_2$ max.

7. Compare the estimated $\dot{V}O_2$ max score to the norms listed in table 10.1.

Equations

MEN (30–65 YEARS)

$\dot{V}O_2$ max (mL • kg^{-1} • min^{-1}) = 139.168 – (0.3877 × age in years)
– (0.1692 × body weight in lbs) – (3.2649 × 1.0-mile walk time in min)
– (0.1565 × heart rate in beats per min)

WOMEN (30–79 YEARS)

$\dot{V}O_2$ max (mL • kg^{-1} • min^{-1}) = 132.853 – (0.3877 × age in years)
– (0.1692 × body weight in lbs) – (3.2649 × 1.0-mile walk time in min)
– (0.1565 × heart rate in beats per min)

MEN (18–29 YEARS)

$\dot{V}O_2$ max (mL • kg^{-1} • min^{-1}) = 97.660 – (0.0957 × body weight in lbs)
– (1.4537 × 1.0-mile walk time in min) – (0.1194 × heart rate in beats per min)

WOMEN (18–29 YEARS)

$\dot{V}O_2$ max (mL • kg^{-1} • min^{-1}) = 88.768 – (0.0957 × body weight in lbs)
– (1.4537 × 1.0-mile walk time in min) – (0.1194 × heart rate in beats per min)

Sample Calculations

Gender: _Female_

Age: _35 years_

Body weight: _138 lbs_

Post-walking heart rate: _118 bpm_

1.0-mile walk time: _15:54 min:sec_

Step 1: Convert time to minutes.
54 sec / 60 sec = 0.9 min
Therefore,
15:54 min:sec = 15.9 min

Step 2: Calculate the predicted $\dot{V}O_2$ max.
$\dot{V}O_2$ max (mL • kg^{-1} • min^{-1})
= 132.853 – (0.3877 × 35 years)
– (0.1692 × 138 lbs) – (3.2649
× 15.9 min) – (0.1565 × 118 bpm)
= 25.6 mL • kg^{-1} • min^{-1}

Step 3: Compare the predicted $\dot{V}O_2$ max score from the Rockport Fitness Walking Test to the norms in table 10.1.

A score of 25.6 mL • kg^{-1} • min^{-1} would be classified as Poor for a 30- to 39-year-old woman in table 10.1.

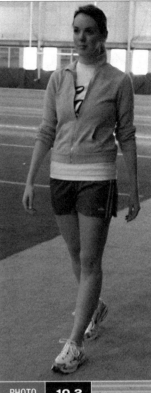

PHOTO **10.2**

Subject walking on the track to complete the Rockport Fitness Walking Test.

TABLE	10.1	Men's and women's aerobic fitness classifications.

Men		Age (years)					
CATEGORY	MEASURE	13–19	20–29	30–39	40–49	50–59	60+
I. Very Poor	$\dot{V}O_2$ max (mL • kg⁻¹ • min⁻¹)	<35.0	<33.0	<31.5	<30.2	<26.1	<20.5
II. Poor	$\dot{V}O_2$ max (mL • kg⁻¹ • min⁻¹)	35.0–38.3	33.0–36.4	31.5–35.4	30.2–33.5	26.1–30.9	20.5–26.0
III. Fair	$\dot{V}O_2$ max (mL • kg⁻¹ • min⁻¹)	38.4–45.1	36.5–42.4	35.5–40.9	33.6–38.9	31.0–35.7	26.1–32.2
IV. Good	$\dot{V}O_2$ max (mL • kg⁻¹ • min⁻¹)	45.2–50.9	42.5–46.4	41.0–44.9	39.0–43.7	35.8–40.9	32.3–36.4
V. Excellent	$\dot{V}O_2$ max (mL • kg⁻¹ • min⁻¹)	51.0–55.9	46.5–52.4	45.0–49.4	43.8–48.0	41.0–45.3	36.5–44.2
VI. Superior	$\dot{V}O_2$ max (mL • kg⁻¹ • min⁻¹)	>56.0	>52.5	>49.5	>48.1	>45.4	>44.3

Women		Age (years)					
CATEGORY	MEASURE	13–19	20–29	30–39	40–49	50–59	60+
I. Very Poor	$\dot{V}O_2$ max (mL • kg⁻¹ • min⁻¹)	<25.0	<23.6	<22.8	<21.0	<20.2	<17.5
II. Poor	$\dot{V}O_2$ max (mL • kg⁻¹ • min⁻¹)	25.0–30.9	23.6–28.9	22.8–26.9	21.0–24.4	20.2–22.7	17.5–20.1
III. Fair	$\dot{V}O_2$ max (mL • kg⁻¹ • min⁻¹)	31.0–34.9	29.0–32.9	27.0–31.4	24.5–28.9	22.8–26.9	20.2–24.4
IV. Good	$\dot{V}O_2$ max (mL • kg⁻¹ • min⁻¹)	35.0–38.9	33.0–36.9	31.5–35.6	29.0–32.8	27.0–31.4	24.5–30.2
V. Excellent	$\dot{V}O_2$ max (mL • kg⁻¹ • min⁻¹)	39.0–41.9	37.0–40.9	35.7–40.0	32.9–36.9	31.5–35.7	30.3–31.4
VI. Superior	$\dot{V}O_2$ max (mL • kg⁻¹ • min⁻¹)	>42.0	>41.0	>40.1	>37.0	>35.8	>31.5

Source: Cooper, Kenneth H. *The Aerobics Way.* Toronto: Bantam Books, 1977, pp. 280–281. Printed with permission of Kenneth H. Cooper, MD, MPH, www.cooperaerobics.com, and J.B. Lipponcott via Copyright Clearance Center.

ROCKPORT FITNESS WALKING TEST FORM

Name _____   Date _____

Gender: _____

Age (years): _____

Body weight (lbs): _____

Post-walking heart rate (bpm): _____

Time to complete the 1.0-mile walk (min:sec): _____

1. Time (in min:sec) to complete the 1.0-mile walk = _____ min

2. Predicted $\dot{V}O_2$ max (mL $\cdot$ kg^{-1} $\cdot$ min^{-1}) = _____

3. Classification = _____ (see table 10.1)

EXTENSION ACTIVITIES

Name _____   Date _____

Use the following data and table 10.1 to answer the questions below.

Gender: _Male_____

Age: _19 years_____

Body weight: _185 lbs_____

Post-walking heart rate: _130 bpm_____

1.0-mile walk time _14:46 min:sec___

1. Calculate the subject's predicted $\dot{V}O_2$ max from the Rockport Fitness Walking Test.

   $\dot{V}O_2$ max = _____ (mL $\cdot$ kg^{-1} $\cdot$ min^{-1})

2. Classify the subject's predicted $\dot{V}O_2$ max from the Rockport Fitness Walking Test (see table 10.1).

   Classification = _____

EXTENSION QUESTIONS

1. What are some common mistakes that may occur in administering this lab?

2. Identify possible sources of error in this lab.

3. Assess the practicality of using this lab in the field.

4. Research the reliability and/or validity of this lab using online resources, journal articles, and other credible sources.

REFERENCES

1. Cramer, J. T., and Coburn, J. W. Fitness testing protocols and norms. In *NSCA's Essentials of Personal Training,* eds. R. W. Earle and T. R. Baechle. Champaign, IL: Human Kinetics, 2005, pp. 218–263.

2. Dolgener, F. A., Hensley, L. D., Marsh, J. J., and Fjelstul, J. K. Validation of the Rockport fitness walking test in college males and females. *Res. Q. Exerc. Sport.* 65: 152–158, 1994.

3. Fenstermaker, K. L., Plowman, S. A., and Looney, M. A. Validation of the Rockport fitness walking test in females 65 years and older. *Res. Q. Exerc. Sport.* 63: 322–327, 1992.

4. George, J. D., Fellingham, G. W., and Fisher, A. G. A modified version of the Rockport fitness walking test for college men and women. *Res. Q. Exerc. Sport.* 69: 205–209, 1998.

5. Kline, G. M., Porcari, J. P., Hintermeister, R., Freedson, P. S., Ward, A., McCarron, R. F., Ross, J., and Rippe, J. M. Estimation of VO_2max from a one-mile track walk, gender, age and body weight. *Med. Sci. Sports Exerc.* 19: 253–259, 1987.

6. Ryan, E.D., and Cramer, J. T., Fitness testing protocols and norms. In *NSCA's Essentials of Personal Training,* eds. R. W. Earle and T. R. Baechle, 2nd edition. Champaign, IL: Human Kinetics, 2012, pp. 201–250.

BACKGROUND

The 12-minute run test is a field test designed to predict maximal oxygen consumption rate ($\dot{V}O_2$ max) by measuring the distance completed in 12 minutes of running (or walking). Although walking is allowed during this test, the objective is to cover as much distance as possible in 12 minutes. A faster pace (speed) during the test will result in a greater distance covered, and, therefore, a higher predicted $\dot{V}O_2$ max. After the test is complete and the distance is recorded, it is used in the following regression equation[2] to predict $\dot{V}O_2$ max:

$$\dot{V}O_2 \text{ max (mL} \cdot \text{kg}^{-1} \cdot \text{min}^{-1}) = (0.0268 \times \text{distance in meters completed in 12 minutes}) - 11.3$$

r (correlation coefficient) = 0.897

The 12-minute run test was originally established based on an early study by Balke,[1] which led to the development of the regression equation used in this laboratory to predict $\dot{V}O_2$ max.[2] Based on the linear relationship between running velocity (from 150 to 300 m $\cdot$ min^{-1}) and steady-state $\dot{V}O_2$, Balke[1] found that a 12-minute "best effort" run closely estimated the $\dot{V}O_2$ max from a constant speed, graded walk test. When Cooper[2] developed the regression equation to predict $\dot{V}O_2$ max using the 12-minute run, a correlation coefficient of r = 0.897 was reported. Since then, Safrit et al.[8] have reported validity coefficients ranging from r = 0.28 to 0.94 for measured $\dot{V}O_2$ max versus predicted $\dot{V}O_2$ max from the 12-minute run test. It was later suggested, however, that the variation among these correlations may have resulted from the type of criterion $\dot{V}O_2$ max test performed.[6] Nevertheless, most studies have agreed that $\dot{V}O_2$ max can be accurately predicted with the 12-minute run test.[2,4,5,6,8,9]

KNOW THESE TERMS & ABBREVIATIONS

- $\dot{V}O_2$ max = maximal oxygen consumption rate
- regression equations = statistical methods that are developed and used to relate two or more variables
- correlation coefficient (r) = a numerical measure of the degree to which two variables are linearly related (a number between −1 and 1)

PROCEDURES[7]

1. Have the subject(s) warm up by walking and/or jogging for 5 minutes prior to the test.
2. Instruct the subject to run (or walk if necessary) as far as possible in 12 minutes. Emphasize that a faster speed will result in a higher predicted $\dot{V}O_2$ max.
3. Measure the distance completed in 12 minutes and record it (in meters) on worksheet 11.1.
4. Use the regression equation below to predict $\dot{V}O_2$ max.
5. Compare the estimated $\dot{V}O_2$ max score to the norms listed in table 11.1.

Equation

$\dot{V}O_2 \max$ (mL • kg⁻¹ • min⁻¹) = (0.0268 × distance in meters completed in 12 minutes) − 11.3

Sample Calculations

Gender: *Female*

Age: *22 years*

12-minute run distance: *1.1 miles*

Common conversion factors: 1.0 mile = 1,609.3 meters
1.0 yard = 0.9144 meter
1.0 foot = 0.3048 meter

Step 1: Convert distance in miles to meters.
1.1 miles × 1,609.3 meters = 1,770.2 meters completed in 12 minutes

Step 2: Calculate the predicted $\dot{V}O_2$max.
$\dot{V}O_2 \max$ = (0.0268 × 1,770.2) − 11.3 = 36.1 mL • kg⁻¹ • min⁻¹

Step 3: Compare the predicted $\dot{V}O_2$ max score from the 12-minute run to the norms in table 11.1.

A score of 36.1 mL • kg⁻¹ • min⁻¹ would be classified as Good for a 20- to 29-year-old woman in table 11.1.

TABLE 11.1   Men's and women's aerobic fitness classifications.

Men		Age (years)					
CATEGORY	MEASURE	13–19	20–29	30–39	40–49	50–59	60+
I. Very Poor	$\dot{V}O_2$ max (mL • kg⁻¹ • min⁻¹)	<35.0	<33.0	<31.5	<30.2	<26.1	<20.5
II. Poor	$\dot{V}O_2$ max (mL • kg⁻¹ • min⁻¹)	35.0–38.3	33.0–36.4	31.5–35.4	30.2–33.5	26.1–30.9	20.5–26.0
III. Fair	$\dot{V}O_2$ max (mL • kg⁻¹ • min⁻¹)	38.4–45.1	36.5–42.4	35.5–40.9	33.6–38.9	31.0–35.7	26.1–32.2
IV. Good	$\dot{V}O_2$ max (mL • kg⁻¹ • min⁻¹)	45.2–50.9	42.5–46.4	41.0–44.9	39.0–43.7	35.8–40.9	32.3–36.4
V. Excellent	$\dot{V}O_2$ max (mL • kg⁻¹ • min⁻¹)	51.0–55.9	46.5–52.4	45.0–49.4	43.8–48.0	41.0–45.3	36.5–44.2
VI. Superior	$\dot{V}O_2$ max (mL • kg⁻¹ • min⁻¹)	>56.0	>52.5	>49.5	>48.1	>45.4	>44.3

Women		Age (years)					
CATEGORY	MEASURE	13–19	20–29	30–39	40–49	50–59	60+
I. Very Poor	$\dot{V}O_2$ max (mL • kg⁻¹ • min⁻¹)	<25.0	<23.6	<22.8	<21.0	<20.2	<17.5
II. Poor	$\dot{V}O_2$ max (mL • kg⁻¹ • min⁻¹)	25.0–30.9	23.6–28.9	22.8–26.9	21.0–24.4	20.2–22.7	17.5–20.1
III. Fair	$\dot{V}O_2$ max (mL • kg⁻¹ • min⁻¹)	31.0–34.9	29.0–32.9	27.0–31.4	24.5–28.9	22.8–26.9	20.2–24.4
IV. Good	$\dot{V}O_2$ max (mL • kg⁻¹ • min⁻¹)	35.0–38.9	33.0–36.9	31.5–35.6	29.0–32.8	27.0–31.4	24.5–30.2
V. Excellent	$\dot{V}O_2$ max (mL • kg⁻¹ • min⁻¹)	39.0–41.9	37.0–40.9	35.7–40.0	32.9–36.9	31.5–35.7	30.3–31.4
VI. Superior	$\dot{V}O_2$ max (mL • kg⁻¹ • min⁻¹)	>42.0	>41.0	>40.1	>37.0	>35.8	>31.5

Source: Cooper, Kenneth H. *The Aerobics Way.* Toronto: Bantam Books, 1977, pp. 280–281. Printed with permission of Kenneth H. Cooper, MD, MPH, www.cooperaerobics.com, and J.B. Lipponcott via Copyright Clearance Center.

12-MINUTE RUN TEST FORM

Worksheet 11.1

Name _____   Date _____

Gender: _____

1. Distance (in meters) completed in 12 minutes = _____

2. $\dot{V}O_2$ max $(mL \cdot kg^{-1} \cdot min^{-1})$ = (0.0268 × distance in meters completed in 12 minutes) − 11.3 = _____

3. Classification = _____ (see table 11.1)

EXTENSION ACTIVITIES

Worksheet 11.2

Name _____   Date _____

Use the following data and table 11.1 to answer the questions below.

Gender: _Male_

Age: _35 years_

12-minute run distance: _5,300 ft_

1. Calculate the subject's predicted $\dot{V}O_2$max from the 12-minute run test.

   $\dot{V}O_2$ max = _____ $mL \cdot kg^{-1} \cdot min^{-1}$

2. Classify the subject's predicted $\dot{V}O_2$max from the 12-minute run test (see table 11.1).

   Classification = _____

3. On the graph below, draw the expected relationship between the distance run in 12 minutes and $\dot{V}O_2$ max.

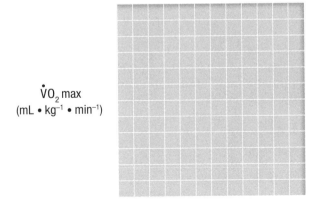

$\dot{V}O_2$ max
$(mL \cdot kg^{-1} \cdot min^{-1})$

12-minute run distance

EXTENSION QUESTIONS

1. What are some common mistakes that may occur in administering this lab?

2. Identify possible sources of error in this lab.

3. Assess the practicality of using this lab in the field.

4. Research the reliability and/or validity of this lab using online resources, journal articles, and other credible sources.

REFERENCES

1. Balke, B. A simple field test for the assessment of physical fitness. Report 63-6 Civil Aeromedical Research Institute. Oklahoma City: Federal Aviation Agency, 1963.

2. Cooper, K. H. A means of assessing maximal oxygen intake. *J. Am. Med. Assoc.* 203: 135–138, 1968.

3. Cramer, J. T., and Coburn, J. W. Fitness testing protocols and norms. In *NSCA's Essentials of Personal Training*, eds. R. W. Earle and T. R. Baechle. Champaign, IL: Human Kinetics, 2005, pp. 218–263.

4. Drinkard, B., McDuffie, J., McCann, S., Uwaifo, G. I., Nicholson, J., and Yanovski, J. A. Relationships between walk/run performance and cardiorespiratory fitness in adolescents who are overweight. *Phys. Ther.* 81: 1889–1896, 2001.

5. Jessup, G. T., Tolson, H., and Terry, J. W. Prediction of maximal oxygen intake from Astrand-Rhyming test, 12-minute run, and anthropometric variables using stepwise multiple regression. *Am. J. Phys. Med.* 53: 200–207, 1974.

6. McCutcheon, M. C., Sticha, S. A., Giese, M. D., and Nagle, F. J. A further analysis of the 12-minute run prediction of maximal aerobic power. *Res. Q. Exerc. Sport.* 61: 280–283, 1990.

7. Ryan, E.D., and Cramer, J. T., Fitness testing protocols and norms. In *NSCA's Essentials of Personal Training*, eds. R. W. Earle and T. R. Baechle, 2nd edition. Champaign, IL: Human Kinetics, 2012, pp. 201–250.

8. Safrit, M. J., Hooper, L. M., Ehlert, S. A., Costa, M. G., and Patterson, P. The validity generalization of distance run tests. *Can. J. Sport Sci.* 13: 188–196, 1988.

9. Wanamaker, G. S. A study of the validity and reliability of the 12-minute run under selected motivational conditions. *Am. Correct Ther. J.* 24: 69–72, 1970.

BACKGROUND

The 1.5-mile run test provides a simple method for estimating a person's maximal oxygen consumption rate ($\dot{V}O_2$ max) by measuring the elapsed time during 1.5 miles of running (or walking). Walking is allowed during this test; however, the objective is to complete the 1.5-mile distance as quickly as possible. A faster pace (speed) during the test will result in a lower time to complete the 1.5 miles, and, therefore, a higher predicted $\dot{V}O_2$ max. The following gender-specific regression equations have been developed[1] to predict $\dot{V}O_2$ max using body weight (kg) and the 1.5-mile run time (min):

MEN

$\dot{V}O_2$ max (mL $\cdot$ kg^{-1} $\cdot$ min^{-1}) = 91.736 − (0.1656 × body weight in kg) − (2.767 × 1.5-mile run time in minutes)

R (multiple correlation coefficient) = 0.90

SEE (standard error of estimate) = 2.8 mL $\cdot$ kg^{-1} $\cdot$ min^{-1}

WOMEN

$\dot{V}O_2$ max (mL $\cdot$ kg^{-1} $\cdot$ min^{-1}) = 88.020 − (0.1656 × body weight in kg) − (2.767 × 1.5-mile run time in minutes)

R (multiple correlation coefficient) = 0.90

SEE (standard error of estimate) = 2.8 mL $\cdot$ kg^{-1} $\cdot$ min^{-1}

The standard error of estimate values associated with these equations represents approximately 6.0% of $\dot{V}O_2$ max.

KNOW THESE TERMS & ABBREVIATIONS

- R = multiple correlation coefficient; a numerical measure of how well a dependent variable can be predicted from a combination of independent variables (a number between −1 and 1)
- SEE = standard error of estimate; a measure of the accuracy of the predictions made using a regression equation
- $\dot{V}O_2$ max = maximal oxygen consumption rate

PROCEDURES[2]

1. Measure body weight (in kilograms) on a scale.
2. Have the subject(s) warm up by walking and/or jogging for 5 minutes prior to the test.
3. Instruct the subject to run (or walk if necessary) as fast as possible for 1.5 miles (2.4 kilometers). Emphasize that a faster speed will result in a higher predicted $\dot{V}O_2$ max.

4. Measure the time it takes to complete the 1.5 miles and record it (in minutes) on worksheet 12.1.

5. Use one of the regression equations below to predict $\dot{V}O_2$ max.

6. Compare the estimated $\dot{V}O_2$ max score to the norms listed in table 12.1.

Equations

MEN

$\dot{V}O_2$ max (mL • kg⁻¹ • min⁻¹) = 91.736 – (0.1656 × body mass in kg) – (2.767 × 1.5-mile run time in min)

WOMEN

$\dot{V}O_2$ max (mL • kg⁻¹ • min⁻¹) = 88.020 – (0.1656 × body mass in kg) – (2.767 × 1.5-mile run time in min)

Sample Calculations

Gender: _Female_

Age: _28 years_

Body weight: _54 kg_

1.5-mile run time: _12:24 min:sec_

Step 1: Convert time to minutes.

24 sec ÷ 60 sec = 0.4 min

Therefore,

12:24 min:sec = 12.4 min

Step 2: Calculate the predicted $\dot{V}O_2$ max.

$\dot{V}O_2$ max = 88.020 – (0.1656 × 54 kg) – (2.767 × 12.4 min)

= 44.8 mL • kg⁻¹ • min⁻¹

Step 3: Compare the predicted $\dot{V}O_2$ max score from the 12-minute run to the norms in table 12.1.

A score of 44.8 mL • kg⁻¹ • min⁻¹ would be classified as Superior for a 20- to 29-year-old woman in table 12.1.

Men's and women's aerobic fitness classifications.	TABLE	12.1

Men		Age (years)					
CATEGORY	MEASURE	13–19	20–29	30–39	40–49	50–59	60+
I. Very Poor	$\dot{V}O_2$ max (mL • kg^{-1} • min^{-1})	<35.0	<33.0	<31.5	<30.2	<26.1	<20.5
II. Poor	$\dot{V}O_2$ max (mL • kg^{-1} • min^{-1})	35.0–38.3	33.0–36.4	31.5–35.4	30.2–33.5	26.1–30.9	20.5–26.0
III. Fair	$\dot{V}O_2$ max (mL • kg^{-1} • min^{-1})	38.4–45.1	36.5–42.4	35.5–40.9	33.6–38.9	31.0–35.7	26.1–32.2
IV. Good	$\dot{V}O_2$ max (mL • kg^{-1} • min^{-1})	45.2–50.9	42.5–46.4	41.0–44.9	39.0–43.7	35.8–40.9	32.3–36.4
V. Excellent	$\dot{V}O_2$ max (mL • kg^{-1} • min^{-1})	51.0–55.9	46.5–52.4	45.0–49.4	43.8–48.0	41.0–45.3	36.5–44.2
VI. Superior	$\dot{V}O_2$ max (mL • kg^{-1} • min^{-1})	>56.0	>52.5	>49.5	>48.1	>45.4	>44.3

Women		Age (years)					
CATEGORY	MEASURE	13–19	20–29	30–39	40–49	50–59	60+
I. Very Poor	$\dot{V}O_2$ max (mL • kg^{-1} • min^{-1})	<25.0	<23.6	<22.8	<21.0	<20.2	<17.5
II. Poor	$\dot{V}O_2$ max (mL • kg^{-1} • min^{-1})	25.0–30.9	23.6–28.9	22.8–26.9	21.0–24.4	20.2–22.7	17.5–20.1
III. Fair	$\dot{V}O_2$ max (mL • kg^{-1} • min^{-1})	31.0–34.9	29.0–32.9	27.0–31.4	24.5–28.9	22.8–26.9	20.2–24.4
IV. Good	$\dot{V}O_2$ max (mL • kg^{-1} • min^{-1})	35.0–38.9	33.0–36.9	31.5–35.6	29.0–32.8	27.0–31.4	24.5–30.2
V. Excellent	$\dot{V}O_2$ max (mL • kg^{-1} • min^{-1})	39.0–41.9	37.0–40.9	35.7–40.0	32.9–36.9	31.5–35.7	30.3–31.4
VI. Superior	$\dot{V}O_2$ max (mL • kg^{-1} • min^{-1})	>42.0	>41.0	>40.1	>37.0	>35.8	>31.5

Source: Cooper, Kenneth H. *The Aerobics Way.* Toronto: Bantam Books, 1977, pp. 280–281. Printed with permission of Kenneth H. Cooper, MD, MPH, www.cooperaerobics.com, and J.B. Lipponcott via Copyright Clearance Center.

Worksheet 12.1 1.5-MILE RUN TEST FORM

Name _____ Date _____

Gender: _____

Age (years): _____

Body weight (kg): _____

1. Time (in min:sec) to complete the 1.5-mile run = _____ min

2. Equation for men:
   $\dot{V}O_2$ max (mL • kg^{-1} • min^{-1}) = 91.736 – (0.1656 × body weight in kg)
   – (2.767 × 1.5-mile run time in min) = _____

   Equation for women:
   $\dot{V}O_2$ max (mL • kg^{-1} • min^{-1}) = 88.020 – (0.1656 × body weight in kg)
   – (2.767 × 1.5-mile run time in min) = _____

3. Classification = _____ (table 12.1)

Name _____   Date _____

Use the following data and table 12.1 to answer the questions below.

Gender: _Male_

Age: _18 years_

Body weight: _82 kg_

1.5-mile run time: _13:45 min:sec_

1. Calculate the subject's predicted $\dot{V}O_2$ max from the 1.5-mile run test.

   $\dot{V}O_2$ max = _____ mL • kg^{-1} • min^{-1}

2. Classify the subject's predicted $\dot{V}O_2$ max from the 1.5-mile run test (table 12.1).

   Classification = _____

3. On the graph below, draw the expected relationship between 1.5-mile run times and $\dot{V}O_2$ max.

$\dot{V}O_2$ max
(mL • kg^{-1} • min^{-1})

1.5-mile run time

EXTENSION QUESTIONS

1. What are some common mistakes that may occur in administering this lab?

2. Identify possible sources of error in this lab.

3. Assess the practicality of using this lab in the field.

4. Research the reliability and/or validity of this lab using online resources, journal articles, and other credible sources.

REFERENCES

1. George, J. D., Vehrs, P. R., Allsen, P. E., Fellingham, G. W., and Fisher, A. G. VO$_2$max estimation from a sub-maximal 1-mile track jog for fit college-age individuals. *Med. Sci. Sports Exerc.* 81: 401–406, 1993.

2. Heyward, V. H. *Advanced Fitness Assessment and Exercise Prescription,* 7th edition. Champaign, IL: Human Kinetics, 2014.

Metabolic Equations to Estimate Oxygen Consumption Rate and Energy Expenditure for Walking, Running, and Leg Cycle Ergometry

Lab 13

BACKGROUND

Aerobic exercise training is important for individuals seeking to improve endurance capacity, reduce cardiovascular disease risk factors, and/or manage body weight.[3] The effectiveness of aerobic exercise training depends on the frequency, duration, intensity, and mode of exercise and is most effective when tailored to the needs of the individual. Exercise prescriptions can be designed based on heart rate, oxygen consumption rate ($\dot{V}O_2$), metabolic equivalents of task (METs), or ratings of perceived exertion (RPEs).[3] When prescribing exercise using $\dot{V}O_2$ or METs, it is necessary to know the oxygen cost of the activity. From this, the estimated energy expenditure (expressed in kilocalories per minute, or kcal·min^{-1}) associated with the activity can be calculated. The $\dot{V}O_2$ and energy expenditure of physical activity can be measured directly, as described in Lab 6. However, it is also possible to estimate the oxygen cost (expressed in milliliters of oxygen per kilogram of body weight per minute, or mL • kg^{-1} • min^{-1}) from a compendium of physical activities[1] or by using metabolic equations.[2,3]

In this laboratory, the $\dot{V}O_2$ and energy expenditure associated with walking, running, and leg cycle ergometry will be estimated from metabolic equations from the ACSM.[2,3]

KNOW THESE TERMS & ABBREVIATIONS

- MET = metabolic equivalent of task; a measure of the energy cost of exercise defined as the ratio of the metabolic cost of the exercise (mL • kg^{-1} • min^{-1}) to a reference metabolic cost (resting = 3.5 mL • kg^{-1} • min^{-1})
- $\dot{V}O_2$ = oxygen consumption rate

EQUATIONS

1. Each equation has a resting component that is always 3.5 mL • kg • min^{-1} (1 MET), a horizontal component, and a vertical/resistance component. Note that there is an additional 3.5 mL • kg^{-1} • min^{-1} value in the leg cycle ergometry equation, which represents the cost of unloaded cycling *above and beyond* the resting component.

2. Speed is expressed in m • min^{-1}. To convert miles per hour (mph) to m • min^{-1}, multiply mph × 26.8.

3. Grade is expressed in decimal format (i.e., 10% grade = 0.10).

4. Work rate is expressed in kgm • min^{-1}. Work rate = resistance (kg) × revolutions per minute (rpm) × flywheel distance (m). The flywheel distance on a Monark cycle ergometer is 6 m.

5. Body weight is expressed in kg.

Note: The metabolic equations are designed to estimate $\dot{V}O_2$ during steady-state submaximal exercise only. The accuracy of the equations deteriorates when they are used outside the speeds or work rates for which they were designed. The walking equation is most accurate for speeds of 50–100 m • min^{-1} (1.9–3.7 mph). The running equation is most accurate for speeds greater than 134 m • min^{-1} (5 mph). The cycle ergometry equation is most accurate for work rates of 300–1,200 kgm·min^{-1} (50–200 W).[3]

Walking

$\dot{V}O_2$ (mL • kg^{-1} • min^{-1}) = 3.5 + (0.1 x speed) + (1.8 x speed x grade)

Running

$\dot{V}O_2$ (mL • kg^{-1} • min^{-1}) = 3.5 + (0.2 x speed) + (0.9 x speed x grade)

Leg Cycle Ergometry

$\dot{V}O_2$ (mL • kg^{-1} • min^{-1}) = 3.5 + 3.5 + (1.8 x (work rate / body weight))

Caloric Expenditure Rate

CER = $\dot{V}O_2$ (mL • kg^{-1} • min^{-1}) x body weight (kg) ÷ 1000 x 4.9

SAMPLE CALCULATIONS

Subject Information

Gender: _Female_

Age: _33 yrs_

Body weight: _55 kg_

Height: _160 cm_

$\dot{V}O_2$ max: _42 mL • kg^{-1} • min^{-1}_

Walking

The subject walked for 45 minutes at 3.2 mph (3.2 × 26.8 = 85.8 m • min^{-1}) and a 3% grade and would like to know the energy cost of this exercise in kcals. How many kcals did she burn?

$\dot{V}O_2$ (mL • kg^{-1} • min^{-1}) = 3.5 + (0.1 x 85.8) + (1.8 x 85.8 x 0.03)

$\dot{V}O_2$ (mL • kg^{-1} • min^{-1}) = 3.5 + 8.6 + 4.6 = 16.7 mL • kg^{-1} • min^{-1}

CER = $\dot{V}O_2$ (mL • kg^{-1} • min^{-1}) x body weight (kg) ÷ 1000 x 4.9

CER = 16.7 mL • kg^{-1} • min^{-1} x 55 kg ÷ 1000 x 4.9 = 4.5 kcal • min^{-1}

4.5 kcal • min^{-1} x 45 min = 202.5 kcal

Running

The subject would like to run at 65% of her $\dot{V}O_2$ max. At what velocity (in mph) would she need to run if running on a 0% grade?

target $\dot{V}O_2$ max = 42 mL • kg^{-1}·min^{-1} x 0.65 = 27.3 mL • kg^{-1} • min^{-1}

27.3 = 3.5 + (0.2 x speed) + (0.9 x speed x 0.0)

27.3 = 3.5 + 0.2 x speed + 0.0

23.8 = 0.2 x speed

119 = speed in m • min^{-1}

119.0 m • min^{-1} ÷ 26.8 = 4.4 mph

Leg Cycle Ergometry

You've prescribed 1,200 kcal • wk^{-1} of cycle ergometry exercise for this subject. She would like to perform three 40-minute sessions per week. At what workload (W) will she need to work in order to fulfill your exercise prescription?

1,200 kcal • wk^{-1} ÷ 3 days = 400 kcal • session $^{-1}$

400 kcal ÷ 40 min = 10 kcal • min^{-1}

10 kcal • min^{-1} = $\dot{V}O_2$ (mL • kg^{-1} • min^{-1}) x 55 kg ÷ 1000 x 4.9

$\dot{V}O_2$ = 37.1 (mL • kg^{-1} • min^{-1})

37.1 = 3.5 + 3.5 + 1.8 x (work rate / 55 kg)

30.1 = 1.8 x (work rate / 55 kg)

16.7 = work rate / 55 kg

work rate = 920 kgm • min^{-1}

920.0 kgm • min^{-1} ÷ 6.12 = 150.3 W

Worksheet 13.1 METABOLIC EQUATIONS TO ESTIMATE OXYGEN CONSUMPTION RATE

Name _____ Date _____

Gender: _____

Age (years): _____

Body weight (kg): _____

Height (cm): _____

$\dot{V}O_2$ max = _____ $mL \cdot kg^{-1} \cdot min^{-1}$

Note: Recall grade is expressed in decimal format: i.e., 3% grade = 0.03; 10% grade = 0.10.

Walking

_____ $mL \cdot kg^{-1} \cdot min^{-1}$ = 3.5 + (0.1 x _____ speed in $m \cdot min^{-1}$) + (1.8 x _____ speed in $m \cdot min^{-1}$ x _____ grade)

Running

_____ $mL \cdot kg^{-1} \cdot min^{-1}$ = 3.5 + (0.2 x _____ speed in $m \cdot min^{-1}$) + (0.9 x _____ speed in $m \cdot min^{-1}$ x _____ grade)

Leg Cycle Ergometry

_____ $mL \cdot kg^{-1} \cdot min^{-1}$ = 3.5 + 3.5 + (1.8 x (_____ work rate in $kgm \cdot min^{-1}$ / _____ body weight in kg))

Worksheet **13.2**

Name _____   Date _____

Gender: _____

Age (years): _____

Body weight (kg): _____

Height (cm): _____

$\dot{V}O_2$ max = _____ mL • kg^{-1} • min^{-1}

Walking Equation

At what speed would you have to walk in order to burn 300 kcals in 50 minutes if the treadmill is at 0% grade?

1. Calculate the kcals burned per minute.

    total kcals burned ÷ minute spent exercising = _____ kcals • min^{-1}

2. Calculate the $\dot{V}O_2$ (mL • kg^{-1} • min^{-1}) associated with this caloric expenditure rate.

    kcal • min^{-1} = $\dot{V}O_2$ (mL • kg^{-1} • min^{-1}) x body weight (kg) ÷ 1000 x 4.9

    _____ kcal • min^{-1} = $\dot{V}O_2$ (mL • kg^{-1} • min^{-1}) x _____ kg ÷ 1000 x 4.9

    _____ = $\dot{V}O_2$ mL • kg^{-1} • min^{-1}

3. Calculate the speed you'd need to walk in order to achieve this $\dot{V}O_2$ (mL • kg^{-1} • min^{-1}).

    $\dot{V}O_2$ (mL • kg^{-1} • min^{-1}) = 3.5 + (0.1 x speed) + (1.8 x speed x grade)

    _____ mL • kg^{-1} • min^{-1} = 3.5 + (0.1 x speed) + 0.0

    speed = _____ m • min^{-1}

Running Equation

You would like to run at 75% of your $\dot{V}O_2$ max for 30 minutes. At what speed would you need to run and what is the energy expenditure (i.e., kcals) associated with completing this exercise? Assume the treadmill grade is 2%.

1. Calculate 75% of your $\dot{V}O_2$ max.

    75% $\dot{V}O_2$ max = $\dot{V}O_2$ max x 0.75 = _____ mL • kg^{-1} • min^{-1}

2. Calculate the speed needed to achieve this $\dot{V}O_2$.

    $\dot{V}O_2$ (mL • kg^{-1} • min^{-1}) = 3.5 + (0.2 x speed) + (0.9 x speed x grade)

    _____ mL • kg^{-1} • min^{-1} = 3.5 + (0.2 x speed) + (0.9 x speed x 0.02)

    _____ = (0.2 x speed) + (0.018 x speed)

    speed = _____ m • min^{-1}

3. Calculate the energy expenditure in kcals associated with this exercise.

kcal • min^{-1} = $\dot{V}O_2$ (mL • kg^{-1} • min^{-1}) x body weight (kg) ÷ 1000 x 4.9

kcal • min^{-1} = _____ mL • kg^{-1} • min^{-1} x _____ kg ÷ 1000 x 4.9

energy expenditure rate = _____ kcal • min^{-1}

Leg Cycle Ergometry Equation

What would your oxygen consumption rate ($\dot{V}O_2$) and energy expenditure rate (kcals • min^{-1}) be if you cycled at 70 revolutions per minute (rpm) at a resistance of 2.0 kg on a Monark bicycle ergometer?

1. Calculate the work rate.

work rate (kgm • min^{-1}) = resistance (kg) x rpms x flywheel distance (m)

work rate (kgm • min^{-1}) = _____ kg x _____ rpm x _____ m

work rate = _____ kgm·min^{-1}

2. Calculate the $\dot{V}O_2$ associated with cycling at this work rate.

$\dot{V}O_2$ (mL • kg^{-1} • min^{-1}) = 3.5 + 3.5 + (1.8 x (work rate ÷ body weight))

$\dot{V}O_2$ (mL • kg^{-1} • min^{-1}) = 7.0 + (1.8 x (_____ kgm • min^{-1} / _____ kg))

$\dot{V}O_2$ = _____ mL • kg^{-1} • min^{-1}

3. Calculate the energy expenditure rate associated with this $\dot{V}O_2$.

kcal • min^{-1} = $\dot{V}O_2$ (mL • kg^{-1} • min^{-1}) x body weight (kg) ÷ 1000 x 4.9

kcal • min^{-1} = _____ mL • kg^{-1} • min^{-1} x _____ kg ÷ 1000 x 4.9

energy expenditure rate = _____ kcal • min^{-1}

REFERENCES

1. Ainsworth, B. E., Haskell, W. L., Herrmann, S. D., Meckes, N., Bassett Jr., D. R., Tudor-Locke, C., Greer, J. L., Vezina, J., Whitt-Glover, M. C., and Leon, A. S. 2011 Compendium of Physical Activities: a second update of codes and MET values. *Med. Sci. Sports Exerc.* 43:1575–1581, 2011.

2. Glass, S., and Dwyer, G. B., eds. *ACSM's Metabolic Calculations Handbook*. Philadelphia: Lippincott Williams & Wilkins, 2007.

3. Pescatello, L. S., Arena, R., Riebe, D., and Thompson, P. D., eds. *ACSM's Guidelines for Exercise Testing and Prescription*, 9th edition. Baltimore: Wolters Kluwer/ Lippincott Williams & Wilkins, 2014.

Unit 3

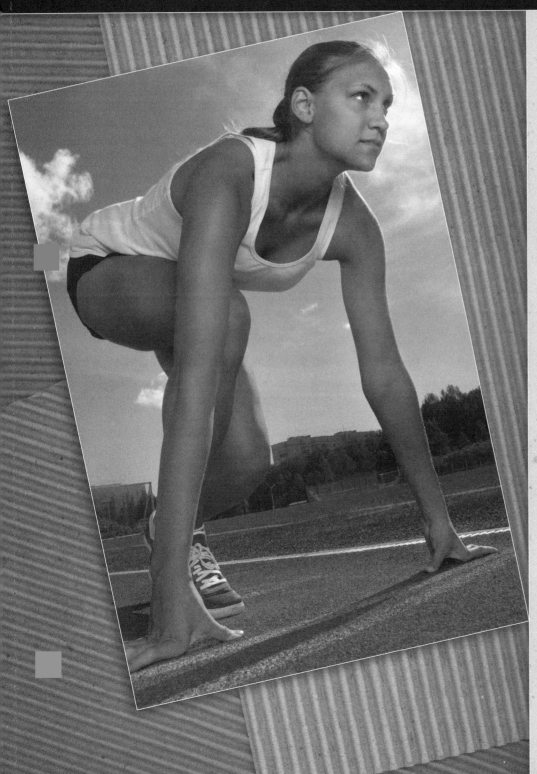

FATIGUE THRESHOLDS

BACKGROUND

Theoretically, the gas exchange threshold (GET) and ventilatory threshold (VT) estimate the exercise intensity above which anaerobic adenosine triphosphate (ATP) production must support aerobic metabolism.[2] Thus, in theory, exercise intensities below the GET and VT are nonfatiguing and are maintained from aerobic ATP production only, while those above these thresholds are fatiguing and utilize anaerobic plus aerobic ATP production. The GET and VT usually occur at approximately 50% to 60% of the maximal oxygen consumption rate ($\dot{V}O_2$ max) in untrained to moderately trained individuals, but occur at 80% of $\dot{V}O_2$ max or above in highly trained endurance athletes.[5] Typically, there is no difference in exercise intensity between the GET and VT because they share a common underlying mechanism. The GET results from excess carbon dioxide (CO_2) generated from bicarbonate buffering of lactic acid produced through anaerobic ATP production during intense exercise. The VT, however, represents the ventilatory response to the excess CO_2. Thus, the excess CO_2 from lactic acid buffering underlies both the GET and VT.

The GET and VT have been used as measures of aerobic fitness in clinical populations including patients with HIV[8] and cystic fibrosis,[9] as well as endurance athletes such as marathon runners.[4,7] The GET and VT have also been used to assess the effectiveness of endurance training programs.[3] Endurance athletes with high GET and VT values can maintain a high percentage (fraction) of their $\dot{V}O_2$ max for a long time without fatigue. Thus, an athlete with high GET and VT values can maintain a faster pace than a competitor with lower values and, therefore, perform better in endurance events. In fact, some elite distance runners with very high GET and VT values can maintain a race pace that corresponds to approximately 90% of their $\dot{V}O_2$ max for the entire duration of a marathon.

The respiratory compensation point (RCP) defines the threshold above which the volume of expired air (called minute ventilation = $\dot{V}_E$) increases at a greater rate than the volume of CO_2 produced ($\dot{V}CO_2$).[1] The RCP represents the hyperventilation that occurs when the blood bicarbonate buffering system is overwhelmed by lactic acid production, which results in an elevated drive for ventilation. The RCP occurs at an exercise intensity above the GET and VT, and typically at about 80% to 90% of $\dot{V}O_2$ max in untrained to moderately trained individuals. One of the primary applications of the GET, VT, and RCP is to demarcate the exercise intensity domains (moderate, heavy, and severe intensity domains). The GET and VT demarcate the moderate domain from the heavy domain, while the RCP demarcates the heavy domain from the severe domain. Thus, exercise intensities below the GET and VT are within the moderate domain, those greater than the GET and VT but less than the RCP are within the heavy domain, and intensities greater than the RCP are within the severe domain.

The GET, VT, and RCP are estimated from expired gas samples collected during an incremental test to exhaustion. Lab 6 describes the characteristics of typical incremental tests to exhaustion, the methods used to collect expired gas samples, and the procedures for calculating the variables used to determine the GET, VT, and RCP. Briefly, during the incremental test to exhaustion, the subject breathes through a two-way valve to collect expired gas samples, which then are analyzed by a metabolic cart (refer back to photos 6.1 and 6.2) to determine the volume of O_2 consumed ($\dot{V}O_2$ in L • min^{-1}), volume of CO_2 produced ($\dot{V}CO_2$ in L • min^{-1}), and minute ventilation ($\dot{V}_E$ in L • min^{-1}). As the exercise intensity increases, more O_2 is consumed ($\dot{V}O_2$ increases) for ATP production, a greater volume of CO_2 is produced ($\dot{V}CO_2$ increases), and $\dot{V}_E$ increases. The $\dot{V}CO_2$ and $\dot{V}_E$ increase linearly with exercise intensity until the GET and VT are reached. Above the GET and VT, disproportionate increases in $\dot{V}CO_2$ and $\dot{V}_E$, relative to $\dot{V}O_2$, occur as a result of the accelerated contribution of anaerobic energy to metabolism and lactate production. The GET and VT are defined as the $\dot{V}O_2$ values that correspond to the "breakpoints" (nonlinear increases) in the $\dot{V}CO_2$ versus $\dot{V}O_2$ and $\dot{V}_E$ versus $\dot{V}O_2$ relationships, respectively (see figures 14.1 and 14.2).

The RCP is determined by plotting the $\dot{V}_E$ versus $\dot{V}CO_2$ relationship. It is defined as the $\dot{V}O_2$ value that corresponds to the "breakpoint" (nonlinear increase) in the $\dot{V}_E$ versus $\dot{V}CO_2$ relationship (see figure 14.3).

In this laboratory, the GET, VT, and RCP will be determined from gas exchange variables using visual inspection of the relationships for $\dot{V}CO_2$ versus $\dot{V}O_2$, $\dot{V}_E$ versus $\dot{V}O_2$, and $\dot{V}_E$ versus $\dot{V}CO_2$, respectively.

KNOW THESE TERMS & ABBREVIATIONS

- ATP = adenosine triphosphate
- $\dot{V}_E$ = volume of gas expired or minute ventilation
- $\dot{V}CO_2$ = volume of CO_2 produced
- $\dot{V}O_2$ = oxygen consumption rate, an indirect measure of aerobic energy production

---

Method for determining the gas exchange threshold (GET). **FIGURE** **14.1**

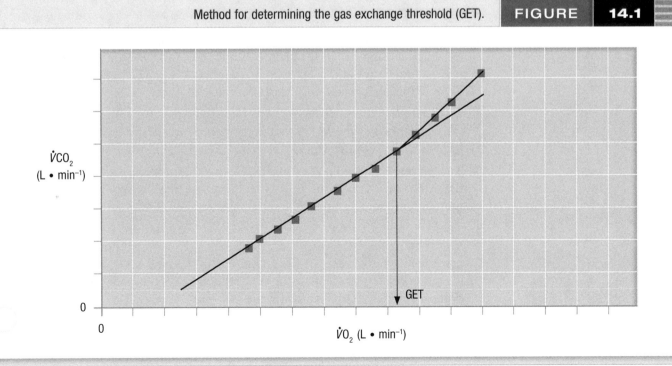

| FIGURE | 14.2 | Method for determining the ventilatory threshold (VT). |

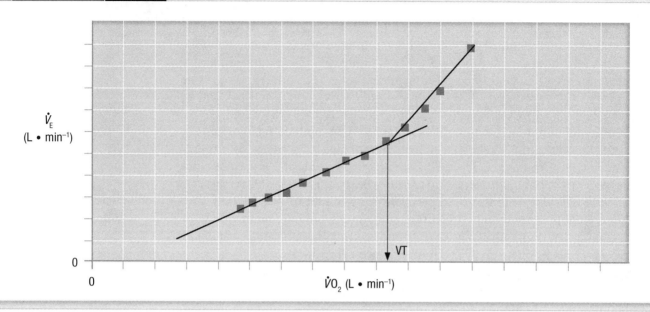

- $\dot{V}O_2$ max = maximal oxygen consumption rate
- VT = ventilatory threshold, an estimation of the exercise intensity above which anaerobic ATP production must supplement aerobic metabolism
- GET = gas exchange threshold, an estimation of the exercise intensity above which anaerobic ATP production must supplement aerobic metabolism
- RCP = respiratory compensation point, the threshold above which $\dot{V}_E$ increases at a greater rate than CO_2

PROCEDURES

1. The subject will perform a maximal cycle ergometer or treadmill test to exhaustion using one of the protocols in Lab 6 (table 6.2). Throughout the test, gas exchange and ventilatory parameters ($\dot{V}O_2$, $\dot{V}CO_2$, and $\dot{V}_E$) will be analyzed using a metabolic cart (refer back to photos 6.1, 6.3, and 6.4).

2. To determine the GET, $\dot{V}CO_2$ is plotted versus $\dot{V}O_2$ (figure 14.1). The GET is defined as the $\dot{V}O_2$ value that corresponds to the breakpoint (nonlinear increase) in the $\dot{V}CO_2$ versus $\dot{V}O_2$ relationship (figure 14.1).

3. To determine the VT, $\dot{V}_E$ is plotted versus $\dot{V}O_2$ (figure 14.2). The VT is defined as the $\dot{V}O_2$ value that corresponds to the breakpoint (nonlinear increase) in the $\dot{V}_E$ versus $\dot{V}O_2$ relationship (figure 14.2).

4. To determine the RCP, $\dot{V}_E$ is plotted versus $\dot{V}CO_2$ (figure 14.3). The RCP is defined as the $\dot{V}O_2$ value that corresponds to the breakpoint (nonlinear increase) in the $\dot{V}_E$ versus $\dot{V}CO_2$ relationship (figure 14.3). For the RCP, it is then necessary to identify the $\dot{V}O_2$ value that corresponds to this breakpoint from the data provided by the metabolic cart.

5. The "breakpoint" in the relationships can be determined through visual inspection.[6] For example, the GET can be estimated by looking at the $\dot{V}CO_2$ versus $\dot{V}O_2$ plot and identifying the data point where the $\dot{V}CO_2$ values begin

| Method for determining the respiratory compensation point (RCP). | FIGURE | 14.3 |

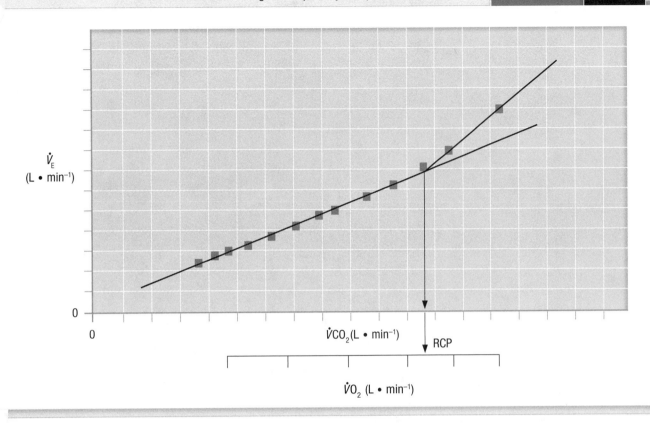

to increase in a nonlinear fashion. The GET is then defined as the $\dot{V}O_2$ value that corresponds to that data point (figure 14.1). The same method is used to identify the VT from the $\dot{V}_E$ versus $\dot{V}O_2$ relationship (figure 14.2). The RCP is the $\dot{V}O_2$ value that corresponds to the data point at the nonlinear increase in the $\dot{V}_E$ versus $\dot{V}CO_2$ relationship (figure 14.3).

Sample Calculations

In this laboratory, estimations of the GET, VT, and RCP will be accomplished from visual inspection of the relationships among the gas exchange and ventilatory parameters.

1. Using the data plotted on worksheet 14.1, visually identify the breakpoint in the $\dot{V}CO_2$ versus $\dot{V}O_2$ relationship and estimate the GET as the $\dot{V}O_2$ value on the x-axis that corresponds to the breakpoint.

   GET = _____ $L \cdot min^{-1}$

2. Using the data plotted on worksheet 14.2, visually identify the breakpoint in the $\dot{V}_E$ versus $\dot{V}O_2$ relationship and estimate the VT as the $\dot{V}O_2$ value on the x-axis that corresponds to the breakpoint.

   VT = _____ $L \cdot min^{-1}$

3. Using the data plotted on worksheet 14.3, visually identify the breakpoint in the $\dot{V}_E$ versus $\dot{V}CO_2$ relationship and estimate the RCP as the $\dot{V}O_2$ value that corresponds to the $\dot{V}CO_2$ value on the x-axis at the breakpoint.

   RCP = _____ $L \cdot min^{-1}$

Worksheet **14.1** GAS EXCHANGE THRESHOLD (GET)

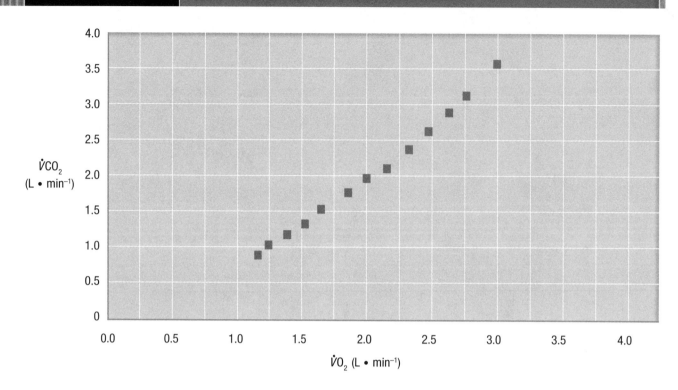

Worksheet **14.2** VENTILATORY THRESHOLD (VT)

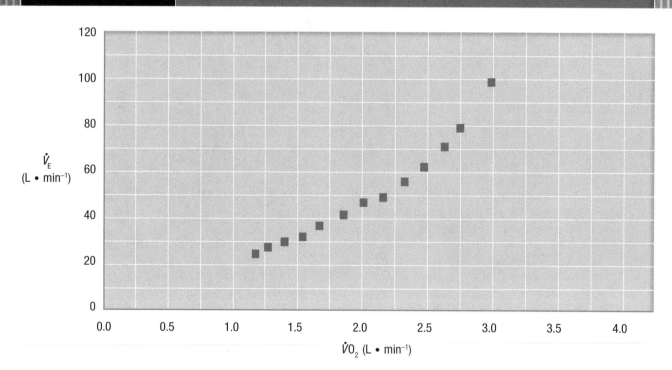

RESPIRATORY COMPENSATION POINT (RCP)

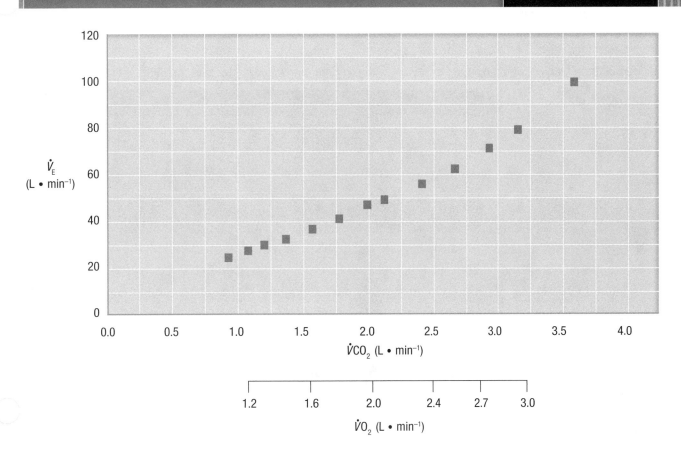

Worksheet 14.4 | EXTENSION ACTIVITIES

Name _____ Date _____

Using the three blank charts provided, graph the following data, and visually estimate the GET, VT, and RCP.

Time (min)	$\dot{V}O_2$ (L·min⁻¹)	$\dot{V}CO_2$ (L·min⁻¹)	$\dot{V}_E$ (L·min⁻¹)
1:00	1.16	0.91	24.53
2:00	1.25	1.06	27.68
3:00	1.38	1.18	30.03
4:00	1.53	1.35	32.55
5:00	1.65	1.55	37.47
6:00	1.84	1.76	42.00
7:00	1.99	2.97	47.61
8:00	2.15	2.11	49.54
9:00	2.31	2.38	56.18
10:00	2.46	2.64	62.71
11:00	2.62	2.90	71.33
12:00	2.74	3.13	79.36
13:00	2.98	3.57	99.76

Chart for estimating GET

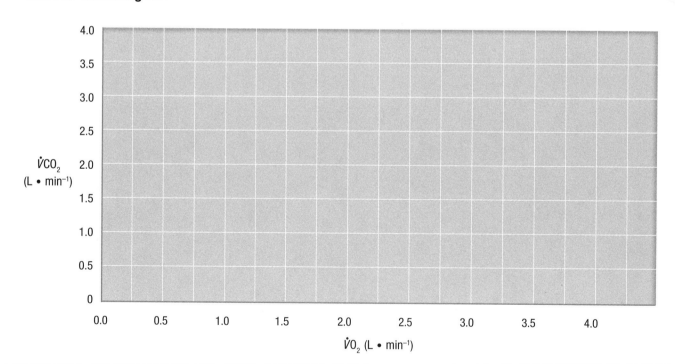

GET ($\dot{V}CO_2$ versus $\dot{V}O_2$) = _____ L · min⁻¹

Chart for estimating VT

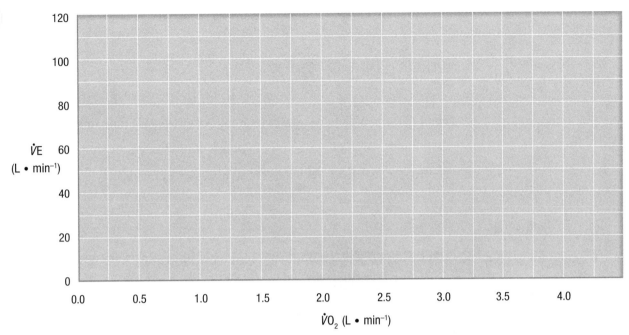

VT ($\dot{V}_E$ versus $\dot{V}O_2$) = _____ L • min^{-1}

Chart for estimating RCP

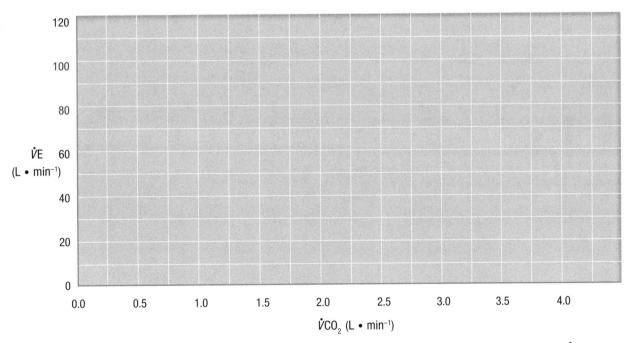

RCP ($\dot{V}_E$ versus $\dot{V}CO_2$) = _____ L • min^{-1}. For the RCP, use the data to determine the $\dot{V}O_2$ value that corresponds to the $\dot{V}CO_2$ value at the RCP.

EXTENSION QUESTIONS

1. Why is the GET important to endurance athletes?

2. Which is greater, the VT or RCP? Why?

3. The GET and VT demarcate which exercise intensity domains?

4. The RCP demarcates which exercise intensity domains?

REFERENCES

1. Beaver, W. L., Wasserman, K., and Whipp, B. J. A new method for detecting anaerobic threshold by gas exchange. *J Appl. Physiol.* 60: 2050–2027, 1986.

2. Bergstrom, H. C., Housh, T. J., Zuniga, J. M., Traylor, D. A., Camic, C. L., Lewis Jr., R. W., Schmidt, R. J., and Johnson, G. O. The relationship among critical power determined from a 3-min all-out test, respiratory compensation point, gas exchange threshold, and ventilatory threshold. *Res. Q. Exerc. Sport.* 84: 232–238, 2013.

3. Jones, A. M., and Carter, H. The effects of endurance training on parameters of aerobic fitness. *Sports Med.* 29: 373–386, 2000.

4. Maffulli, N., Testa, V., and Gapasso, G. Anaerobic threshold determination in master endurance runners. *J. Sports Med. Phys. Fitness* 34: 242–249, 1994.

5. Malek, M. H., Housh, T. J., Coburn, J. W., Schmidt, R. J., and Beck, T. W. Cross-validation of ventilatory threshold prediction equations on aerobically trained men and women. *J. Strength Cond. Res.* 21: 29–33, 2007.

6. Orr, G. W., Green, H. J., Hughson, R. L., and Bennett, G. W. A computer linear regression model to determine ventilatory anaerobic threshold. *J. Appl. Physiol.* 53: 1345–1352, 1982.

7. Tanaka, K., and Matsuura, Y. Marathon performance, anaerobic threshold, and onset of blood lactate accumulation. *J. Appl. Physiol.* 57: 640–643, 1984.

8. Tesiorowski, A. M., Harris, M., Chan, K. J., Thompson, C. R., and Montaner, J. S. Anaerobic threshold and random venous lactate levels among HIV-positive patients on antiretroviral therapy. *J. Acquir. Immune Defic. Syndr.* 31: 250–251, 2002.

9. Thin, A. G., Linnane, S. J., McKone, E. F., Freaney, R., Fitzgerald, M. X., Gallagher, C. G., and McLoughlin, P. Use of the gas exchange threshold to noninvasively determine the lactate threshold in patients with cystic fibrosis. *Chest* 121: 1761–1770, 2002.

BACKGROUND

Theoretically, the ventilatory threshold (VT) is an estimation of the exercise intensity above which anaerobic adenosine triphosphate (ATP) production must supplement aerobic metabolism. Thus, in theory, exercise intensities below the VT are non-fatiguing and are maintained from aerobic ATP production only, while those above the VT are fatiguing and utilize anaerobic plus aerobic ATP production. Typically, the VT occurs at approximately 50% to 60% of maximal oxygen consumption rate ($\dot{V}O_2$ max) in untrained to moderately trained individuals, but 80% of $\dot{V}O_2$ max or above in highly trained endurance athletes.[4]

The VT has been used as a measure of aerobic fitness in clinical populations including patients with HIV[6] and cystic fibrosis,[7] as well as endurance athletes such as marathon runners.[3,5] The VT has also been used to assess the effectiveness of endurance training programs.[1]

Endurance athletes with a high VT can maintain a high percentage (fraction) of their $\dot{V}O_2$ max for a long time without fatigue. Thus, an athlete with a high VT can maintain a faster race pace than a competitor with a lower VT and, therefore, perform better in endurance events. In fact, some elite distance runners with very high VT values can maintain a race pace that corresponds to approximately 90% of their $\dot{V}O_2$ max for the entire duration of a 26.2-mile marathon.

The VT is estimated from expired gas samples collected during an incremental test to exhaustion (see Lab 14). During the test, the subject breathes through a two-way valve to collect expired gas samples, which are then analyzed by a metabolic cart (see photo 15.1) to determine the volume of oxygen consumed ($\dot{V}O_2$ in L • min^{-1}) and the volume of gas expired, called minute ventilation or $\dot{V}_E$. As the exercise intensity increases, more oxygen is consumed per minute ($\dot{V}O_2$ increases) for ATP production, and a greater volume of gas is expired. The $\dot{V}_E$ increases linearly with exercise intensity ($\dot{V}O_2$) until the VT is reached. Above the VT, there is a disproportionate increase in $\dot{V}_E$ (relative to $\dot{V}O_2$) as a result of the accelerated contribution of anaerobic energy to the metabolism. The VT is defined as the $\dot{V}O_2$ value (L • min^{-1}) that corresponds to the "breakpoint" (nonlinear increase) in the $\dot{V}_E$ versus $\dot{V}O_2$ relationship (see figure 15.1).

Direct determination of the VT in a laboratory setting requires a metabolic cart to analyze expired

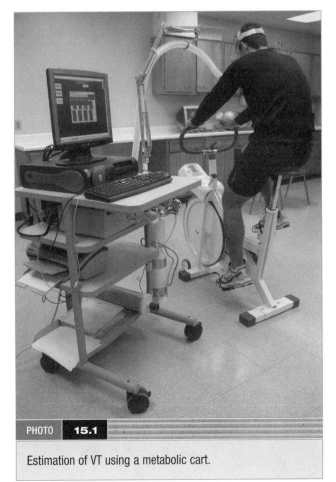

PHOTO 15.1

Estimation of VT using a metabolic cart.

| FIGURE | 15.1 | Method for determining the ventilatory threshold (VT). |

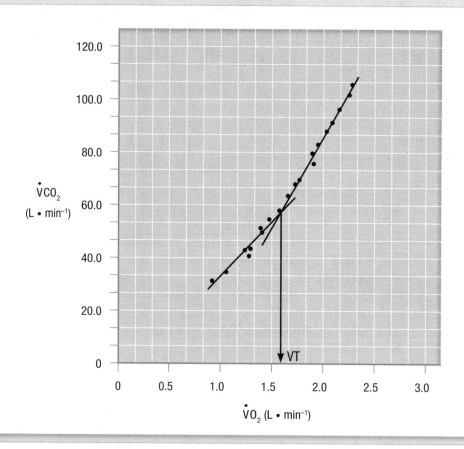

gas samples collected during the incremental test to exhaustion. In this laboratory, however, the VT for adult males and females can be estimated using a multiple regression equation that utilizes only age and height as predictor variables.[2]

KNOW THESE TERMS & ABBREVIATIONS

- ATP = adenosine triphosphate
- $\dot{V}_E$ = volume of gas expired per minute or minute ventilation
- $\dot{V}O_2$ = oxygen consumption rate, an indirect measure of aerobic energy production
- $\dot{V}O_2$ max = maximal oxygen consumption rate
- VT = ventilatory threshold, an estimation of the exercise intensity above which anaerobic ATP production must supplement aerobic metabolism

PROCEDURES

1. Record the subject's age in years and height in cm (inches × 2.54) on worksheet 15.1.
2. Use the equation on the following page and worksheet 15.1 to calculate the VT.

Equation[2]

VT (L • min^{-1}) = (0.024 $\times$ height in cm) – (0.0074 $\times$ age in years) – 2.43

R (multiple correlation coefficient) = 0.651

SEE (standard error of estimate) = 0.316 L • min^{-1}

Note: This equation is used for both males and females.

Sample Calculation

Age: _____21_____

Height: _70 inches (or 177.8 cm)_

VT (L • min^{-1}) = (0.024 $\times$ 177.8) – (0.0074 $\times$ 21) – 2.43 = 1.68 L • min^{-1}

Worksheet 15.1 — NON-EXERCISE-BASED ESTIMATION OF VENTILATORY THRESHOLD FORM

Name _____ Date _____

Age: _____ yrs

Height: _____ cm

VT $(L \cdot min^{-1})$ = (0.024 × height in cm) − (0.0074 × age in years) − 2.43 = _____

Worksheet 15.2 — EXTENSION ACTIVITIES

Name _____ Date _____

Use the following data to answer the questions below.

Age: _23 years_

Height: _182 cm_

$\dot{V}O_2$ max: _3.3 L · min⁻¹_

1. Calculate the VT.

   VT = _____ $L \cdot min^{-1}$

2. What percent of $\dot{V}O_2$ max is this VT value?

   VT = _____ % $\dot{V}O_2$ max

EXTENSION QUESTIONS

1. What are some common mistakes that may occur in administering this lab?

2. Identify possible sources of error in this lab.

3. Assess the practicality of using this lab in the field.

4. Research the reliability and/or validity of this lab using online resources, journal articles, and other credible sources.

REFERENCES

1. Jones, A. M., and Carter, H. The effects of endurance training on parameters of aerobic fitness. *Sports Med.* 29: 373–386, 2000.

2. Jones, N. L., Makrides, L., Hitchcock, C., Chypchar, T., and McCartney, N. Normal standards for an incremental progressive cycle ergometer test. *Am. Rev. Respir. Dis.* 131: 700–708, 1985.

3. Maffulli, N., Testa, V., and Gapasso, G. Anaerobic threshold determination in master endurance runners. *J. Sports Med. Phys. Fitness* 34: 242–249, 1994.

4. Malek, M. H., Housh, T. J., Coburn, J. W., Schmidt, R. J., and Beck, T. W. Cross-validation of ventilatory threshold prediction equations on aerobically trained men and women. *J. Strength Cond. Res.* 21: 29–33, 2007.

5. Tanaka, K., and Matsuura, Y. Marathon performance, anaerobic threshold, and onset of blood lactate accumulation. *J. Appl. Physiol.* 57: 640–643, 1984.

6. Tesiorowski, A. M., Harris, M., Chan, K. J., Thompson, C. R., and Montaner, J. S. Anaerobic threshold and random venous lactate levels among HIV-positive patients on antiretroviral therapy. *J. Acquir. Immune Defic. Syndr.* 31: 250–251, 2002.

7. Thin, A. G., Linnane, S. J., McKone, E. F., Freaney R., Fitzgerald, M. X., Gallagher, C. G., and McLoughlin, P. Use of the gas exchange threshold to noninvasively determine the lactate threshold in patients with cystic fibrosis. *Chest* 121: 1761–1770, 2002.

BACKGROUND

Theoretically, the Critical Power (CP) cycle ergometer test estimates three parameters of physical working capacity:[1,2,3,4] (1) the maximal power output that can be maintained for an extended period of time without fatigue, called the CP; (2) the total amount of work that can be accomplished using only stored energy sources (creatine phosphate, glycogen, and oxygen bound to myoglobin) within the activated muscles, called the anaerobic work capacity (AWC); and (3) the time to exhaustion, or time limit (TL), during continuous cycle ergometry at any power output greater than the CP. The CP test uses linear mathematical modeling of the relationship between the total work accomplished at different power outputs and the corresponding TL values to simultaneously estimate the CP, AWC, and TL at any power output greater than the CP (figure 16.1).

Critical Power. The CP is an estimate of the maximal power output during cycle ergometry that can be maintained for an extended period of time without fatigue and is, conceptually, analogous to the anaerobic threshold.[4] The anaerobic threshold is one of three primary physiological factors (along with $\dot{V}O_2$max and economy of movement) that contribute to performance in endurance events. The anaerobic threshold is typically determined from the measurement of blood lactate levels (the lactate threshold) or expired gas samples (the gas exchange threshold and ventilatory threshold). The CP, however, can be estimated using only a cycle ergometer and stopwatch and, therefore, does not require oxygen and carbon dioxide analyzers or invasive blood-sampling procedures.

Anaerobic Work Capacity. The AWC is an estimate of the total amount of work that can be accomplished using only stored energy sources within the activated muscles, such as creatine phosphate, glycogen, and oxygen bound to myoglobin.[1,4,5] Because it is not dependent upon the level of oxygen supply to the muscles,[4] the AWC represents anaerobic ATP production capabilities, and it has been shown to be correlated with mean power from the Wingate Test[5] (see Lab 29). The ability to perform high-intensity, short-duration sports and activities such as weightlifting, 100–400 meter runs, 100–200 meter swims, gymnastics, basketball, football, and speed skating relies primarily on the anaerobic production of ATP to fuel muscle contraction. Thus, the CP test provides estimates of physical working capacity associated with both aerobic (the CP) and anaerobic (the AWC) ATP production.

Time to Exhaustion or Time Limit. There is a negative, curvilinear (asymptotic) relationship between power output and time to exhaustion that is called the power output versus TL curve (figure 16.1a). Based on his or her levels of aerobic and anaerobic fitness, each individual is characterized by a unique power output versus TL curve. That is, some individuals can

Curvilinear power output versus time limit relationship during cycle ergometry.   **FIGURE**   **16.1**

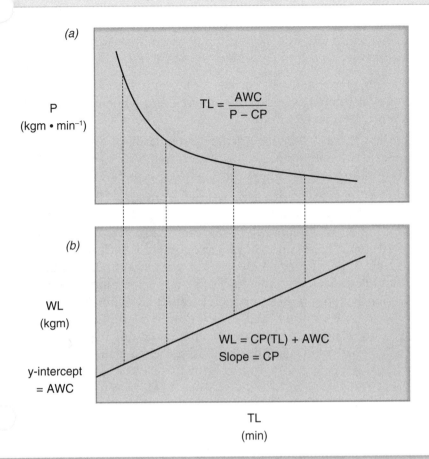

Figure 16.1a represents the negative, curvilinear power output (P) versus time limit (TL) relationship during cycle ergometry and provides the equation that can be used to estimate the TL for any P greater than the CP. Please note that, theoretically, any P ≤ CP can be maintained indefinitely without exhaustion. In reality, however, the CP can often be maintained for an extended period of time (usually > 30 minutes), but not indefinitely. Figure 16.1b represents the linear relationship between work limit (WL) and TL, and provides the equation that can be used to estimate the critical power (CP) and anaerobic work capacity (AWC).

maintain a particular power output for a long time, while other individuals fatigue rapidly at the same power output. The linear mathematical model used to estimate CP and AWC (figure 16.1b) can also be used to derive an individual's power output versus TL curve and, therefore, estimate the time to exhaustion (TL) for any power output that is greater than the CP.[3] Theoretically, the CP is the asymptote of the power output versus TL relationship (figure 16.1a) and, therefore, any power output that is less than the CP should be able to be continued indefinitely. In reality, however, the CP can often be maintained for an extended period of time (usually > 30 minutes), but not indefinitely.[1,3]

KNOW THESE TERMS & ABBREVIATIONS

- ATP = adenosine triphosphate
- AWC = anaerobic work capacity (kgm), defined as the y-intercept of the work limit (WL) versus time limit (TL) relationship (figure 16.1b)
- CP = critical power (kgm • min^{-1}), defined as the slope coefficient of the work limit (WL) versus time limit (TL) relationship (figure 16.1b)
- P = power output (kgm • min^{-1})
- TL = time limit (TL) or time to exhaustion (min)
- WL = work limit (WL) or total work performed (kgm)

PROCEDURES

The CP test will be performed using a Monark cycle ergometer and stopwatch. The three parameters of physical working capacity that will be determined are the CP, AWC, and TL for any power output greater than the CP. Use worksheet 16.1 to record the results of the CP test.

1. Prior to beginning the test: (1) adjust the seat height of the cycle ergometer to allow for near full extension of the subject's legs while pedaling and (2) record a pre-exercise heart rate.

2. Warm-up. The CP test will be preceded by a standardized warm-up protocol that includes 4 minutes of pedaling at 70 rpm with a resistance of 0.5 kg (power output = 210 kgm • min^{-1}).

3. Typically, the CP test involves a series of two or more cycle ergometer workbouts to exhaustion at different power outputs.[1,2,3,4,5] In this laboratory, two (or more) workbouts will be performed at a constant pedaling cadence of 70 rpm. The selection of power outputs for each subject usually ranges from approximately 1050 (2.5 kg resistance) to 2520 kgm • min^{-1} (6.0 kg resistance). See table 16.1. The power outputs should be selected so that the times to exhaustion (TL values in figure 16.1) for the shortest (highest power output) and longest (lowest power output) workbouts range from approximately 1 to 10 minutes and differ by 5 minutes or more.[1,2] For small and/or untrained subjects, the recommended power outputs when using only two workbouts for the CP test are 1260 kgm • min^{-1} (3.0 kg resistance) and 1680 kgm • min^{-1} (4.0 kg resistance). For large and/or trained subjects, as well as experienced cyclists, the recommended power outputs are 1470 kgm • min^{-1} (3.5 kg resistance) and 1890 kgm • min^{-1} (4.5 kg resistance). These power outputs should be viewed as only recommendations. It may be necessary to adjust them up or down to ensure that the subject's actual TL values are between approximately 1 and 10 minutes and differ by 5 minutes or more.[1,2]

TABLE 16.1	Resistance settings and corresponding power outputs at 70 rpm for a Monark cycle ergometer.

Resistance (kg)	Power output (kgm • min^{-1})
1.0	420
1.5	630
2.0	840
2.5	1050
3.0	1260
3.5	1470
4.0	1680
4.5	1890
5.0	2100
5.5	2310
6.0	2520

EXTENSION ACTIVITIES

Name _____   *Date* _____

1. A CP test resulted in the following data:

WL (kgm)	P (kgm $\cdot$ min^{-1})	TL (min)
8500	_____	_____
4500	_____	_____
2700	_____	_____
12000	_____	_____

Given the expected relationships among WL, P, and TL, fill in the blanks with the P and TL values from the randomly ordered choices below.

P (kgm $\cdot$ min^{-1}) = 1260, 1680, 1890, and 2310

TL (min) = 2.38, 1.17, 9.52, and 5.06

2. Given a CP of 1550 kgm $\cdot$ min^{-1} and an AWC of 1900 kgm, what is the estimated TL for a P of 1890 kgm $\cdot$ min^{-1}?

3. Use your own data to calculate the following:

   a. CP = _____ kgm $\cdot$ min^{-1}

   b. AWC = _____ kgm

   c. TL at a P of CP + 200 kgm $\cdot$ min^{-1} = _____ min

EXTENSION QUESTIONS

1. What are some common mistakes that may occur in administering this lab?

2. Identify possible sources of error in this lab.

3. Assess the practicality of using this lab in the field.

4. Research the reliability and/or validity of this lab using online resources, journal articles, and other credible sources.

REFERENCES

1. Hill, D. W. The critical power concept. *Sports Med.* 4: 237–254, 1993.

2. Housh, D. J., Housh, T. J., and Bauge, S. M. A methodological consideration for the determination of critical power and anaerobic work capacity. *Res. Q. Exerc. Sport* 61: 406–409, 1990.

3. Housh, D. J., Housh, T. J., and Bauge, S. M. The accuracy of the critical power test for predicting time to exhaustion during cycle ergometry. *Ergonomics* 32: 997–1004, 1989.

4. Moritani, T., Nagata, A., deVries, H. A., and Muro, M. Critical power as a measure of physical work capacity and anaerobic threshold. *Ergonomics* 24: 339–350, 1981.

5. Nebelsick-Gullett, L. J., Housh, T. J., Johnson, G. O., and Bauge, S. M. A comparison between methods of measuring anaerobic work capacity. *Ergonomics* 31: 1413–1419, 1988.

BACKGROUND

A single workbout test for estimating critical power (CP), anaerobic work capacity (AWC), and the time to exhaustion (or time limit = TL) at any power output (P) greater than the CP has been developed[1,2,6] as an alternative to the procedures described in Lab 16. The original CP test[5] required two to five exhaustive workouts. A protocol that requires only a single workbout reduces the time required for the subject and improves the practicality of the CP test. This test, called the CP 3-minute all-out test (CP_{3min}), involves pedaling a cycle ergometer at a maximal effort for 3 minutes against a resistance determined by multiplying the subject's body weight (in kg) by 0.045.[1]

The CP from the 3-minute all-out test is defined as the asymptote (a line whose distance to a given curve tends to 0) of the power output versus TL curve (figure 17.1) and is calculated as the mean power output over the last 30 seconds of the test (figure 17.2). The AWC is the area under the curve from 0 to 150 seconds (figure 17.3) and reflects the total amount of work that can be performed above CP, using only stored energy sources within the active muscle (i.e., creatine phosphate, glycogen, and the oxygen bound to myoglobin).[4,5] When both CP and AWC are known, the TL for any power output greater than the CP can be estimated from the power output versus TL relationship using the equation TL = AWC/(P–CP) (see Lab 16 for the derivation of this equation). The salient feature of the CP_{3min} test is that both aerobic (CP) and anaerobic (AWC) capabilities can be determined from a single, all-out workbout using only a cycle ergometer, stopwatch, and scale.

The negative, curvilinear power output (P) versus time limit (TL) relationship during cycle ergometry, with the equation that can be used to estimate the TL for any P greater than the CP.   **FIGURE 17.1**

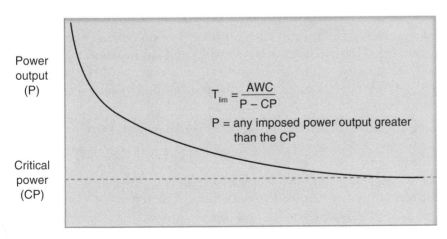

$$T_{lim} = \frac{AWC}{P - CP}$$

P = any imposed power output greater than the CP

KNOW THESE TERMS & ABBREVIATIONS

- ○ AWC = anaerobic work capacity (expressed in kgm or J), determined from the equation $AWC = 2.5 \min (MP_{0-150} - CP)$
- ○ CP = critical power (expressed in $kgm \cdot min^{-1}$ or W), defined as the average power output over the last 30 seconds of the test
- ○ J = joule; standard unit of work
- ○ P = power output ($kgm \cdot min^{-1}$ or W)
- ○ TL = time to exhaustion or time limit
- ○ W = watts

PROCEDURES

The CP_{3min} test will be performed using a Monark cycle ergometer, a stopwatch, and a scale. Three parameters, the CP, AWC, and TL for any power output greater than the CP, will be determined from this test. Worksheet 17.1 (see p. 131) should be used to record the subject's data from the CP_{3min} test.

1. Prior to beginning the test: (a) Record the subject's body weight in kg. (b) Determine the resistance to be used for the CP_{3min} test by multiplying the subject's body weight in kg by 4.5% or 0.045 (resistance = body weight [kg] × 0.045). [*Note:* The resistance for the CP_{3min} test may also be set based on the training status of the subject where the resistance is set at 3% (body weight [kg] × 0.03), 4% (body weight [kg] × 0.04), or 5% (body weight [kg] × 0.05) of body weight for recreationally active subjects, anaerobic/aerobic athletes, or endurance athletes, respectively.[3]] The example calculations for this lab, however, will be performed using a resistance setting calculated by multiplying body weight by 4.5%. (c) Adjust the seat height of the cycle ergometer to allow for near full extension of the subject's legs while pedaling.

2. Warm-up. The CP_{3min} test will be preceded by a standardized warm-up that includes 5 minutes of pedaling at 70 rev·min⁻¹ and a resistance of 1 kg (power output = 420 kgm·min⁻¹ or ~70W). After the warm-up, the subject should rest for 5 minutes. During the rest period, instruct the subject to give an all-out effort throughout the entire duration of the test by maintaining a pedaling cadence that is as high as possible at all times.

3. The CP_{3min} test should begin with 3 minutes of unloaded cycling at 70 rev·min⁻¹. During the last 5 seconds of the unloaded phase, the cadence should be increased to 110 rev·min⁻¹. At the command "Go" the subject should pedal as fast as possible and the resistance should be increased to 0.045 kg per kg of body weight within the first 2 to 3 seconds of the test.

4. Once the resistance has been set, begin the 3-minute test. During this time, the rev·min⁻¹ should be recorded on worksheet 17.1 every 5 seconds from the display on the front of the cycle ergometer. Throughout the test, the tester will encourage the subject to give a maximal effort and monitor the resistance setting and elapsed time. See figure 17.2 for a plot of the power output vs. time relationship for a typical CP_{3min} test.

5. Cool-down: After the CP_{3min} test, have the subject continue to pedal for 2 to 3 minutes (or longer if the subject desires) with no resistance.

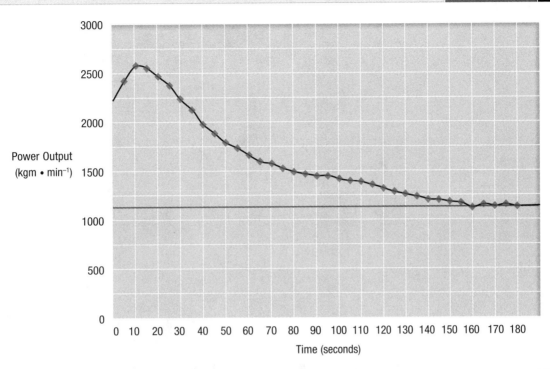

Example of the power output vs time relationship for a CP_{3min} test. **FIGURE** **17.2**

A number of software packages are available that interface with the Monark cycle ergometer and can be used to record the power output during the CP_{3min}. If the software is available, power output can be recorded continuously and expressed as 5-second averages. The software packages typically report values in SI units (International System of Units). The standard unit of power in the SI system is the watt (W). To convert the CP (kgm • min⁻¹) to W, divide kgm • min⁻¹ by 6.12 (kgm • min⁻¹ / 6.12 = W). The standard unit of work in the SI system the joule (J). The AWC (kgm) can be expressed in J by multiplying the kgm value by 9.807 (kgm x 9.807 = J).

Sample Calculations

Calculate CP and AWC from the CP_{3min} test.

Use the equation $TL = \dfrac{AWC}{(P-CP)}$ to estimate the TL for any power output greater than the CP.

Body weight (kg): ___72 kg___

Resistance: body weight (kg) x 0.045
(rounded to the nearest 0.25 kg): ___3.25 kg___

The data in table 17.1 are used to estimate CP, AWC, and TL from the CP_{3min} test.

Calculate the power output at each 5-second interval for the 3-minute test

Calculating power output:

> kgm • min⁻¹ = 3.25 kg of resistance x 6 m (this is a constant associated with the flywheel for the Monark cycle ergometer) x the 5-second pedal cadence in rev·min⁻¹.

| TABLE | 17.1 | Results for calculations of 5-second power outputs. |

seconds	resistance	x	6	x	rev • min^{-1}	=	kgm • min^{-1}
1–5	3.25	x	6	x	147	=	2867
6–10	3.25	x	6	x	157	=	3062
11–15	3.25	x	6	x	155	=	3023
16–20	3.25	x	6	x	150	=	2925
21–25	3.25	x	6	x	144	=	2808
26–30	3.25	x	6	x	136	=	2652
31–35	3.25	x	6	x	129	=	2516
36–40	3.25	x	6	x	120	=	2340
41–45	3.25	x	6	x	114	=	2223
46–50	3.25	x	6	x	109	=	2126
51–55	3.25	x	6	x	105	=	2048
56–60	3.25	x	6	x	101	=	1970
61–65	3.25	x	6	x	97	=	1892
66–70	3.25	x	6	x	96	=	1872
71–75	3.25	x	6	x	93	=	1814
76–80	3.25	x	6	x	90	=	1755
81–85	3.25	x	6	x	89	=	1736
86–90	3.25	x	6	x	88	=	1716
91–95	3.25	x	6	x	88	=	1716
96–100	3.25	x	6	x	86	=	1677
101–105	3.25	x	6	x	85	=	1658
106–110	3.25	x	6	x	84	=	1638
111–115	3.25	x	6	x	82	=	1599
116–120	3.25	x	6	x	80	=	1560
121–125	3.25	x	6	x	78	=	1521
126–130	3.25	x	6	x	77	=	1502
131–135	3.25	x	6	x	75	=	1463
136–140	3.25	x	6	x	73	=	1424
141–145	3.25	x	6	x	73	=	1424
146–150	3.25	x	6	x	72	=	1404
151–155	3.25	x	6	x	71	=	1385
156–160	3.25	x	6	x	68	=	1326
161–165	3.25	x	6	x	70	=	1365
166–170	3.25	x	6	x	69	=	1346
171–175	3.25	x	6	x	70	=	1365
176–180	3.25	x	6	x	69	=	1346

Calculate CP (express the CP as kgm·min⁻¹ and W)

Calculate the mean power output over the last 30 seconds of the test (150 to 180 seconds). Table 17.2 shows the results.

CP (kgm • min⁻¹) = 1385 + 1326 + 1365 + 1346 + 1365 + 1346 = 8133 / 6 = 1356 kgm • min⁻¹

Convert kgm • min⁻¹ to W (kgm • min⁻¹ / 6.12)

CP (W) = 1356 kgm • min⁻¹ / 6.12 = 222 W

Results for calculations of mean power output for the final 30 seconds of the test. **TABLE 17.2**

seconds	resistance	x	6	x	rev • min⁻¹	=	kgm • min⁻¹
151–155	3.25	x	6	x	71	=	1385
156–160	3.25	x	6	x	68	=	1326
161–165	3.25	x	6	x	70	=	1365
166–170	3.25	x	6	x	69	=	1346
171–175	3.25	x	6	x	70	=	1365
176–180	3.25	x	6	x	69	=	1346
					Mean	=	1356

Calculate AWC

Express the AWC in kgm and J.

(1) Calculate the mean power output over the first 150 seconds of the test (MP_{0-150}).

Table 17.3 shows the results.

MP_{0-150} = 1998 kgm

(2) AWC = 2.5 min x (the mean power output from 0 to 150 s [MP_{0-150}] – CP)

MP_{0-150} = 1998 kgm·min⁻¹

CP = 1356 kgm·min⁻¹

AWC = 2.5 min x (1998 kgm·min⁻¹ – 1356 kgm·min⁻¹)

AWC = 1605 kgm

Convert AWC to J (kgm x 9.807).

AWC (J) = 1605 x 9.807 = 15,740 J

Calculate the TL

If a subject's CP = 1356 kgm • min⁻¹ and AWC = 1603 kgm, what is the estimated TL at a P of 1550 kgm • min⁻¹?

$$TL = \frac{AWC}{(P - CP)}$$

$$TL = \frac{1605}{(1550 - 1356)} = 8.27 \text{ minutes}$$

| TABLE | 17.3 | Results of the mean power output over the first 150 seconds of the test (MP_{0-150}). |

seconds	resistance	x	6	x	rev • min^{-1}	=	kgm • min^{-1}
1–5	3.25	x	6	x	147	=	2867
6–10	3.25	x	6	x	157	=	3062
11–15	3.25	x	6	x	155	=	3023
16–20	3.25	x	6	x	150	=	2925
21–25	3.25	x	6	x	144	=	2808
26–30	3.25	x	6	x	136	=	2652
31–35	3.25	x	6	x	129	=	2516
36-40	3.25	x	6	x	120	=	2340
41-45	3.25	x	6	x	114	=	2223
46–50	3.25	x	6	x	109	=	2126
51–55	3.25	x	6	x	105	=	2048
56–60	3.25	x	6	x	101	=	1970
61–65	3.25	x	6	x	97	=	1892
66–70	3.25	x	6	x	96	=	1872
71–75	3.25	x	6	x	93	=	1814
76–80	3.25	x	6	x	90	=	1755
81–85	3.25	x	6	x	89	=	1736
86–90	3.25	x	6	x	88	=	1716
91–95	3.25	x	6	x	88	=	1716
96–100	3.25	x	6	x	86	=	1677
101–105	3.25	x	6	x	85	=	1658
106–110	3.25	x	6	x	84	=	1638
111–115	3.25	x	6	x	82	=	1599
116–120	3.25	x	6	x	80	=	1560
121–125	3.25	x	6	x	78	=	1521
126–130	3.25	x	6	x	77	=	1502
131–135	3.25	x	6	x	75	=	1463
136–140	3.25	x	6	x	73	=	1424
141–145	3.25	x	6	x	73	=	1424
146–150	3.25	x	6	x	72	=	1404
					Mean	=	1998

RESULTS OF THE CRITICAL POWER 3-MINUTE TEST

Worksheet **17.1**

Name _____   *Date*

Body weight (kg): _____ x 0.045 = resistance (kg): _____

seconds	resistance	x	6	x	rev • min^{-1}	=	kgm • min^{-1}
1–5		x	6	x		=	
6–10		x	6	x		=	
11–15		x	6	x		=	
16–20		x	6	x		=	
21–25		x	6	x		=	
26–30		x	6	x		=	
31–35		x	6	x		=	
36–40		x	6	x		=	
41–45		x	6	x		=	
46–50		x	6	x		=	
51–55		x	6	x		=	
56–60		x	6	x		=	
61–65		x	6	x		=	
66–70		x	6	x		=	
71–75		x	6	x		=	
76–80		x	6	x		=	
81–85		x	6	x		=	
86–90		x	6	x		=	
91–95		x	6	x		=	
96–100		x	6	x		=	
101–105		x	6	x		=	
106–110		x	6	x		=	
111–115		x	6	x		=	
116–120		x	6	x		=	
121–125		x	6	x		=	
126–130		x	6	x		=	
131–135		x	6	x		=	
136–140		x	6	x		=	
141–145		x	6	x		=	
146–150		x	6	x		=	
151–155		x	6	x		=	
156–160		x	6	x		=	
161–165		x	6	x		=	
166–170		x	6	x		=	
171–175		x	6	x		=	
176–180		x	6	x		=	

CP (kgm • min^{-1}) = _____ kgm • min^{-1}

CP (W) = CP (kgm • min^{-1}) _____ / 6.12 = _____ W

AWC (kgm) = _____ kgm

AWC (J) = AWC (kgm) _____ x 9.807 = _____ J

Worksheet 17.2 | EXTENSION ACTIVITIES

(1) On the graph below, draw the expected relationship between power output and time for the CP_{3min} test and indicate the time periods used to calculate the CP and AWC.

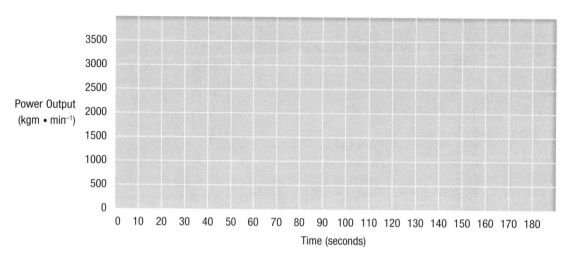

(2) Rocky (who weighs 190 lbs) performed a CP_{3min} all-out test.

A. Determine the resistance used for this test (body weight [kg] x 0.045). Round the resistance to the nearest 0.25 kg. Record your answer in the chart below.

Resistance (kg) = _____ (body weight [kg]) x 0.045)

seconds	resistance	x	6	x	rev • min⁻¹	=	kgm • min⁻¹
151–155		x	6	x	70	=	
156–160		x	6	x	72	=	
161–165		x	6	x	71	=	
166–170		x	6	x	69	=	
171–175		x	6	x	71	=	
176–180		x	6	x	70	=	

B. Use the resistance calculated for part A and the pedal revolution data provided in the table in part A to calculate the power output for each 5-second interval over the last 30 seconds of the test. Record your answers for each 5-second interval in the table above.

C. Calculate CP from the data in the table above. Express CP in kgm • min⁻¹ and W.

CP = mean power output over the final 30 seconds of the test = _____ kgm • min⁻¹

_____ kgm • min⁻¹ / 6.12 = _____ W

D. Calculate AWC using the CP calculated for Part C and a mean power output for the first 150 seconds of the test (MP_{0-150}) of 2570 kgm • min⁻¹. Express AWC in kgm and J.

AWC = 2.5 x (MP_{0-150} − CP)

AWC = 2.5 x (_____ kgm • min⁻¹ − _____ kgm • min⁻¹)

AWC = _____ kgm

_____ kgm x 9.807 = _____ J

E. Using the CP and AWC values calculated for parts C and D, what is the estimated TL for a power output of 1950 kgm • min⁻¹ using the equation

$$TL = \frac{AWC}{(P - CP)}$$

TL = _____ kgm / (1950 kgm • min⁻¹ – _____ kgm • min⁻¹)

TL = _____ minutes

(3) Use your own data from a CP_{3min} test to calculate the following:

a. CP = _____ kgm • min⁻¹ = _____ W

b. AWC = _____ kgm = _____ J

c. TL at a power output of CP + 150 kgm • min⁻¹ = _____ min

EXTENSION QUESTIONS

1. What are some common mistakes that may occur in administering this lab?

2. Identify possible sources of error in this lab.

3. Assess the practicality of using this lab in the field.

4. Research the reliability and validity of this lab using online resources, journal articles, and other credible sources.

REFERENCES

1. Bergstrom, H. C., Housh, T. J., Zuniga, J. M., Camic, C. L., Traylor, D. A., Schmidt, R. J., and Johnson, G. O. A new single workbout test to estimate critical power and anaerobic work capacity. *J. Strength Cond. Res.* 26: 656–663, 2012.

2. Burnley, M., Doust, J. H., and Vanhatalo, A. A 3-min all-out test to determine peak oxygen uptake and the maximal steady state. *Med. Sci. Sports Exerc.* 38: 1995–2003, 2006.

3. Clark, I. E., Murray, S. R., and Pettitt, R. W. Alternative procedures for the three-minute all-out exercise test. *J. Strength Cond. Res.* 27: 2104–2112, 2013.

4. Hill, D. W. The critical power concept. *Sports Med.* 4: 237–254, 1993.

5. Moritani, T, Nagata, A, deVries, H. A., and Muro, M. Critical power as measure of physical work capacity and anaerobic threshold. *Ergonomics* 24: 335-339, 1981.

6. Vanhatalo, A., Doust, J. H., and Burnley, M. Determination of critical power using a 3-min all-out cycling test. *Med. Sci. Sports Exerc.* 39: 548–555, 2007.

BACKGROUND

The critical velocity (CV) test is a treadmill analog of the critical power (CP) test for cycle ergometry (see Lab 16). The CV test estimates three parameters of physical working capacity[1-5]: (1) the maximal running velocity that can be maintained for an extended period of time without fatigue, called the CV; (2) the total running distance that can be accomplished using only stored energy sources within the activated muscles (such as creatine phosphate, glycogen, and oxygen bound to myoglobin), called the anaerobic running capacity (ARC); and (3) the time to exhaustion or time limit (TL) during continuous running at any velocity greater than the CV. The CV test uses linear mathematical modeling of the relationship between the total running distance (TD) at different velocities and the corresponding TL values to simultaneously estimate the CV, ARC, and TL at any velocity greater than the CV (figures 18.1a and b; see figures 18.2a and b for sample calculations of TL, CV, and ARC).

Curvilinear velocity (V) versus time limit (TL) relationship. **FIGURE** **18.1**

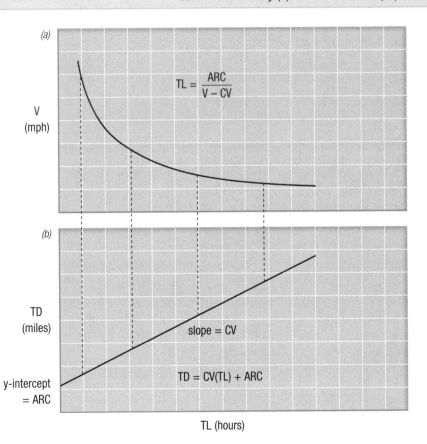

(a)

$$TL = \frac{ARC}{V - CV}$$

V (mph)

(b)

TD (miles)

slope = CV

TD = CV(TL) + ARC

y-intercept = ARC

TL (hours)

Figure 18.1a represents the negative, curvilinear velocity (V) versus time limit (TL) curve during treadmill running and provides the equation that can be used to estimate the TL for any V. Please note that, theoretically, any V less than or equal to the critical velocity (CV) can be maintained indefinitely without exhaustion. In reality, however, the CV can often be maintained for an extended period of time (usually >30 minutes), but not indefinitely. Figure 18.1b represents the linear relationship between total distance (TD) and TL and provides the equation that can be used to estimate the CV and anaerobic running capacity (ARC).

FIGURE **18.2** Graphic representation of sample calculations for the CV (7.44 mph), the ARC (0.09 miles), and the TL (0.02 hours) at 12 mph.

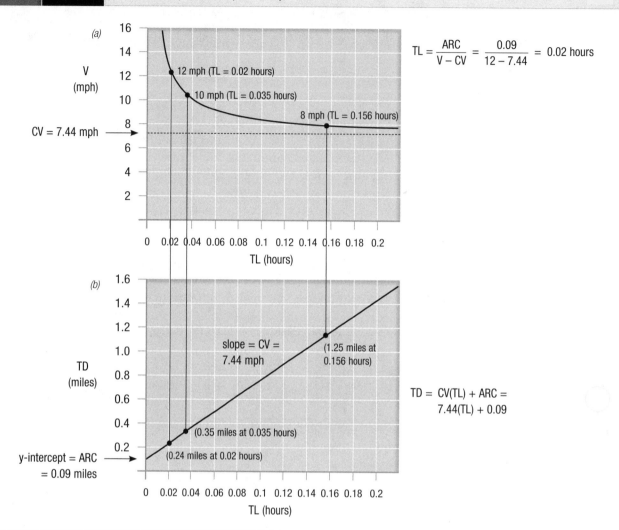

$$TL = \frac{ARC}{V - CV} = \frac{0.09}{12 - 7.44} = 0.02 \text{ hours}$$

$$TD = CV(TL) + ARC = 7.44(TL) + 0.09$$

Critical Velocity (CV)

The CV is an estimate of the maximal running velocity that can be maintained for an extended period of time without fatigue and is, conceptually, analogous to the anaerobic threshold.[2,4] The anaerobic threshold is one of three primary physiological factors (along with $\dot{V}O_2$ max and economy of movement) that contribute to performance in endurance events. The anaerobic threshold is typically determined from the measurement of blood lactate levels (the lactate threshold) or expired gas samples (the gas exchange threshold or ventilatory threshold; see Lab 14). A salient feature of the CV test, however, is that it requires only a treadmill and stopwatch.

Anaerobic Running Capacity (ARC)

The ARC is an estimate of the total distance that can be run using only stored energy sources within the activated muscles, such as creatine phosphate, glycogen, and oxygen bound to myoglobin.[3]

Theoretically, the ARC represents the capacity to produce ATP from anaerobic metabolic pathways. Thus, the CV test provides estimates of the physical working capacity associated with both aerobic (the CV) and anaerobic (the ARC) ATP production.

Time to Exhaustion or Time Limit (TL)

There is a negative, curvilinear (asymptotic) relationship between running velocity and TL that is called the running velocity versus TL curve (figure 18.1a). Based on fitness level, each individual has a unique running velocity versus TL curve. The linear mathematical model used to estimate CV and ARC (figure 18.1b) can also be used to derive an individual's running velocity versus TL curve and, therefore, an equation to predict TL for any velocity greater than the CV. Theoretically, the CV is the asymptote of the running velocity versus TL curve (figure 18.1a), and any running velocity less than or equal to the CV should thus be able to be maintained indefinitely. In reality, however, the CV can often be maintained for an extended period of time (often >30 minutes) but not indefinitely.[2,4,5]

KNOW THESE TERMS & ABBREVIATIONS

- CV = critical velocity (mph), defined as the slope coefficient of the total distance (TD) versus TL relationship (figure 18.1b).
- ARC = anaerobic running capacity (miles), defined as the y-intercept of the TD versus TL relationship (figure 18.1b).
- V = velocity (mph)
- TL = time limit (TL) or time to exhaustion (hours)

PROCEDURES (see photo 18.1)

The CV test will be performed using a treadmill and stopwatch. The three parameters of physical working capacity that will be determined are the (1) CV, (2) ARC, and (3) TL for any running velocity greater than the CV.

1. Warm-up. Prior to the warm-up, record a pre-exercise heart rate. The CV test will be preceded by a warm-up that includes 3 minutes of walking at 3.5–4.0 mph and then 3 minutes of jogging at about 6.0 mph.

2. Prior to beginning each run, have the subject practice getting on and off the treadmill three to four times to become familiar with the running velocity greater than the CV.

3. Typically, the CV test involves a series of two or more treadmill runs at different velocities.[1,3,4] In this laboratory, two (or more) treadmill runs will be performed. The selection of velocities for each subject usually ranges from approximately 8.0 to 14.0 mph. The treadmill always stays at zero percent grade. The velocities should be selected so that the

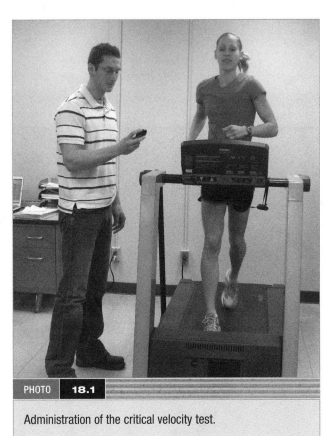

PHOTO **18.1**

Administration of the critical velocity test.

TL values (figure 18.2) for the shortest (highest velocity) and longest (lowest velocity) runs range from approximately 2 to 12 minutes[4] and differ by 5 minutes or more. For untrained subjects, the recommended velocities when using only two treadmill runs for the CV test are 8 and 10 mph. For trained subjects, as well as experienced runners, the recommended velocities are 10 and 12 mph. These velocities should be viewed only as recommendations, and it may be necessary to adjust them up or down to ensure that the actual TL values are between approximately 2 and 12 minutes and differ by 5 minutes or more.[4]

4. After warming up, practicing getting on and off the treadmill, and resting for a two-minute period, the subject straddles the running treadmill (which is set at the appropriate velocity) and holds on to the handrails. For the test, the subject is instructed to run as long as possible and then grasp the handrails when exhausted.

5. Have the subject begin running on the treadmill and release the handrails when comfortable (usually 2–3 seconds after getting on the treadmill). Timing for the run begins when the handrails are released.

6. It is recommended that two spotters stand beside and behind the treadmill to ensure the subject's stability while running.

7. Give verbal encouragement throughout the run, and record the TL when the subject grasps the handrails to signal exhaustion.[1,2,3,5]

8. Cool-down. After each exhaustive run, the subject walks on the treadmill at 3.0 mph (or slower) as long as the subject desires.

9. No more than two exhaustive treadmill runs at different velocities should be performed by an individual on a single day. If a second run is to be performed during the same laboratory visit, have the subject rest (following the cool-down) until the heart rate returns to within 10 beats per minute of the pre-exercise level to ensure that the subject is fully recovered before performing the second run. This usually takes at least 30 minutes.

Sample Calculations

The following are sample calculations of CV and ARC, along with the derivation of the equation used to estimate the TL for any running velocity greater than the CV.

1. Calculate the TD for each of the two or more treadmill runs by multiplying the running V (mph) by the TL (hours).

   First run
   V = 10 mph
   TL = 2 minutes and 6 seconds = 0.035 hours
   TD = 0.35 miles

   Second run
   V = 8 mph
   TL = 9 minutes and 22 seconds = 0.156 hours
   TD = 1.25 miles

2. Use a simple linear regression analysis (y = b(x) + a) to characterize the relationship for the TD (miles) values for the two treadmill runs versus the corresponding TL values (figure 18.2b). Many handheld calculators, or software (such as Microsoft Excel and others) for PC and Macintosh computers, can be used to perform simple linear regression. The slope coefficient and y-intercept values for the linear TD versus TL relationship are the CV and ARC, respectively (figure 18.2b).

	TD VALUES	**TL VALUES**
First run (10 mph)	0.35 miles	0.035 hours
Second run (8 mph)	1.25 miles	0.156 hours

Simple linear regression equation:

TD = 7.44(TL) + 0.09

Thus, CV = 7.44 mph and ARC = 0.09 miles.

3. The linear regression analysis used to determine the CV and ARC for each subject is also used to derive the equation to estimate the TL for any velocity that is greater than CV (figure 18.2a). The equation is derived by equalizing the two mathematical expressions for determining the TD. That is,

TD = V(TL) = CV(TL) + ARC

Thus,

CV(TL) + ARC = V(TL)

ARC = V(TL) − CV(TL)

ARC = TL(V − CV)

$$\frac{ARC}{V - CV} = \frac{TL(V - CV)}{V - CV}$$

$$TL = \frac{ARC}{V - CV}$$

Using figure 18.2a, if a subject's CV = 7.44 mph and ARC = 0.09 miles, what is the subject's TL at a V of 12 mph?

$$TL = \frac{0.09}{12 - 7.44} = 0.02 \text{ hours (1.2 minutes)}$$

Worksheet 18.1 CRITICAL VELOCITY TEST FORM

Name _____ Date _____

Pre-exercise heart rate _____

Velocity (V)

Velocity 1 = _____ mph

Velocity 2 = _____ mph

Velocity 3 (if used) = _____ mph

Velocity 4 (if used) = _____ mph

Time limit (TL)

Velocity 1 = _____ hours

Velocity 2 = _____ hours

Velocity 3 = _____ hours

Velocity 4 = _____ hours

Total distance (TD)

Velocity 1 = V _____ (mph) × TL _____ (hours) = TD _____ miles

Velocity 2 = V _____ × TL _____ = TD _____ miles

Velocity 3 = V _____ × TL _____ = TD _____ miles

Velocity 4 = V _____ × TL _____ = TD _____ miles

TD versus TL relationship

Use linear regression analysis to determine the equation that describes the TD versus TL relationship: TD = CV(TL) + ARC (see figure 18.2b).

CV = _____ mph

ARC = _____ miles

Equation for estimating the TL at any V greater than the CV (see figure 18.2a)

$$TL = \frac{ARC}{V - CV} = \text{_____ hours}$$

Name _____   *Date* _____

1. A CV test resulted in the following data:

TD (miles)	V (mph)	TL (hours)
1.64	_____	_____
1.44	_____	_____
0.75	_____	_____
0.70	_____	_____

   Given the expected relationships among TD, V, and TL, fill in the blanks with the V and TL values from the randomly ordered choices below:

   > V (mph) = 11.0, 12.0, 10.5, and 11.5
   >
   > TL (hours) = 0.065, 0.131, 0.156, and 0.058

2. Given a CV of 8.7 mph and an ARC of 0.07 miles, what is the estimated TL for a V of 10.5 mph?

3. Use your own data to calculate the following:

   a. CV = _____ mph

   b. ARC = _____ miles

   c. TL at a V of CV + 3.0 mph = _____ hours

REFERENCES

1. Housh, T. J., Cramer, J. T., Bull, A. J., Johnson, G. O., and Housh, D. J. The effect of mathematical modeling on critical velocity. *Eur. J. Appl. Physiol.* 84: 469–475, 2001.

2. Housh, T. J., Johnson, G. O., McDowell, S. L., Housh, D. J., and Pepper, M. Physiological responses at the fatigue threshold. *Int. J. Sports Med.* 12: 305–308, 1991.

3. Housh, T. J., Johnson, G. O., McDowell, S. L., Housh, D. J., and Pepper, M. The relationship between anaerobic running capacity and peak plasma lactate. *J. Sports Med. Phys. Fitness* 32: 117–122, 1992.

4. Hughson, R. L., Orok, C. J., and Staudt, L. E. A high velocity treadmill running test to assess endurance running potential. *Int. J. Sports Med.* 5: 23–25, 1984.

5. Pepper, M. L., Housh, T. J., and Johnson, G. O. The accuracy of the critical velocity test for predicting time to exhaustion during treadmill running. *Int. J. Sports Med.* 13: 121–124, 1992.

BACKGROUND

The purpose of this lab is to describe the procedures for performing the Critical Velocity (CV) test on a running track. The CV test estimates three parameters of physical working capacity[1–5]: (1) the maximal running velocity that can be maintained for an extended period of time without fatigue, called the CV; (2) the total distance that can be run using only stored energy sources within the activated muscles (creatine phosphate, glycogen, and oxygen bound to myoglobin), called the anaerobic running capacity (ARC); and (3) the time to exhaustion or time limit (TL) during continuous running at any velocity (V) greater than the CV. The CV test uses linear mathematical modeling of the relationship between the total distance (TD) at different velocities and the corresponding TL values to simultaneously estimate the CV, ARC, and TL at any velocity greater than the CV (figure 19.1).

Critical Velocity (CV). The CV is an estimate of the maximal running velocity that can be maintained for an extended period of time without fatigue and is conceptually analogous to the anaerobic threshold.[2,4] The anaerobic threshold is one of three primary physiological factors (along with $\dot{V}O_2$ max and economy of movement) that contribute to performance in endurance events. The anaerobic threshold is typically determined from the measurement of blood lactate levels (the lactate threshold) or expired gas samples (the gas exchange threshold or ventilatory threshold; see Lab 14). A salient feature of the critical velocity for track running test, however, is that it requires only a running track, markers (e.g., orange cones, reflective tape) placed at 100-meter intervals around the track, and a stopwatch.

Anaerobic Running Capacity (ARC). The ARC is an estimate of the total distance that can be run using only stored energy sources within the activated muscles such as creatine phosphate, glycogen, and oxygen bound to myoglobin.[3] Theoretically, the ARC represents the capacity to produce ATP from anaerobic metabolic pathways. Thus, the CV test provides estimates of physical working capacity associated with both aerobic (the CV) and anaerobic (ARC) ATP production.

Time to Exhaustion or Time Limit (TL). There is a negative, curvilinear (asymptotic) relationship between V and TL that is called the V versus TL curve (figure 19.1a). Based on fitness level, each individual has a unique V versus TL curve. The linear mathematical model used to estimate CV and ARC (figure 19.1b) can also be used to derive an individual's V versus TL curve and, therefore, an equation to predict the person's TL for any V greater than the CV. Theoretically, the CV is the asymptote of the V versus TL curve (figure 19.1a) and, thus, any V ≤ CV should be able to be continued indefinitely. In reality, however, the CV can often be maintained for an extended period of time (usually > 30 minutes), but not indefinitely.[2,4,5]

FIGURE 19.1 Curvilinear velocity (V) versus time limit (TL) relationship.

Figure 19.1a represents the negative, curvilinear velocity (V) versus time limit (TL) relationship and provides the equation that can be used to estimate the TL for any V. Please note that, theoretically, any V less than the critical velocity (CV) can be maintained indefinitely without exhaustion. In reality, however, the CV can often be maintained for an extended period of time (usually > 30 minutes), but not indefinitely. Figure 19.1b represents the linear relationship between total distance (TD) and TL, and provides the equation that can be used to estimate the CV and anaerobic running capacity (ARC).

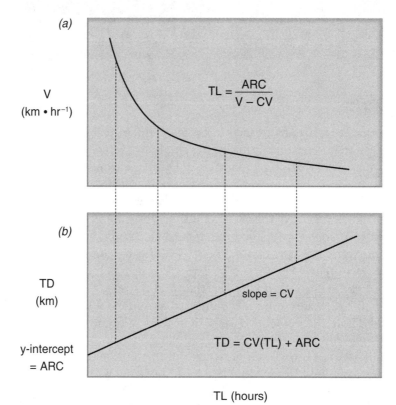

(a)

V
(km • hr^{-1})

$$TL = \frac{ARC}{V - CV}$$

(b)

TD
(km)

slope = CV

$$TD = CV(TL) + ARC$$

y-intercept
= ARC

TL (hours)

KNOW THESE TERMS & ABBREVIATIONS

○ CV = critical velocity (km • hr^{-1}), defined as the slope coefficient of the total distance (TD) versus TL relationship (figure 19.1b)

○ ARC = anaerobic running capacity (km), defined as the y-intercept of the total distance (TD) versus TL relationship (figure 19.1b)

○ V = velocity (km • hr^{-1})

○ TL = time to exhaustion or time limit (TL) (hours)

PROCEDURES (see photo 19.1)

The CV test can be performed on either a 400-meter or a 200-meter track (or other length tracks with appropriate modifications for time splits). The equipment required for the test includes stopwatches and two or four markers that will be placed at 100-meter increments around the track. Four markers are used for a 400-meter track, and two markers are used for a 200-meter track. The three parameters of physical working capacity that will be determined are the CV, ARC, and TL for any running V greater than the CV.

1. As stated previously, an important feature of the CV test is that it uses very little equipment. The test does, however, require two (or more) exhaustive runs, each of which is performed at a different constant velocity. To achieve constant velocities during the runs, the subjects will be required to reach 100-meter intervals on the track at designated

time points, or splits. For example, with a 400-meter track, four markers are placed at 100-meter intervals around the track. If a subject is required to run at a velocity of 18 km • hr^{-1} (11.18 mph), he or she should reach the first marker (i.e., 100 meters away from the starting line) in 20 seconds, the second marker in 40 seconds, the third marker in 60 seconds, and the starting line in 80 seconds (figure 19.2). Figure 19.2 shows the 100-meter time splits required for four different velocities. It is important to note that the same time splits can be used for a 200-meter track. With a 200-meter track, however, only two markers (one at the starting line and another one 100 meters away from the starting line) are used. For untrained subjects, the recommended 100-meter time splits when using only two runs for the CV test are 30 seconds (12 km • hr^{-1} or 7.45 mph) and 20 seconds (18 km • hr^{-1} or 11.18 mph). For trained subjects or experienced runners, the recommended 100-meter time splits are 25 seconds (14.4 km • hr^{-1} or 8.94 mph) and 15 seconds (24 km • hr^{-1} or 14.91 mph).

2. Warm-up. Prior to the warm-up, record a pre-exercise heart rate. The CV test should be preceded by a warm-up that includes 3 minutes of walking and then 3 minutes of jogging at a comfortable pace around the track.

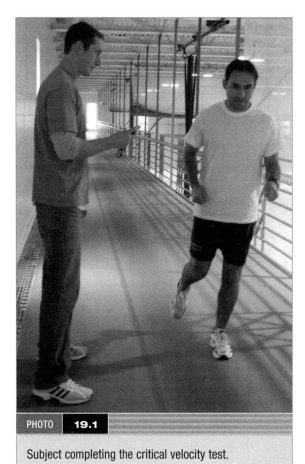

PHOTO **19.1**

Subject completing the critical velocity test.

Example of the marker locations for the critical velocity (CV) test with a 400-meter track. **FIGURE** **19.2**

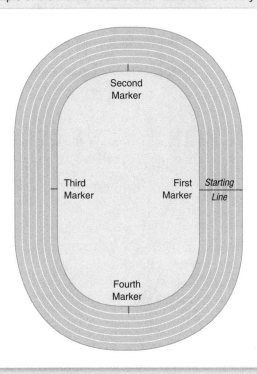

The 100-meter time splits are shown. Note that the CV test can also be performed with a 200-meter track, in which case only two markers would be used (one at the starting line, and another one that is 100 meters away from the starting line).

100-meter time splits for four running velocities:

15-second time splits = 24 km • hr^{-1} or 14.91 mph

20-second time splits = 18 km • hr^{-1} or 11.18 mph

25-second time splits = 14.4 km • hr^{-1} or 8.94 mph

30-second time splits = 12 km • hr^{-1} or 7.45 mph

3. Following the warm-up and a 2-minute rest period, instruct the subject that during the test, he or she should run at the designated time splits for as long as possible. The run ends when the subject cannot maintain the designated split time.

4. When the subject is ready to begin the test, have him or her start a stopwatch and run toward the first marker to complete the first time split. If the subject is unable to accomplish any of the first four time splits, he or she should stop the test and rest until his or her heart rate is within 10 beats per minute of the resting heart rate. The test should then be restarted at a lower velocity.

5. For each run, the subject continues until he or she can no longer complete the designated time splits. The number of time splits completed is recorded on worksheet 19.1. The TL is then calculated with the following equation:

   TL = number of time splits (each 100 meters) successfully completed
   × duration (in seconds) of each split

   For example, if the subject ran 20-second time splits and was able to complete eight splits, then the TL was 160 seconds (8 time splits × 20 seconds per split), or 0.044 hours. The corresponding TD can then be calculated with the following equation:

   TD = number of time splits successfully completed × distance (in meters) of each split

   Thus, the TD for this example would be 800 meters (8 time splits × 100 meters per split), or 0.8 km.

6. Cool-down. After each exhaustive run, have the subject walk around the track at a comfortable pace for as long as desired.

7. No more than two exhaustive runs at different velocities (time splits) should be performed on a single day. If a second run is to be performed on the same day, have the subject rest (following the cool-down) until his or her heart rate returns to within 10 beats per minute of the pre-exercise level to ensure that the individual is fully recovered before performing the second run. This usually takes at least 30 minutes.

Sample Calculations

Calculations of CV and ARC, as well as the derivation of the equation used to estimate the TL for any V greater than the CV, follow.

1. Calculate the TL and TD for each of the two or more track runs at different velocities.

   FIRST RUN
   100 meter time split = 20 seconds (18 km • hr^{-1})
   Number of time splits successfully completed = 8
   TL = 8 time splits × 20 seconds per split = 160 seconds = 0.044 hours
   TD = 8 time splits × 100 meters per split = 800 meters = 0.8 km

SECOND RUN

100 meter time split = 30 seconds (12 km • hr⁻¹)

Number of time splits successfully completed = 14

TL = 14 time splits × 30 seconds per split = 420 seconds = 0.117 hours

TD = 14 time splits × 100 meters per split = 1400 meters = 1.4 km

2. Use a simple linear regression analysis (y = b(x) + a) to characterize the relationship for the TD (km) values for the two track runs versus the corresponding TL (hours) values (figure 19.3b). Simple linear regression can be performed using many handheld calculators or software (such as Microsoft Excel and others) for PC and Macintosh computers. The slope coefficient and y-intercept values for the linear TD versus TL relationship are the CV and ARC, respectively (figure 19.3b).

	TD (km)	TL (hours)
First run (20-second time splits)	0.8	0.044
Second run (30-second time splits)	1.4	0.117

Simple linear regression equation: TD = 8.22(TL) + 0.44

Thus,

CV = 8.22 km • hr⁻¹ and ARC = 0.44 km.

3. The linear regression analysis used to determine the CV and ARC for each subject is also used to derive the equation to estimate the TL for any velocity that is greater than CV (figure 19.3a). The equation is derived by equalizing the two mathematical expressions for determining the TD. That is,

TD = V(TL) = CV(TL) + ARC

Thus,

CV(TL) + ARC = V(TL)

ARC = V(TL) − CV(TL)

ARC = TL(V − CV)

$$\frac{ARC}{(V - CV)} = \frac{TL(V - CV)}{(V - CV)}$$

$$TL = \frac{ARC}{V - CV}$$

If a subject's CV = 8.22 km • hr⁻¹ and ARC = 0.44 km, what is his or her TL at a velocity of 16 km • hr⁻¹?

$$TL = \frac{0.44}{16 - 8.22} = 0.057 \text{ hours (3.42 minutes)}$$

FIGURE 19.3 Graphic representation of sample calculations for critical velocity (CV = 8.22 km • hr⁻¹), anaerobic running capacity (ARC = 0.44 km), and the estimated time limit (TL = 0.057 hours) at 16 km • hr⁻¹.

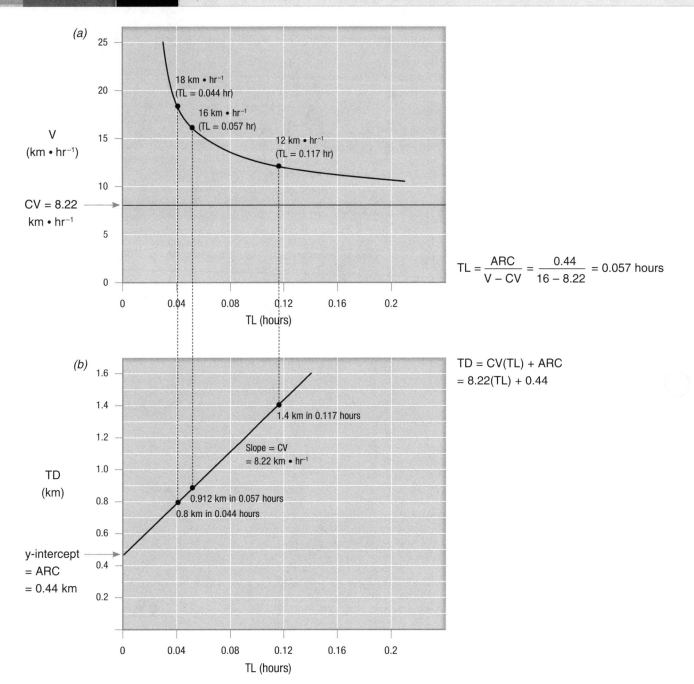

CRITICAL VELOCITY FOR TRACK RUNNING TEST FORM   Worksheet **19.1**

Name _____   *Date* _____

Pre-exercise Heart Rate _____

Velocity (V)   **Time splits**

Velocity 1: _____ km • hr^{-1} _____ sec

Velocity 2: _____ km • hr^{-1} _____ sec

Velocity 3 (if used): _____ km • hr^{-1} _____ sec

Velocity 4 (if used): _____ km • hr^{-1} _____ sec

Time Limit (TL)

Velocity 1: Number of splits completed _____ × _____ seconds per split = _____ seconds ÷ 3600 = _____ hours

Velocity 2: Number of splits completed _____ × _____ seconds per split = _____ seconds ÷ 3600 = _____ hours

Velocity 3: Number of splits completed _____ × _____ seconds per split = _____ seconds ÷ 3600 = _____ hours

Velocity 4: Number of splits completed _____ × _____ seconds per split = _____ seconds ÷ 3600 = _____ hours

Total Distance (TD)

Velocity 1: Number of splits completed _____ × 100 meters per split = _____ m ÷ 1000 = _____ km

Velocity 2: Number of splits completed _____ × 100 meters per split = _____ m ÷ 1000 = _____ km

Velocity 3: Number of splits completed _____ × 100 meters per split = _____ m ÷ 1000 = _____ km

Velocity 4: Number of splits completed _____ × 100 meters per split = _____ m ÷ 1000 = _____ km

TD vs. TL Relationship

Use linear regression analysis to determine the equation that describes the TD vs. TL relationship:
TD = CV(TL) + ARC (see figure 19.3b)

CV = _____ km • hr^{-1}

ARC = _____ km

Equation for estimating the TL at any V greater than the CV (see figure 19.3a)

$$TL = \frac{ARC}{V - CV} = \underline{\hspace{3cm}} \text{ hours}$$

Worksheet 19.2 | EXTENSION ACTIVITIES

Name _____ Date _____

1. A critical velocity for track running test resulted in the following data:

TD (km)	V (km • hr⁻¹)	TL (hours)
2.64	_____	_____
2.32	_____	_____
1.20	_____	_____
1.12	_____	_____

Given the expected relationships among TD, V, and TL, fill in the blanks with the V and TL values from the randomly ordered choices below.

   V (km • hr⁻¹) = 18.5, 16.9, 19.3, 17.7

   TL (hours) = 0.065, 0.058, 0.131, 0.156

2. Given a CV of 15.94 km • hr⁻¹ and an ARC of 0.19 km, what is the estimated TL for a V of 18.0 km • hr⁻¹?

3. Use your own data to calculate the following:

   a. CV = _____ km • hr⁻¹

   b. ARC = _____ km

   c. TL at a V of CV + 2.0 km • hr⁻¹ = _____ hours

EXTENSION QUESTIONS

1. What are some common mistakes that may occur in administering this lab?

2. Identify possible sources of error in this lab.

3. Assess the practicality of using this lab in the field.

4. Research the reliability and/or validity of this lab using online resources, journal articles, and other credible sources.

REFERENCES

1. Housh, T. J., Cramer, J. T., Bull, A. J., Johnson, G. O., and Housh, D. J. The effect of mathematical modeling on critical velocity. *Eur. J. Appl. Physiol.* 84: 469–475, 2001.

2. Housh, T. J., Johnson, G. O., McDowell, S. L., Housh, D. J., and Pepper, M. Physiological responses at the fatigue threshold. *Int. J. Sports Med.* 12: 305–308, 1991.

3. Housh, T. J., Johnson, G. O., McDowell, S. L., Housh, D. J., and Pepper, M. The relationship between anaerobic running capacity and peak plasma lactate. *J. Sports Med. Phys. Fitness* 32: 117–122, 1992.

4. Hughson, R. L., Orok, C. J., and Staudt, L. E. A high velocity treadmill running test to assess endurance running potential. *Int. J. Sports Med.* 5: 23–25, 1984.

5. Pepper, M. L., Housh, T. J., and Johnson, G. O. The accuracy of the critical velocity test for predicting time to exhaustion during treadmill running. *Int. J. Sports Med.* 13: 121–124, 1992.

Physical Working Capacity at the Heart Rate Threshold Test

BACKGROUND

Theoretically, the physical working capacity at the heart rate threshold (PWC_{HRT}) test provides an estimate of the maximal power output during cycle ergometry that can be maintained for a very long period of time (4 to 8 hours) with no increase in heart rate (e.g., a steady-state heart rate).[1,2] The PWC_{HRT} test is most applicable to situations where assessing the ability to perform long-term, submaximal physical activity is more important than defining a subject's maximal exercise capacity (such as maximal oxygen consumption rate, $\dot{V}O_2$ max). Potential applications of the PWC_{HRT} test include assessing the physical working capacity of workers in industrial settings where strenuous labor is performed for 8 or more hours per day, evaluating the effectiveness of endurance-training programs in a variety of populations including the elderly, and examining the training status of ultra-endurance athletes such as triathletes or long-distance cyclists.[1,3] Furthermore, the submaximal protocol used to determine the PWC_{HRT} makes it appropriate for assessing aerobic fitness in subjects where maximal exercise testing may be contraindicated, such as the elderly or clinical populations.

The PWC_{HRT} test involves performing two or more 8-minute workbouts at different submaximal power outputs. This lab will describe the procedures for estimating the PWC_{HRT} using two workbouts performed on the same day. Three or four workbouts, however, can also be used if the PWC_{HRT} test is completed over two or more days. During each workbout, heart rate (HR) is recorded and the slope coefficient for the HR versus time relationship is determined. The power output values are then plotted as a function of the slope coefficients for the HR versus time relationships, and the y-intercept is defined as the PWC_{HRT} (see figure 20.1b, page 156). Salient features of the PWC_{HRT} test are that it requires only submaximal exercise, and it can be performed using only a cycle ergometer, stopwatch, and heart rate monitoring system.

KNOW THESE TERMS & ABBREVIATIONS

- HR = heart rate (bpm)
- PWC_{HRT} = physical working capacity at the heart rate threshold (watts), defined as the y-intercept of the power output versus HR slope coefficient relationship (figure 20.1b)
- $\dot{V}O_2$ max = maximal oxygen consumption rate

PROCEDURES (see photos 20.1 and 20.2)

The PWC_{HRT} test will be performed using a Monark cycle ergometer, heart rate monitoring system, and stopwatch.

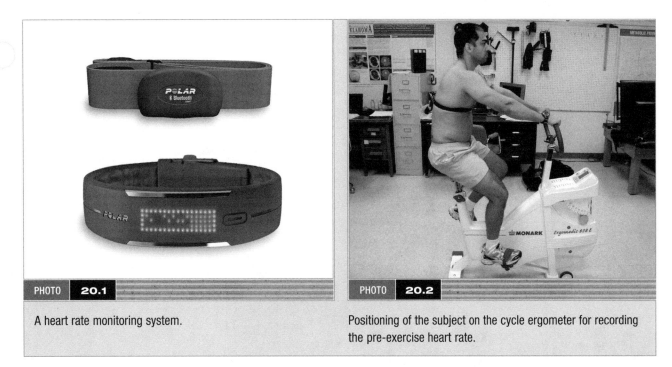

PHOTO	20.1

A heart rate monitoring system.

PHOTO	20.2

Positioning of the subject on the cycle ergometer for recording the pre-exercise heart rate.

1. Prior to beginning the test: (1) adjust the seat height of the cycle ergometer to allow for near full extension of the subject's legs while pedaling, (2) fit the subject with a heart rate monitoring system (see photo 20.1), and (3) record a pre-exercise heart rate (see photo 20.2).

2. Warm-up: The PWC_{HRT} test should be preceded by a standardized warm-up protocol that includes 4 minutes of pedaling at 70 rpm at a resistance of 0.5 kg (power output = 34 watts).

3. The PWC_{HRT} test involves two to four cycle ergometer workbouts at different power outputs.[1,2,3] Each workbout is performed at a constant pedaling cadence of 70 rpm, and the selection of power outputs for each subject usually ranges from approximately 52 (0.75 kg resistance) to 223 (3.25 kg resistance) watts.[2,3] See table 20.1. The power outputs should be selected low enough so that the subject is able to complete the full 8 minutes for each workbout, but high enough to elicit a positive slope in the HR versus time relationship. Record the selected power outputs on worksheet 20.1. For small or untrained subjects, the recommended power outputs for the PWC_{HRT} test are between 52 (0.75 kg resistance) and 137 (2.0 kg resistance) watts. For large or trained subjects, as well as experienced cyclists, the recommended power outputs are between 137 (2.0 kg resistance) and 223 (3.25 kg resistance) watts. These power outputs, however, should be viewed as only recommendations. It may be necessary to adjust them up or down to ensure that the HR versus time slope coefficient is positive and the subject is able to complete the entire 8-minute workbout.

4. Following the warm-up and a 2-minute rest period, have the subject begin to pedal at 70 rpm, and set the resistance (power output) to the appropriate level as quickly as possible during the first few seconds of the workbout.

TABLE	20.1	Resistance settings and corresponding power outputs at 70 rpm for a Monark cycle ergometer.

Resistance (kg)	Power output (watts)
0.50	34
0.75	52
1.00	69
1.25	86
1.50	103
1.75	120
2.00	137
2.25	154
2.50	172
2.75	189
3.00	206
3.25	223
3.50	240
3.75	257
4.00	275

5. Once the resistance is set, begin to time the workbout with a stopwatch.

6. Give the subject verbal encouragement to maintain the 70 rpm cadence. Record a HR on worksheet 20.1 at the end of minutes 4, 5, 6, 7 and 8. HR data should not be collected during the first 3 minutes to allow for the initial cardiac adjustment to exercise.

7. Cool-down. After each workbout, allow the subject to continue to pedal for 2 to 3 minutes (or longer if the subject desires) with no resistance.

8. The two workbouts at different power outputs can be performed on a single day. If a second workbout is to be performed during the same laboratory visit, have the subject rest (following the cool-down) until the heart rate returns to within 10 beats per minute of the pre-exercise level to ensure that the individual is fully recovered before performing the second workbout. This usually takes at least 30 minutes.

Sample Calculations

1. Use simple linear regression analysis ($y = b(x) + a$) to calculate the slope coefficient for the HR versus time relationship for each workbout (figure 20.1a). Simple linear regression can be performed using many handheld calculators or software (such as Microsoft Excel and others) for PC and Macintosh computers.

TIME (min)	Workbout 1 HR (bpm)	Workbout 2 HR (bpm)
1	HR data not recorded to allow for the	
2	initial cardiac adjustment to exercise	
3	↓	↓
4	138	154
5	140	158
6	143	163
7	146	166
8	149	172

For workbout 1, enter the x-values as 4, 5, 6, 7, and 8, and the y-values as 138, 140, 143, 146, and 149.

> Workbout 1 simple linear regression equation: HR = 2.8 (time) + 126.4
> Thus, workbout 1 HR versus time slope coefficient = 2.8 bpm • min^{-1}

For workbout 2, enter the x-values as 4, 5, 6, 7, and 8, and the y-values as 154, 158, 163, 166, and 172.

> Workbout 2 simple linear regression equation: HR = 4.4 (time) + 136.2
> Thus, workbout 2 HR versus time slope coefficient = 4.4 bpm • min^{-1}

2. Use simple linear regression analysis $(y = b(x) + a)$ to calculate the y-intercept (i.e., the PWC_{HRT}) for the power output versus HR slope coefficient relationship (figure 20.1b).

	HR versus time slope coefficient (bpm • min^{-1})	Power output (watts)
Workbout 1	2.8	125
Workbout 2	4.4	175

Simple linear regression equation: Power output = 31.3 (HR versus time slope coefficient) + 37.5.

Thus, the estimated maximal power output that can be maintained with no change in HR over time (PWC_{HRT}) = 37.5 watts.

| FIGURE | 20.1 | Description of the method for estimating the physical working capacity at the heart rate threshold (PWC_{HRT}). |

(a) The heart rate (HR) data are plotted as a function of time for various power outputs on a cycle ergometer. (b) The slope coefficients from (a) are plotted for each of the power outputs, and the PWC_{HRT} is estimated as the y-intercept value.

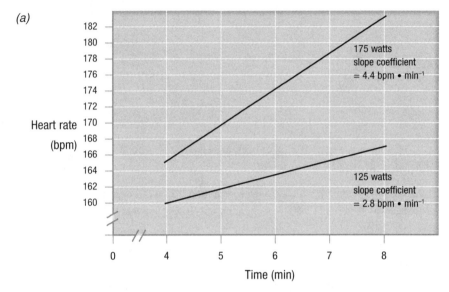

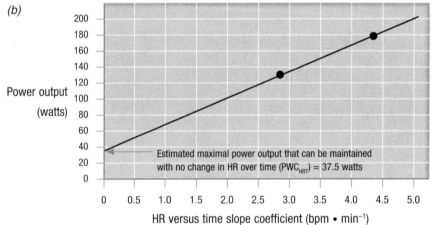

PHYSICAL WORKING CAPACITY AT THE HEART RATE THRESHOLD (PWC$_{HRT}$) TEST FORM	Worksheet **20.1**

Name _____   *Date* _____

Seat height _____

Pre-exercise heart rate _____ bpm

Power Output

Workbout 1: _____ kg of resistance × 420 [70 rpm (constant pedal cadence) × 6 meters (constant that defines the distance the flywheel travels each pedal revolution)] / 6.12 = _____ watts

Workbout 2: _____ kg of resistance × 420 / 6.12 = _____ watts

Workbout 3 (if used): _____ kg of resistance × 420 / 6.12 = _____ watts

Workbout 4 (if used): _____ kg of resistance × 420 / 6.12 = _____ watts

Time (min)	Workbout 1 HR (bpm)	Workbout 2 HR (bpm)	Workbout 3 HR (bpm)	Workbout 4 HR (bpm)
1	Do not collect HR data for the first 3 minutes to allow for the initial cardiac adjustment to exercise.			
2				
3				
4	_____	_____	_____	_____
5	_____	_____	_____	_____
6	_____	_____	_____	_____
7	_____	_____	_____	_____
8	_____	_____	_____	_____

HR Versus Time Slope Coefficient

Use linear regression analysis to determine the slope coefficient for the HR versus time relationship for each workbout: y = b(x) + a

Workbout 1: _____ bpm • min^{-1}

Workbout 2: _____ bpm • min^{-1}

Workbout 3 (if used): _____ bpm • min^{-1}

Workbout 4 (if used): _____ bpm • min^{-1}

Use linear regression analysis to determine the y-intercept (i.e., PWC$_{HRT}$) of the power output versus HR slope coefficient relationship:

Power output = b(HR slope coefficient) + PWC$_{HRT}$ (see figure 20.1b).

PWC$_{HRT}$ = _____ watts

Worksheet 20.2 | EXTENSION ACTIVITIES

Name _____ Date _____

1. Two subjects performed four separate 8-minute workbouts on a cycle ergometer at the following power outputs: workbout 1 = 125 watts, workbout 2 = 150 watts, workbout 3 = 175 watts, and workbout 4 = 200 watts. The HR responses for each subject and workbout are shown below:

SUBJECT A

Time (min)	Workbout 1 HR (bpm)	Workbout 2 HR (bpm)	Workbout 3 HR (bpm)	Workbout 4 HR (bpm)
4	137	140	154	163
5	140	143	158	167
6	142	146	163	173
7	146	150	168	179
8	148	153	172	184

SUBJECT B

Time (min)	Workbout 1 HR (bpm)	Workbout 2 HR (bpm)	Workbout 3 HR (bpm)	Workbout 4 HR (bpm)
4	155	163	169	170
5	159	168	174	175
6	161	172	181	182
7	164	177	188	188
8	168	183	193	196

Which subject has the higher PWC_{HRT}? subject A or subject B (circle the correct choice)

2. Describe two advantages of the PWC_{HRT} test when compared to a $\dot{V}O_2$ max test.

3. Use your own data to calculate your PWC_{HRT}.

EXTENSION QUESTIONS

1. What are some common mistakes that may occur in administering this lab?

2. Identify possible sources of error in this lab.

3. Assess the practicality of using this lab in the field.

4. Research the reliability and/or validity of this lab using online resources, journal articles, and other credible sources.

REFERENCES

1. Perry, S. R., Housh, T. J., Johnson, G. O., Ebersole, K. T., and Bull, A. J. Heart rate and ratings of perceived exertion at the physical working capacity at the heart rate threshold. *J. Strength Cond. Res.* 15: 225–229, 2001.

2. Wagner, L. L., and Housh, T. J. A proposed test for determining physical working capacity at the heart rate threshold. *Res. Q. Exerc. Sport* 64: 361–364, 1993.

3. Weir, L. L., Weir, J. P., Housh, T. J., and Johnson, G. O. Effect of an aerobic training program on physical working capacity at heart rate threshold. *Eur. J. Appl. Physiol.* 75: 351–356, 1997.

Physical Working Capacity at the Rating of Perceived Exertion Threshold Test

BACKGROUND

Theoretically, the physical working capacity at the rating of perceived exertion threshold (PWC_{RPE}) test provides an estimate of the maximal power output that can be maintained for an extended period of time without an increase in the perception of effort during cycle ergometry.[3] The PWC_{RPE} test uses the rating of perceived exertion (RPE, 6–20) scale developed by Borg[1,2] (see figure 21.1) to assess the overall perception of effort during cycle ergometry at various submaximal power outputs. Thus, the submaximal protocol used to determine the PWC_{RPE} makes it appropriate for assessing aerobic fitness in subjects where maximal exercise testing may be contraindicated, such as the elderly or clinical populations. In addition, the PWC_{RPE} test is most applicable to situations where assessing the ability to perform long-term, submaximal physical activity is more important than defining a subject's maximal exercise capacity (such as maximal oxygen consumption rate, $\dot{V}O_2$ max).

FIGURE	21.1	Borg rating of perceived exertion (RPE).[1,2]

THE SCALE

No exertion at all	6
	7
Extremely light	8
Very light	9
	10
Light	11
	12
Somewhat hard	13
	14
Hard (heavy)	15
	16
Very hard	17
	18
Extremely hard	19
Maximal exertion	20

Borg RPE Scale®

©Gunnar Borg, 1970, 1985, 1998, 2004.

INSTRUCTIONS to the Borg-RPE Scale®

During the work we want you to rate your perception of exertion, i.e., how heavy and strenuous the exercise feels to you and how tired you are. The perception of exertion is mainly felt as strain and fatigue in your muscles and as breathlessness, or aches in the chest. All work requires some effort, even if this is only minimal. This is true also if you only move a little, e.g., walking slowly.

   Use this scale from 6 to 20, with 6 meaning "No exertion at all" and 20 meaning "maximal exertion."

6   "No exertion at all" means that you don't feel any exertion whatsoever, e.g., no muscle fatigue, no breathlessness or difficulties breathing.

9   "Very light" exertion, as taking a shorter walk at your own pace.

13   A "somewhat hard" work, but it still feels OK to continue.

15   It is "hard" and tiring, but continuing isn't terribly difficult.

17   "Very hard." This is very strenuous work. You can still go on, but you really have to push yourself and you are very tired.

19   An "extremely" strenuous level. For most people this is the most strenuous work they have ever experienced.

Try to appraise your feeling of exertion and fatigue as spontaneously and as honestly as possible, without thinking about what the actual physical load is. Try not to underestimate and not to overestimate your exertion. It's your own feeling of effort and exertion that is important, not how this compares with other people's. Look at the scale and the expressions and then give a number. Use any number you like on the scale, not just one of those with an explanation behind it.

Any questions?

Note: For correct use of the scale, the exact design and instructions given in Borg's folders must be followed.

The PWC$_{RPE}$ test involves performing two or more 8-minute workbouts at different submaximal power outputs. This lab will describe the procedures for estimating the PWC$_{RPE}$ using two workbouts performed on the same day. Three or four workbouts, however, can also be used if the PWC$_{RPE}$ test is completed over two or more days. During each workbout, RPE values are recorded and the slope coefficient for the RPE versus time relationship is determined. The power output values are then plotted as a function of the slope coefficients for the RPE versus time relationships, and the y-intercept is defined as the PWC$_{RPE}$ (see figure 21.2b, p. 164). Salient features of the PWC$_{RPE}$ test are that it requires only submaximal exercise, and it can be performed using only a cycle ergometer, stopwatch, and RPE scale.

KNOW THESE TERMS & ABBREVIATIONS

- PWC$_{RPE}$ = physical working capacity at the rating of perceived exertion threshold (watts), defined as the y-intercept of the power output versus RPE slope coefficient relationship (figure 21.2b)
- RPE = rating of perceived exertion
- $\dot{V}O_2$ max = maximal oxygen consumption rate

PROCEDURES (see photo 21.1)

The PWC$_{RPE}$ test will be performed using a Monark cycle ergometer, stopwatch, and RPE scale.

1. Prior to beginning the test: (1) adjust the seat height of the cycle ergometer to allow for near full extension of the subject's legs while pedaling, and (2) record a pre-exercise heart rate on worksheet 21.1.

2. Warm-up: The PWC$_{RPE}$ test should be preceded by a standardized warm-up protocol that includes 4 minutes of pedaling at 70 rpm at a resistance of 0.5 kg (power output = 34 watts).

3. The PWC$_{RPE}$ test involves two to four cycle ergometer workbouts at different power outputs.[3] Each workbout is performed at a constant pedaling cadence of 70 rpm, and the selection of power outputs for each subject usually ranges from approximately 52 (0.75 kg resistance) to 223 (3.25 kg resistance) watts.[3] See table 21.1. The power outputs should be low enough that the subject is able to complete the full 8 minutes for each workbout, but high enough to elicit a positive slope in the RPE versus time relationship. For small or untrained subjects, the recommended power outputs for the PWC$_{RPE}$ test are between 52 (0.75 kg resistance) and 137 (2.0 kg resistance) watts. For large or trained subjects, as well as experienced cyclists, the recommended power outputs are between 137 (2.0 kg resistance) and 223 (3.25 kg resistance) watts. These power outputs, however, should be viewed as only recommendations. It may

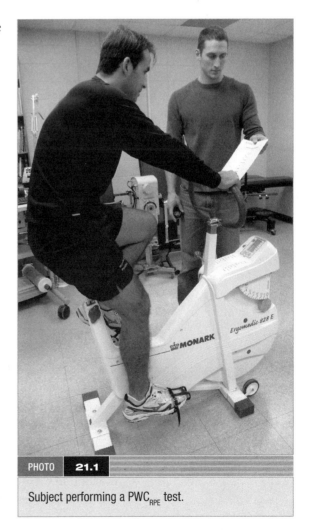

PHOTO **21.1**

Subject performing a PWC$_{RPE}$ test.

TABLE 21.1	Resistance settings and corresponding power outputs at 70 rpm for a Monark cycle ergometer.

Resistance (kg)	Power output (watts)
0.50	34
0.75	52
1.00	69
1.25	86
1.50	103
1.75	120
2.00	137
2.25	154
2.50	172
2.75	189
3.00	206
3.25	223
3.50	240
3.75	257
4.00	275

be necessary to adjust them up or down to ensure that the RPE versus time slope coefficient is positive and the subject is able to complete the entire 8-minute workbout.

4. Following the warm-up, have the subject rest for 2 minutes. During this rest period, instruct the subject on how to use the RPE scale shown in figure 21.1. Provide the following instructions: "During the exercise test, we want you to pay close attention to how hard you feel the exercise work rate is. This feeling should reflect your total amount of exertion and fatigue, combining all sensations and feelings of physical stress, effort, and fatigue. Don't concern yourself with any one factor, such as leg pain, shortness of breath, or exercise intensity, but try to concentrate on your total, inner feeling of exertion. Try not to underestimate or overestimate your feelings of exertion; be as accurate as you can."

5. After the 2-minute rest period, have the subject begin to pedal at 70 rpm, and set the resistance (power output) to the appropriate level as quickly as possible during the first few seconds of the workbout.

6. Once the resistance is set, begin to time the workbout with a stopwatch.

7. Give the subject verbal encouragement to maintain the 70 rpm cadence. At the end of minutes 1, 2, 3, 4, 5, 6, 7, and 8, show the subject the RPE scale (figure 21.1), and ask the subject for an RPE value that reflects his or her perception of effort. Record the subject's RPE value on worksheet 21.1.

8. Cool-down. After each workbout, allow the subject to continue to pedal for 2 to 3 minutes (or longer if the subject desires) with no resistance.

9. The two workbouts at different power outputs can be performed on a single day. If a second workbout is to be performed during the same laboratory visit, have the subject rest (following the cool-down) until the heart rate returns to within 10 beats per minute of the pre-exercise level to ensure that he or she is fully recovered before performing the second workbout. This usually takes at least 30 minutes.

Sample Calculations

1. Use simple linear regression analysis $(y = b(x) + a)$ to calculate the slope coefficient for the RPE versus time relationship for each workbout (figure 21.2a). Simple linear regression can be performed using many handheld calculators or software (such as Microsoft Excel and others) for PC and Macintosh computers.

TIME (min)	WORKBOUT 1 RPE values	WORKBOUT 2 RPE values
1	6	8
2	6	9
3	7	10
4	8	11
5	10	11
6	11	12
7	12	14
8	13	17

For workbout 1, enter the x-values as 1, 2, 3, 4, 5, 6, 7, and 8, and the y-values as 6, 6, 7, 8, 10, 11, 12, and 13.

Workbout 1 simple linear regression equation: RPE = 0.7 (time) + 4.9

Thus, for workbout 1, the RPE versus time slope coefficient = 0.7 RPE • min^{-1}.

For workbout 2, enter the x-values as 1, 2, 3, 4, 5, 6, 7, and 8, and the y-values as 8, 9, 10, 11, 11, 12, 14, and 17.

Workbout 2 simple linear regression equation: RPE = 1.1(time) + 6.5

Thus, for workbout 2, the RPE versus time slope coefficient = 1.1 RPE • min^{-1}.

2. Use simple linear regression analysis $(y = b(x) + a)$ to calculate the y-intercept (i.e., the PWC$_{RPE}$) for the power output versus RPE slope coefficient relationship (figure 21.2b).

	RPE VERSUS TIME SLOPE COEFFICIENT (RPE • min^{-1})	POWER OUTPUT (watts)
Workbout 1	0.7	125
Workbout 2	1.1	175

Simple linear regression equation:

Power output = 125 (RPE versus time slope coefficient) + 37.5.

Thus, the estimated power output that can be maintained with no change in RPE (PWC$_{RPE}$) = 37.5 watts.

Description of the method for estimating the physical working capacity at the rating of perceived extension threshold (PWC$_{RPE}$).

(a) The RPE data are plotted as a function of time for various power outputs on a cycle ergometer.
(b) The slope coefficients from (a) are plotted for each of the power outputs, and the PWC$_{RPE}$ is estimated as the y-intercept value.

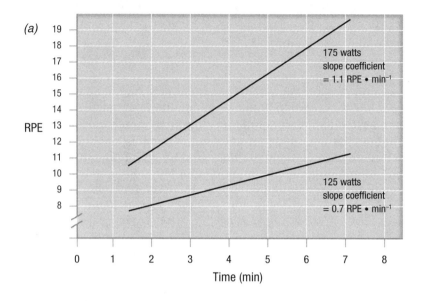

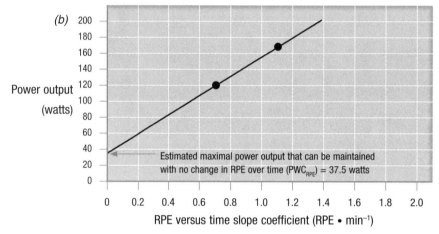

| **PHYSICAL WORKING CAPACITY AT THE RATING OF PERCEIVED EXERTION THRESHOLD (PWC$_{RPE}$) TEST FORM** | Worksheet **21.1** |

Name _____   *Date* _____

Seat height _____

Pre-exercise heart rate _____ bpm

Power Output

Workbout 1: _____ kg of resistance × 420 [70 rpm (constant pedal cadence) × 6 meters (constant that defines the distance the flywheel travels each pedal revolution)] / 6.12 = _____ watts

Workbout 2: _____ kg of resistance × 420 / 6.12 = _____ watts

Workbout 3 (if used): _____ kg of resistance × 420 / 6.12 = _____ watts

Workbout 4 (if used): _____ kg of resistance × 420 / 6.12 = _____ watts

Time (min)	Workbout 1 RPE	Workbout 2 RPE	Workbout 3 RPE	Workbout 4 RPE
1	_____	_____	_____	_____
2	_____	_____	_____	_____
3	_____	_____	_____	_____
4	_____	_____	_____	_____
5	_____	_____	_____	_____
6	_____	_____	_____	_____
7	_____	_____	_____	_____
8	_____	_____	_____	_____

RPE versus Time Slope Coefficient

Use linear regression analysis to determine the slope coefficient for the RPE versus time relationship for each workbout: $y = b(x) + a$

Workbout 1: _____ RPE • min^{-1}

Workbout 2: _____ RPE • min^{-1}

Workbout 3 (if used): _____ RPE • min^{-1}

Workbout 4 (if used): _____ RPE • min^{-1}

Use linear regression analysis to determine the y-intercept (i.e., PWC$_{RPE}$) of the power output versus RPE slope coefficient relationship:

Power output = b (RPE slope coefficient) + PWC$_{RPE}$ (see figure 21.2b).

PWC$_{RPE}$ = _____ watts

Worksheet 21.2 EXTENSION ACTIVITIES

Name _____ Date _____

1. Two subjects performed two separate 8-minute workbouts on a cycle ergometer at the following power outputs: workbout 1 = 150 watts and workbout 2 = 200 watts. The RPE responses for each subject and workbout are shown below:

SUBJECT A

Time (min)	Workbout 1 RPE	Workbout 2 RPE
1	6	8
2	6	9
3	7	9
4	7	10
5	8	11
6	8	12
7	9	13
8	10	14

SUBJECT B

Time (min)	Workbout 1 RPE	Workbout 2 RPE
1	6	8
2	7	9
3	7	11
4	8	12
5	9	14
6	10	15
7	11	17
8	12	19

Which subject has the higher PWC_{RPE}? subject A or subject B (circle the correct choice)

2. Describe two advantages of the PWC_{RPE} test compared to a $\dot{V}O_2$ max test.

3. Use your own data to calculate your PWC_{RPE}.

EXTENSION QUESTIONS

1. What are some common mistakes that may occur in administering this lab?

2. Identify possible sources of error in this lab.

3. Assess the practicality of using this lab in the field.

4. Research the reliability and/or validity of this lab using online resources, journal articles, and other credible sources.

REFERENCES

1. Borg, G. Perceived exertion as an indicator of somatic stress. *Scand. J. Rehabil. Med.* 2: 92–98, 1970.

2. Borg, G. *Borg's perceived exertion and pain scales.* Champaign, IL: Human Kinetics, 1998.

3. Mielke, M., Housh, T. J., Malek, M. H., Beck, T. W., Schmidt, R. J., and Johnson, G. O. Rating of perceived exertion based tests of physical working capacity. *J. Strength Cond. Res.* 22: 293–302, 2008.

Unit 4

MUSCULAR STRENGTH

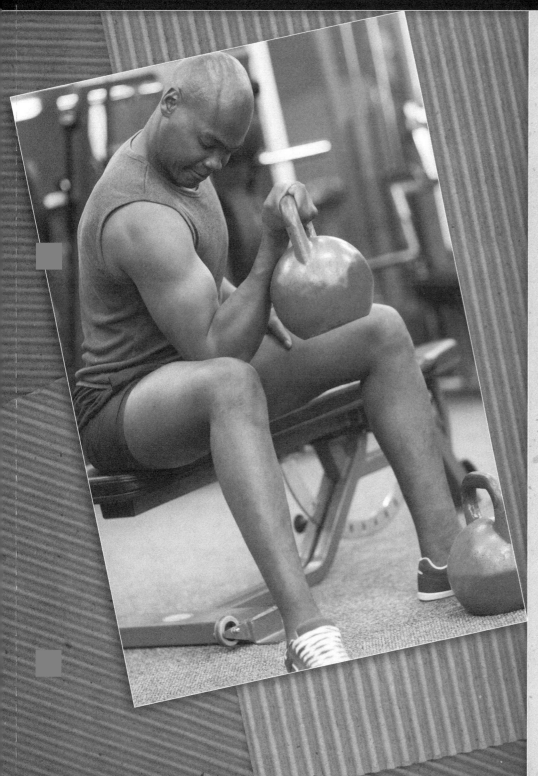

BACKGROUND

The three most common forms of strength testing are isometric, dynamic constant external resistance (DCER), and isokinetic.

Isometric testing typically involves the use of a device (such as a hand-grip dynamometer) that measures force output resulting from muscle actions with the body segment (limb, etc.) in a fixed position (thus, no movement is involved and no mechanical work is performed). *DCER testing* utilizes resistances (such as free weights) that are moved through a range of motion by a body segment.

Both of these forms of strength testing, while fairly easy to administer, have limitations in the scope of the information they yield. With isometric testing, the results are specific to the joint angle and, therefore, are not reflective of force production capabilities for normal movements such as those involved in throwing, kicking, or running. With DCER testing, the resultant strength value is indicative only of the amount of resistance that can be overcome at the weakest point in the range of motion. Thus, greater resistances can be overcome at other points of the movement, but these values remain unassessed. Also, DCER tests typically do not assess force production capabilities at controlled velocities of movement. Yet it is known that peak force output is specific to the velocity of movement.

In contrast to such limitations, *isokinetic testing* provides feedback on all of the above factors. That is, isokinetic testing provides force output values (torques) for every point throughout the movement, and it also allows for control of the velocity of such movements. This involves the use of special equipment that continuously measures and records torques and joint angles as a body segment moves through a range of motion at a preselected velocity controlled by the isokinetic dynamometer (see photo 22.1).

Because of increased dependency on fast-twitch fibers (resulting from a reduction in the contribution of slow-twitch fibers to force production), as velocity of movement increases, peak torque levels during concentric muscle actions typically tend to decrease (figure 22.1). Thus, those who excel in activities requiring high-velocity movements (fastball pitching, shot putting, field goal kicking, sprinting, etc.) do so, in part, because of an ability to develop

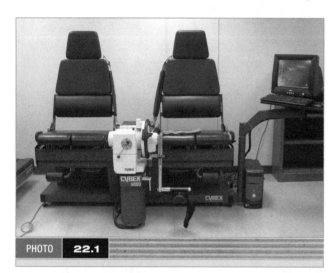

PHOTO 22.1

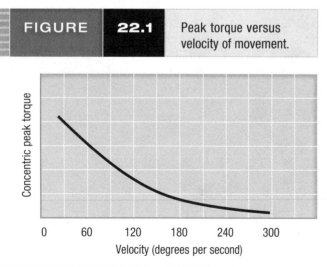

FIGURE 22.1 | Peak torque versus velocity of movement.

high levels of torque during rapid movements. This ability results from a genetically determined high proportion of fast-twitch fibers and/or hypertrophy of fast-twitch fibers induced via resistance training programs.

Analysis of torques and corresponding joint angles demonstrates that force production capabilities are diminished at the extremes of a full range of motion in a movement such as leg extension (figure 22.2). This response pattern underscores the inability to apply maximal overload throughout a DCER-type movement (thus the training effect is compromised).

With repeated "maximal effort" muscle actions, torque production declines as a result of fatigue. Fast-twitch fibers (particularly fast-twitch glycolytic [FG] fibers) tend to become fatigued sooner than slow-twitch fibers. Therefore, the rate at which torque declines during repeated muscle actions reflects, to some degree, the fiber type composition of the muscle group involved. (However, training-induced increases in the oxidative characteristics of any fiber type will slow this rate of torque decline.) Based on this, isokinetic testing can be used to estimate fiber type in the exercised muscle group, even though such results are more correctly reflective of endurance properties rather than twitch rates.[2] To demonstrate the nature of such responses, a protocol of 50 maximal-effort leg extensions is performed at $180° \cdot s^{-1}$ within a one-minute period (figure 22.3).[2]

From this laboratory experience, you will learn the principles underlying the different forms of strength measurement, as well as the contractile response characteristics (and the practical implications of such responses) under the various conditions demonstrated.

KNOW THESE TERMS & ABBREVIATIONS

- isometric testing = measurements of force output resulting from muscle actions with the body segment in a fixed position, which results in no movement or mechanical work performed

- dynamic constant external resistance (DCER) testing = measurements of force utilizing resistances (such as free weights) that are moved through a range of motion by a body segment

- isokinetic testing = measurements of torque (rotary force) for every point in the range of motion at preselected velocities

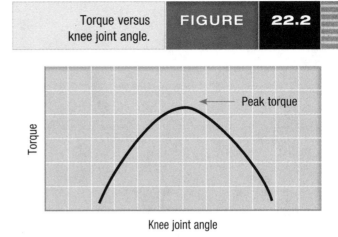

Torque versus knee joint angle.   FIGURE   22.2

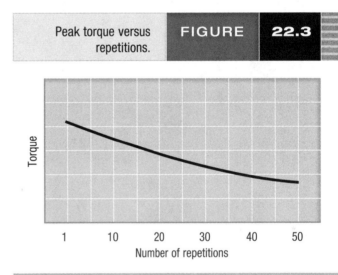

Peak torque versus repetitions.   FIGURE   22.3

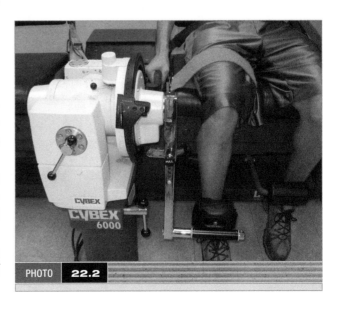

PHOTO   22.2

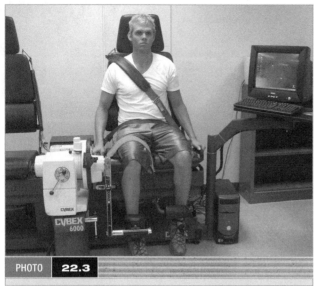

PHOTO **22.3**

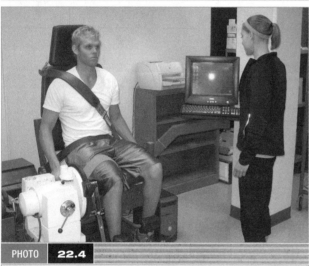

PHOTO **22.4**

PROCEDURES (see photos 22.2–22.4)

1. *Subject Position*
   a. Seat the subject and fasten straps to stabilize the hips and thighs.
   b. Line up the input shaft of the dynamometer with the axis of rotation of the knee joint. Adjust the shin pad so that it is just above the ankle and fastened securely.
   c. The subject should hold on to the handles by the seat of the dynamometer to help maintain upper-body position.

2. *Warm-Up*
   a. The subject should do approximately six repetitions of leg extension and flexion at approximately 50% of maximal effort for the left and right legs at 60, 180, and 300° $\cdot$ s^{-1}.
   b. Allow the subject to rest for approximately 2 minutes following the warm-up.

3. *Testing*
   a. *Isokinetic Peak Torque Test:* For each speed (60, 180, and 300° $\cdot$ s^{-1}), the subject is to perform one set of three maximal-effort leg extension and flexion repetitions. Test both legs.
   b. *Fiber Type Test:* The subject will perform 50 maximal-effort leg extensions (left leg) at 180° $\cdot$ s^{-1} within a 1-minute period. Passive leg flexion recovery should be allowed between the maximal leg extensions.

4. *Cool-Down:* The subject should stretch the quadriceps and hamstring muscles following testing.

5. *Record* the torque values on worksheet 22.1.

Sample Calculations[2]

Percent Decline = ((Initial Peak Torque − Final Peak Torque)/Initial Peak Torque) × 100

Percent Fast-Twitch Fibers = (Percent Decline − 5.2)/0.9

Example:

Percent Decline = ((100 − 50)/100) × 100 = 50%

Percent Fast-Twitch Fibers = (50 − 5.2)/0.9 = 49.8%

ISOKINETIC TEST FORM

Gender _____ *Age* _____ *Body Weight* _____

A. Record peak torque for each limb at each velocity (60, 180, and 300° • s⁻¹). Compare absolute peak torque (ft-lbs) at 60° • s⁻¹ and peak torque at 60° • s⁻¹ expressed as a percentage of body weight (in pounds) to the norms in tables 22.1 and 22.2. Then graph peak torque as a function of velocity (four graphs: one each for leg flexion and leg extension, and right and left legs) and compare to the expected pattern in figure 22.1.

	60° • s⁻¹	Category (absolute)	Category (% body weight)	180° • s⁻¹	300° • s⁻¹
Leg Flexion					
Left					
Right					
Leg Extension					
Left					
Right					

B. Record torque values for the following ratios.

Ratios	60° • s⁻¹	Expected Ratio[1]	180° • s⁻¹	Expected Ratio[1]	300° • s⁻¹	Expected Ratio[1]
Flexion/Extension		0.55–0.65		0.70–0.80		0.80–0.90
Left/Right (Extension)		0.95–1.05		0.95–1.05		0.95–1.05
Left/Right (Flexion)		0.95–1.05		0.95–1.05		0.95–1.05

C. Fiber Type Test (see sample calculations on previous page)

Initial Peak Torque _____

Final Peak Torque _____

Percent Decline _____

Percent Fast-Twitch Fibers _____

See table 22.3 for information concerning the muscle fiber type distribution patterns of males, females, non-athletes, and athletes in various sports.

TABLE	22.1	Norms for peak torque (at 60° • s⁻¹) in ft-lbs (% body weight) for females.

Note: The values without parentheses are in ft-lbs of torque.

The values in parentheses are ft-lbs of torque divided by body weight in pounds.

CATEGORIES

L = Low

F = Fair

A = Average

M = Moderate

H = High

			Females			
AGE		**LEG FLEX**			**LEG EXT**	
18–22	L	14–25	(11–18)		31–54	(23–39)
	F	26–36	(19–26)		55–78	(40–56)
	A	37–47	(27–34)		79–101	(57–73)
	M	48–59	(35–42)		102–127	(74–91)
	H	>59	(>42)		>127	(>91)
23–27	L	16–27	(16–20)		35–58	(25–42)
	F	28–38	(21–28)		59–82	(43–59)
	A	39–49	(29–36)		83–106	(60–76)
	M	50–61	(37–44)		107–131	(77–95)
	H	>61	(>44)		>131	(>95)
28–32	L	14–25	(11–18)		31–54	(23–39)
	F	26–36	(19–26)		55–78	(40–56)
	A	37–47	(27–34)		79–101	(57–73)
	M	48–59	(35–42)		102–127	(74–91)
	H	>59	(>42)		>127	(>91)
33–37	L	12–22	(8–16)		25–48	(18–34)
	F	23–33	(17–24)		49–72	(35–51)
	A	34–45	(25–32)		73–96	(52–68)
	M	46–56	(33–41)		97–121	(69–88)
	H	>56	(>41)		>121	(>88)
38–42	L	10–21	(7–15)		22–44	(16–32)
	F	22–32	(16–23)		45–68	(33–49)
	A	33–43	(24–31)		69–92	(50–66)
	M	44–55	(32–40)		93–117	(67–86)
	H	>55	(>40)		>117	(>86)
43–47	L	9–20	(6–13)		19–42	(14–30)
	F	21–31	(14–22)		43–66	(31–48)
	A	32–42	(23–30)		67–90	(49–65)
	M	43–54	(31–39)		91–115	(66–83)
	H	>54	(>39)		>115	(>83)
48–52	L	7–17	(5–13)		15–38	(10–27)
	F	18–29	(14–21)		39–62	(28–44)
	A	30–40	(22–29)		63–86	(45–62)
	M	41–51	(30–37)		87–111	(63–86)
	H	>51	(>37)		>111	(>86)
53–57	L	5–16	(4–11)		11–34	(8–24)
	F	17–27	(12–20)		35–58	(25–42)
	A	28–38	(21–28)		59–82	(43–59)
	M	39–50	(29–36)		83–107	(60–78)
	H	>50	(>36)		>107	(>78)
58–62	L	4–15	(3–11)		9–32	(7–23)
	F	16–26	(12–19)		33–56	(24–40)
	A	27–37	(20–27)		57–80	(41–57)
	M	38–49	(28–36)		81–105	(58–76)
	H	>49	(>36)		>105	(>76)

Norms for peak torque (at 60° • s⁻¹) in ft-lbs (% body weight) for males.   **TABLE**   **22.2**

Males					
AGE		**LEG FLEX**		**LEG EXT**	
18–22	L	24–42	(14–25)	47–82	(27–49)
	F	43–62	(26–36)	83–120	(50–70)
	A	63–81	(37–47)	121–156	(71–91)
	M	82–100	(48–58)	157–194	(92–113)
	H	>100	(>58)	>194	(>113)
23–27	L	28–47	(17–27)	55–91	(32–52)
	F	48–66	(28–38)	92–128	(53–74)
	A	67–85	(39–50)	129–164	(75–93)
	M	86–105	(51–61)	165–203	(94–119)
	H	>105	(>61)	>203	(>119)
28–32	L	27–45	(15–27)	51–88	(30–51)
	F	46–64	(28–37)	89–124	(52–72)
	A	65–83	(38–48)	125–161	(73–93)
	M	84–103	(49–60)	162–200	(94–116)
	H	>103	(>61)	>200	(>116)
33–37	L	24–42	(14–25)	47–82	(27–49)
	F	43–62	(26–36)	83–120	(50–70)
	A	63–80	(37–47)	121–156	(71–91)
	M	81–100	(48–58)	157–194	(92–113)
	H	>100	(>58)	>194	(>113)
38–42	L	20–38	(12–22)	39–74	(23–43)
	F	39–57	(23–33)	75–111	(44–64)
	A	58–77	(34–45)	112–148	(65–87)
	M	78–96	(46–56)	149–186	(88–108)
	H	>96	(>56)	>186	(>108)
43–47	L	15–34	(9–20)	30–66	(17–39)
	F	35–53	(21–31)	67–103	(40–59)
	A	54–73	(32–42)	104–140	(60–82)
	M	74–92	(43–54)	141–178	(83–104)
	H	>92	(>54)	>178	(>104)
48–52	L	13–31	(8–18)	25–60	(15–35)
	F	32–51	(19–30)	61–98	(36–57)
	A	52–70	(31–41)	99–135	(58–79)
	M	71–90	(42–53)	136–173	(80–101)
	H	>90	(>53)	>173	(>101)
53–57	L	11–30	(6–17)	22–57	(13–33)
	F	31–49	(18–28)	58–95	(34–55)
	A	50–68	(29–40)	96–131	(56–76)
	M	69–88	(41–51)	132–170	(77–99)
	H	>88	(>51)	>170	(>99)
58–62	L	7–25	(4–15)	14–49	(8–29)
	F	26–45	(16–26)	50–87	(30–50)
	A	46–64	(27–37)	88–123	(51–72)
	M	65–83	(38–49)	124–161	(73–95)
	H	>83	(>49)	>161	(>95)

Note: The values without parentheses are in ft-lbs of torque.

The values in parentheses are ft-lbs of torque divided by body weight in pounds.

CATEGORIES

L = Low

F = Fair

A = Average

M = Moderate

H = High

| TABLE | 22.3 | Approximate average percentage of fast-twitch and slow-twitch fibers in the thigh muscles of male and female non-athletes and athletes in various sports. |

Females	% fast-twitch	% slow-twitch
Non-athletes	50	50
800 m runners	40	60
Cross-country skiers	40	60
Cyclists	49	51
Shot-putters and discus throwers	50	50
Long jumpers and high jumpers	52	48
Javelin throwers	60	40
Sprinters	73	27
Males	**% fast-twitch**	**% slow-twitch**
Non-athletes	50	50
Marathon runners	18	82
Swimmers	26	74
Distance runners	30	70
Speed skaters	30	70
Cross-country skiers	37	63
Ice hockey players	40	60
Cyclists	43	57
Shot-putters and discus throwers	63	37
Sprinters and jumpers	64	36
800 m runners	54	46
Weight lifters	53	47
Javelin throwers	52	48
Triathletes	37	63

Adapted from Bowers, R. W., and Fox, E. L. *Sports Physiology,* 3rd ed. Dubuque: Wm. C. Brown, 1988, p. 128–129; McArdle, W. D., Katch, F. I., and Katch, V. L. *Exercise Physiology,* 4th ed. Baltimore: Williams and Wilkins, 1996, p. 333; Wilmore, J. H., and Costill, D. L. *Physiology of Sport and Exercise,* 2nd ed. Champaign: Human Kinetics, 1999, p. 45.

EXTENSION ACTIVITIES   Worksheet **22.2**

Name   *Date*

1. How would a drug that blocked all slow-twitch muscle fibers affect an individual's fatigue curve from repeated maximal concentric isokinetic muscle actions? Plot on the graph below.

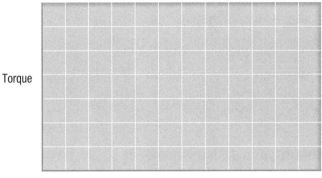

Torque

Number of repetitions

——————— Before the drug

---------------- After the drug

2. What effect would a resistance training program have on the concentric peak torque–velocity curve? Plot on the graph below.

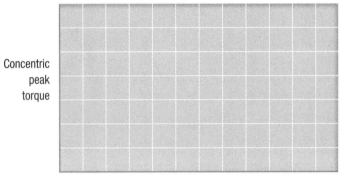

Concentric peak torque

Velocity

——————— Before training

---------------- After training

3. Given the following information: Body weight = 180 lbs

Initial peak torque = 210 ft-lbs

Final peak torque = 72 ft-lbs

Calculate:

a. Peak strength relative to body weight in kilograms.

b. Estimated percent of fast-twitch muscle fibers.

REFERENCES

1. Perrin, D. H. *Isokinetic Exercise and Assessment.* Champaign, IL: Human Kinetics, 1993.

2. Thorstensson, A., and Karlsson, J. Fatigability and fiber composition of human skeletal muscle. *Acta Physiol. Scand.* 98: 318–322, 1976.

BACKGROUND

Isometric hand grip strength is an important component of physical fitness and provides a simple method for characterizing overall body strength.[1,2] The performance of many manual labor activities, such as yard and garden work and lifting and carrying large objects, depends on a certain degree of hand grip strength. Thus, the purpose of this lab is to describe the procedures for measuring isometric hand grip strength with a hand grip dynamometer.

KNOW THESE TERMS & ABBREVIATIONS

- hand grip dynamometer = an instrument that measures isometric hand grip strength, which provides a simple method for characterizing overall body strength
- isometric strength = tension production by a muscle without movement at the joint or shortening of the muscle fibers
- percentile rank = in this lab, a score between 10% and 90% that shows how the subject performed relative to others in the age group. A percentile ranking of 70, for example, indicates that the subject's grip strength is higher than 70% of the others in the age group and lower than 30% of the others in the age group.

PROCEDURES

The isometric hand grip strength test can be performed using a variety of dynamometers (photo 23.1).

1. Prior to beginning the test, adjust the length of the handle on the hand grip dynamometer such that it feels comfortable in the hand. For indi-

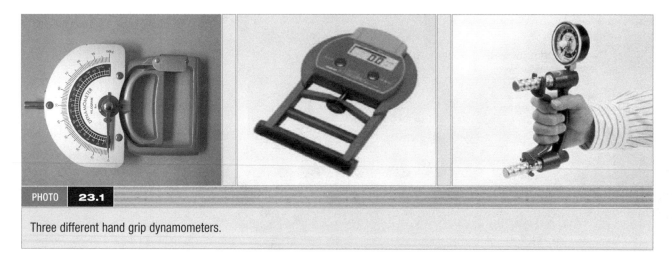

PHOTO **23.1**

Three different hand grip dynamometers.

viduals with very small hands, the handle of the dynamometer should be shortened, while for those with very large hands, the handle should be lengthened.[1]

2. Have the subject hold the hand grip dynamometer in the right hand with the palm facing up and the elbow at approximately 90 degrees (photo 23.2). When ready, the subject should squeeze the dynamometer maximally for 3 seconds. Read the force value (kg) from the dynamometer and record it on worksheet 23.1. Perform the strength test two more times with the right hand, separating the trials by 2 minutes of rest.

3. Repeat the procedures described in step 2 for the left hand.

4. Add the highest strength value (kg) for the right hand to that from the left hand and record the value on worksheet 23.1. Divide the sum by body weight in kg and record this value on worksheet 23.1.

5. Percentile rank norms by age and gender are provided in tables 23.1 through 23.4. Compare the sum of right and left hand grip strength to the values in tables 23.1 and 23.2 based on age and gender. Compare the sum of right and left hand grip strength divided by body weight to the values in tables 23.3 and 23.4 based on age and gender.

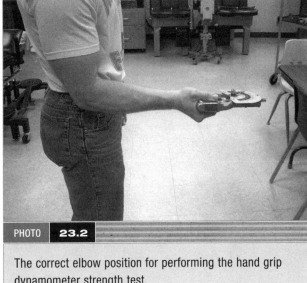

PHOTO **23.2**

The correct elbow position for performing the hand grip dynamometer strength test.

Percentile ranks for sum of grip strengths (kg, right plus left) for males.	TABLE	23.1

Percentile rank	Age (yrs)																
	10	11	12	13	14	15	16	17	18	19	20–24	25–29	30–34	35–39	40–44	45–49	50–59
90	34	42	52	69	89	96	106	111	117	118	122	123	124	123	123	116	110
80	30	37	47	60	80	90	99	105	106	113	115	115	115	115	115	108	102
70	26	34	41	53	72	84	95	99	101	109	110	110	110	109	108	104	96
60	24	32	38	48	66	80	91	93	98	104	105	107	106	106	103	99	93
50	22	29	34	44	61	76	87	89	96	101	102	103	102	102	100	95	89
40	20	26	31	42	58	73	84	85	93	98	99	100	98	98	97	91	85
30	18	23	30	39	54	69	78	81	90	94	94	95	95	93	93	82	81
20	15	21	27	34	49	64	74	76	86	90	89	90	90	88	87	81	75
10	11	16	23	28	39	55	68	70	81	84	80	81	82	79	81	75	66

Adapted from Montoye, H. J., and Lamphiear, D. E. Grip and arm strength in males and females, age 10 to 69. *Research Quarterly for Exercise and Sport*, Vol. 48, pp. 109–120, 1977. Reprinted with permission of the publisher, Taylor & Francis Ltd, www.tandfonline.com.

| TABLE | 23.2 | Percentile ranks for sum of grip strengths (kg, right plus left) for females. |

Percentile rank	Age (yrs)																
	10	11	12	13	14	15	16	17	18	19	20–24	25–29	30–34	35–39	40–44	45–49	50–59
90	30	37	44	49	65	60	58	61	59	63	61	67	65	66	64	64	57
80	25	33	40	44	50	54	53	54	55	59	57	62	60	59	58	57	52
70	22	30	36	41	48	49	49	50	52	54	53	57	57	55	54	53	48
60	20	27	33	38	44	45	48	47	49	50	50	53	53	53	51	52	45
50	18	25	31	36	41	43	43	44	46	48	48	49	49	51	49	49	43
40	17	23	28	34	39	41	41	42	43	46	45	48	47	49	47	47	40
30	15	20	26	32	36	38	39	39	39	42	42	46	44	46	43	44	38
20	14	17	22	30	32	36	36	36	36	39	38	43	41	43	40	40	34
10	10	12	18	26	27	31	33	31	31	36	34	37	36	36	36	34	30

Adapted from Montoye, H. J., and Lamphiear, D. E. Grip and arm strength in males and females, age 10 to 69. *Research Quarterly for Exercise and Sport,* Vol. 48, pp. 109–120, 1977. Reprinted with permission of the publisher, Taylor & Francis Ltd, www.tandfonline.com.

| TABLE | 23.3 | Percentile ranks for ratio of sum of grip strengths to body weight (kg/kg body weight) for males. |

Percentile rank	Age (yrs)															
	10	11	12	13	14	15	16	17	18	19	20–24	25–29	30–34	35–39	40–49	50–59
90	0.89	1.04	1.10	1.20	1.40	1.45	1.56	1.62	1.62	1.75	1.73	1.72	1.64	1.62	1.54	1.39
80	0.83	0.94	0.97	1.13	1.28	1.36	1.49	1.48	1.50	1.54	1.59	1.54	1.52	1.51	1.41	1.30
70	0.76	0.85	0.93	1.03	1.23	1.29	1.43	1.44	1.47	1.44	1.53	1.47	1.45	1.42	1.34	1.22
60	0.69	0.80	0.86	0.98	1.15	1.25	1.39	1.39	1.44	1.36	1.45	1.40	1.39	1.35	1.28	1.19
50	0.65	0.77	0.80	0.93	1.09	1.22	1.30	1.35	1.37	1.33	1.39	1.35	1.33	1.28	1.24	1.14
40	0.62	0.71	0.74	0.86	1.02	1.17	1.19	1.28	1.33	1.29	1.32	1.28	1.29	1.23	1.19	1.10
30	0.52	0.66	0.70	0.80	0.96	1.14	1.14	1.21	1.31	1.24	1.26	1.20	1.24	1.17	1.14	1.03
20	0.45	0.58	0.66	0.77	0.90	1.06	1.09	1.16	1.22	1.17	1.18	1.12	1.18	1.11	1.07	0.98
10	0.38	0.48	0.61	0.65	0.81	0.95	0.98	1.01	1.16	1.12	1.08	1.01	1.10	1.02	0.99	0.89

Adapted from Montoye, H. J., and Lamphiear, D. E. Grip and arm strength in males and females, age 10 to 69. *Research Quarterly for Exercise and Sport,* Vol. 48, pp. 109–120, 1977. Reprinted with permission of the publisher, Taylor & Francis Ltd, www.tandfonline.com.

Percentile ranks for ratio of sum of grip strengths to body weight (kg/kg body weight) for females.	TABLE	23.4

Percentile rank	Age (yrs)															
	10	11	12	13	14	15	16	17	18	19	20–24	25–29	30–34	35–39	40–49	50–59
90	0.71	0.91	0.92	0.96	1.08	1.04	0.98	1.12	1.02	1.10	1.04	1.12	1.05	1.07	1.02	0.90
80	0.65	0.80	0.80	0.86	0.96	0.92	0.94	1.02	0.95	1.04	0.97	1.02	1.00	1.00	0.93	0.83
70	0.62	0.72	0.75	0.81	0.86	0.89	0.84	0.96	0.90	0.94	0.91	0.97	0.94	0.93	0.87	0.78
60	0.57	0.68	0.72	0.79	0.81	0.84	0.79	0.89	0.82	0.85	0.86	0.91	0.89	0.87	0.81	0.71
50	0.54	0.64	0.66	0.73	0.76	0.79	0.76	0.83	0.78	0.80	0.81	0.86	0.83	0.84	0.77	0.68
40	0.50	0.57	0.61	0.68	0.71	0.76	0.73	0.78	0.72	0.77	0.77	0.82	0.78	0.80	0.73	0.63
30	0.46	0.53	0.57	0.65	0.67	0.69	0.71	0.71	0.69	0.74	0.72	0.75	0.72	0.75	0.69	0.59
20	0.42	0.45	0.54	0.63	0.65	0.65	0.65	0.66	0.65	0.69	0.68	0.68	0.66	0.69	0.63	0.52
10	0.32	0.33	0.47	0.52	0.58	0.57	0.57	0.52	0.58	0.64	0.61	0.61	0.60	0.60	0.54	0.48

Adapted from Montoye, H. J., and Lamphiear, D. E. Grip and arm strength in males and females, age 10 to 69. *Research Quarterly for Exercise and Sport,* Vol. 48, pp. 109–120, 1977. Reprinted with permission of the publisher, Taylor & Francis Ltd, www.tandfonline.com.

Sample Calculations

Gender: ___Male___

Age: ___21 years___

Body weight: ___75 kg___

	Trial 1 (kg)	Trial 2 (kg)	Trial 3 (kg)	Max of three trials (kg)
Right hand	50	52	53	53
Left hand	51	50	52	52

Sum of right and left = ___105___ kg

Approximate percentile rank = ___60___ (table 23.1)

Sum of right and left (kg)		Body weight (kg)		Grip strength ratio (kg/kg body weight)
___105___	/	___75___	=	___1.40___

Approximate percentile rank = ___51___ (table 23.3)

Worksheet 23.1 — ISOMETRIC HAND GRIP STRENGTH FORM

Name _____   *Date* _____

Age _____   *Gender* _____

	Trial 1 (kg)	Trial 2 (kg)	Trial 3 (kg)	Max of three trials (kg)
Right hand	_____	_____	_____	_____
Left hand	_____	_____	_____	_____

Sum of right plus left _____

Percentile rank (see tables 23.1 and 23.2) = _____

Sum of right and left (kg)	**Body weight (kg)**	**Grip strength ratio (kg/kg body weight)**
_____ /	_____ =	_____

Percentile rank (see tables 23.3 and 23.4): _____

Worksheet 23.2 — EXTENSION ACTIVITIES

Name _____   *Date* _____

1. Using your own data, report the sum of your right and left hand grip strength scores (kg) and percentile ranking.

2. Using your own data, report the ratio of the sum of your grip strengths to body weight (kg/kg body weight) and percentile ranking.

3. Describe three activities that you regularly perform that depend on possessing a high degree of hand grip strength.

4. Describe three sporting activities that, in part, require a high degree of hand grip strength.

EXTENSION QUESTIONS

1. What are some common mistakes that may occur in administering this lab?

2. Identify possible sources of error in this lab.

3. Assess the practicality of using this lab in the field.

4. Research the reliability and/or validity of this lab using online resources, journal articles, and other credible sources.

REFERENCES

1. Montoye, H. J., and Faulkner, J. A. Determination of the optimum setting of an adjustable grip dynamometer. *Res. Q. Exerc. Sport 35:* 29–36, 1964.

2. Montoye, H. J., and Lamphiear, D. E. Grip and arm strength in males and females, age 10 to 69. *Res. Q. Exerc. Sport 48:* 109–120, 1977.

BACKGROUND

The one-repetition maximum, or 1-RM, refers to the maximum amount of weight that can be lifted one time. The 1-RM is a standard index to quantify muscle strength. A 1-RM determination can be made for any dynamic constant external resistance (DCER; formerly known as isotonic) strength exercise, such as the bench press, leg extension and flexion, leg press, squat, or power clean. In addition, 1-RM testing can be performed using free weights or machine exercises. The procedure is a trial-and-error method where, after a warm-up period, progressively heavier weights are lifted one time until the subject cannot successfully complete the lift of a given weight.[1] The weight is then reduced until the heaviest successful weight is determined.

In performing 1-RM testing for a given exercise it is helpful (but not required) to have subjects with some minimal level of weightlifting experience, because strength exercises are a motor skill that improves with practice. Therefore, a 1-RM value is affected not only by the subject's strength, but also by the subject's skill in performing the task. In addition, prior experience allows subjects to estimate their strength more accurately prior to testing. This estimate helps eliminate unnecessary lifts that are either too easy or too hard, so that the testing is efficient and the effects of fatigue are minimized.

In this laboratory you will learn to perform 1-RM strength testing for bench press and leg press exercises. You will also compare the 1-RM strength values to age- and gender-specific norms. Percentile rank norms for strength relative to body weight (1-RM strength in lbs/body weight in lbs) are provided in tables 24.1 through 24.4 for the bench press and leg press exercises for males and females.

Bench Press

The bench press is a common exercise in both training and testing (see photos 24.1 and 24.2). The motion of the bench press is analogous to a push-up, except the subject lies on his or her back and the resistance is supplied by a barbell or a bench

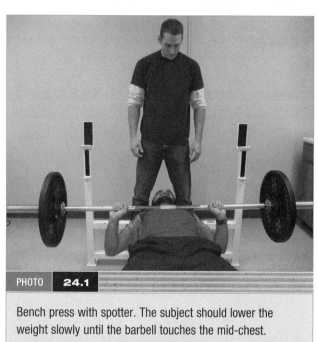

PHOTO **24.1**

Bench press with spotter. The subject should lower the weight slowly until the barbell touches the mid-chest.

PHOTO **24.2**

Bench press with spotter. During ascent and descent the forearms should be vertical to the floor and parallel to each other.

press machine. The pectoral muscles, triceps brachii, and anterior deltoid muscles are the primary muscles involved in the lift. Because the use of a barbell requires that the subject balance the resistance in addition to lifting the weight, the 1-RM from a free weight bench press may be quite different from the 1-RM determined on a machine. Further, because the mechanics of the different machines vary, the 1-RM from the same subject on different machines may also differ substantially. These factors should be kept in mind when interpreting the results relative to the normative values provided in tables 24.1 and 24.2.

					TABLE	24.1
Percentile rank norms for bench press 1-RM relative to body weight by age for males.[3]						

Percentile rank	20–29	30–39	40–49	50–59	60–69
90	1.48	1.24	1.10	0.97	0.89
80	1.32	1.12	1.00	0.90	0.82
70	1.22	1.04	0.93	0.84	0.77
60	1.14	0.98	0.88	0.79	0.72
50	1.06	0.93	0.84	0.75	0.68
40	0.99	0.88	0.80	0.71	0.66
30	0.93	0.83	0.76	0.68	0.63
20	0.88	0.78	0.72	0.63	0.57
10	0.80	0.71	0.65	0.57	0.53

Note: Values are bench press 1-RM in lbs/body weight in lbs.

					TABLE	24.2
Percentile rank norms for bench press 1-RM relative to body weight by age for females.[3]						

Percentile rank	20–29	30–39	40–49	50–59	60–69
90	0.54	0.49	0.46	0.40	0.41
80	0.49	0.45	0.40	0.37	0.38
70	0.42	0.42	0.38	0.35	0.36
60	0.41	0.41	0.37	0.33	0.32
50	0.40	0.38	0.34	0.31	0.30
40	0.37	0.37	0.32	0.28	0.29
30	0.35	0.34	0.30	0.26	0.28
20	0.33	0.32	0.27	0.23	0.26
10	0.30	0.27	0.23	0.19	0.25

Note: Values are bench press 1-RM in lbs/body weight in lbs.

When using free weights, a failed attempt to lift a weight may result in injury if the bar becomes out of control. Therefore, an experienced "spotter" should be ready to help the subject lift the weight when the attempt is clearly going to fail.[2] Most bench press machines do not require the use of a spotter.

For the free weight bench press, the subject should lie supine on the bench with both feet flat on the floor with the buttocks and shoulders in contact with the bench. The subject should grip the barbell with a closed grip. That is, the thumb should wrap around the barbell so that it cannot roll out of the hand. Grip width should be slightly wider than the shoulders and evenly spaced so that the load is the same on each arm. The barbell should then be removed from the bench press racks. The spotter may help the subject by assisting the "liftoff." After the liftoff, the subject should lower the weight slowly until the barbell touches the mid-chest.[2] This should take 1 to 2 seconds. As soon as the barbell touches the chest, the subject should lift it upward until the elbows are locked. During the descent and ascent, the forearms should be parallel to each other and oriented vertical to the floor.[2] After the lift, the spotter may help the subject place the barbell on the racks. Lifts are not acceptable if the barbell bounces off the chest or if the buttocks come off the bench.

Leg Press (see photos 24.3 and 24.4)

The leg press is a machine-based exercise that primarily involves the simultaneous activation of the leg extensors (quadriceps) and thigh extensors (gluteal muscles and hamstrings). There are several different types of machines, and the body position can vary considerably from machine to machine, which will affect the amount of weight that can be lifted. Therefore, as with the bench press, caution should be used when interpreting the normative leg press values in tables 24.3 and 24.4. Most machines allow you to alter the angle between the torso and thigh, and, if possible, this should be set to about 90 degrees.[2]

TABLE   24.3   Percentile rank norms for leg press 1-RM relative to body weight by age for males.[3]

Percentile rank	20–29	30–39	40–49	50–59	60–69
90	2.27	2.07	1.92	1.80	1.73
80	2.13	1.93	1.82	1.71	1.62
70	2.05	1.85	1.74	1.64	1.56
60	1.97	1.77	1.68	1.58	1.49
50	1.91	1.71	1.62	1.52	1.43
40	1.83	1.65	1.57	1.46	1.38
30	1.74	1.59	1.51	1.39	1.30
20	1.63	1.52	1.44	1.32	1.25
10	1.51	1.43	1.35	1.22	1.16

Note: Values are leg press 1-RM in lbs/body weight in lbs.

Percentile rank	20–29	30–39	40–49	50–59	60–69
90	2.05	1.73	1.63	1.51	1.40
80	1.66	1.50	1.46	1.30	1.25
70	1.42	1.47	1.35	1.24	1.18
60	1.36	1.32	1.26	1.18	1.15
50	1.32	1.26	1.19	1.09	1.08
40	1.25	1.21	1.12	1.03	1.04
30	1.23	1.16	1.03	0.95	0.98
20	1.13	1.09	0.94	0.86	0.94
10	1.02	0.94	0.76	0.75	0.84

Percentile rank norms for leg press 1-RM relative to body weight by age for females.[3] **TABLE 24.4**

Note: Values are leg press 1-RM in lbs/body weight in lbs.

At the start of the lift, the feet should be about shoulder-width apart and the toes pointed up or in a slightly "toe out" position. The shoulders and buttocks should be firmly braced against the machine.[2] Most leg press machines have hand grips that the subject can use to help stabilize the torso during the lift. Once positioned, the subject will unrack the weight so that the legs are fully extended (although the legs should not be hyperextended at the start of the lift). From full extension, the subject lowers the weight slowly until the angle at the knee joint reaches approximately 90 degrees (photo 24.3), and then extends the legs and thighs until the legs are again fully extended (photo 24.4). The subject should keep the legs in line with the hips and ankles, so that the legs do not track in (knock-kneed) or out.[2]

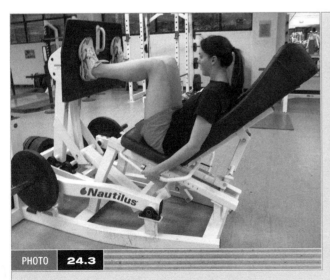

PHOTO **24.3**

Leg press. The subject lowers the weight slowly until the angle at the knee reaches approximately 90 degrees.

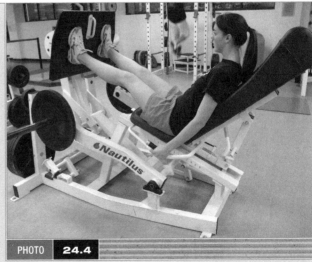

PHOTO **24.4**

Leg press. The subject should keep the legs in line with the hips and ankles.

KNOW THESE TERMS & ABBREVIATIONS

○ DCER = dynamic constant external resistance

○ 1-RM = one-repetition maximum, a standard index to quantify muscle strength that refers to the maximum amount of weight that can be lifted one time

○ leg extensors = the quadriceps, made up of the rectus femoris, vastus lateralis, vastus intermedius, and vastus medialis

○ thigh extensors = the gluteal muscles (gluteus maximus and gluteus medius) and the hamstrings (biceps femoris, semitendinosus, and semimembranosus)

○ hyperextension = extension of a joint beyond the normal range of motion

PROCEDURES (see photos 24.1 to 24.4)

1. Have the subject estimate his or her 1-RM strength and record it on worksheet 24.1.

2. Have the subject perform a general warm-up (3 to 5 minutes) of the body area to be tested.

3. Continue the warm-up by performing eight repetitions at a weight equal to 50% of the estimated 1-RM and three repetitions at 70% of the estimated 1-RM.

4. To determine the 1-RM, perform a single repetition at a heavier weight than that used during the warm-up. The increase in weight should be based on the relative ease or difficulty of the set in the warm-up.

5. Repeat performing single repetitions using progressively heavier weights until a weight is reached that cannot be successfully lifted. Adjust the increases in weight so that increments are approximately evenly spaced and so that at least two single lifts are performed between the weight used in the warm-up and the estimated 1-RM.

6. At failure, decrease the weight to a level approximately midway between the last successful lift and the weight at failure.

7. Repeat using heavier or lighter weights until the desired level of precision is achieved (usually within about 5 lbs) and record the 1-RM weight on worksheet 24.1.

8. Rest intervals between single lifts should be between 1 and 5 minutes.[4,5]

9. Try to determine the 1-RM in about three to five single lifts, excluding warm-up lifts.[1]

10. To increase time efficiency, more than one subject can be tested at a given station, so that one person is performing lifts while the others are resting.

Sample Calculations

Gender: _____Male_____

Body weight: _____180 lbs_____

Age: _____21 years_____

Mode of lift: _____Bench press_____

Estimated 1-RM: _____200 lbs_____

WARM-UP

1. _____8_____ repetitions at _____100_____ lbs (approximately 50% of estimated 1-RM)

2. _____3_____ repetitions at _____140_____ lbs (approximately 70% of estimated 1-RM)

1-RM TESTING

1. *Circle:* (success) failure at _____170_____ lbs

2. *Circle:* (success) failure at _____185_____ lbs

3. *Circle:* success (failure) at _____200_____ lbs

4. *Circle:* (success) failure at _____195_____ lbs

5. *Circle:* success failure at _____ lbs

6. *Circle:* success failure at _____ lbs

7. *Circle:* success failure at _____ lbs

1-RM/body weight: _____195 lbs/180 lbs_____ = _____1.08_____

Percentile rank classification for 1-RM in lbs/body weight in lbs

= _____52nd percentile_____ (see table 24.1)

Worksheet 24.1 | DETERMINATION OF ONE-REPETITION MAXIMUM STRENGTH

Name _____   Date _____

Gender: _____

Body Weight: _____ lbs

Age: _____

Mode of lift: _____

Estimated 1-RM lbs: _____

WARM-UP

1. _____ repetitions at _____ lbs (approximately 50% of estimated 1-RM)

2. _____ repetitions at _____ lbs (approximately 70% of estimated 1-RM)

1-RM TESTING

1. *Circle:*   success   failure   at _____ lbs

2. *Circle:*   success   failure   at _____ lbs

3. *Circle:*   success   failure   at _____ lbs

4. *Circle:*   success   failure   at _____ lbs

5. *Circle:*   success   failure   at _____ lbs

6. *Circle:*   success   failure   at _____ lbs

7. *Circle:*   success   failure   at _____ lbs

1-RM/body weight _____

Percentile rank classification for 1-RM in lbs/body weight in lbs = _____ (see tables 24.1–24.4)

Worksheet **24.2**

Name   *Date*

1. Given the following data, answer the questions below.

    Gender: _____ Female _____

    Age: _____ 22 years _____

    Bench press 1-RM: _____ 70 lbs _____

    Body weight: _____ 150 lbs _____

    Bench press 1-RM in lbs/body weight in lbs: _____

    Percentile rank = _____ (see table 24.2)

2. Given the following data, answer the questions below.

    Gender: _____ Male _____

    Age: _____ 44 years _____

    Leg press 1-RM: _____ 275 lbs _____

    Body weight: _____ 180 lbs _____

    Leg press 1-RM in lbs/body weight in lbs: _____

    Percentile rank = _____ (see table 24.3)

EXTENSION QUESTIONS

1. What are some common mistakes that may occur in administering this lab?

2. Identify possible sources of error in this lab.

3. Assess the practicality of using this lab in the field.

4. Research the reliability and/or validity of this lab using online resources, journal articles, and other credible sources.

REFERENCES

1. Brown, L. E., and Weir, J. P. ASEP Procedures Recommendation I: Accurate assessment of muscular strength and power. *J. Exercise Phys. Online* 4: 1–21, 2001.

2. Graham, J. F. Resistance exercise techniques and spotting. In *Conditioning for Strength and Human Performance,* eds. T. J. Chandler and L. E. Brown. Baltimore: Lippincott Williams & Wilkins, 2008, pp. 182–236.

3. Hoffman, J. *Norms for Fitness, Performance, and Health.* Champaign, IL: Human Kinetics, 2006.

4. Matuszak, M. E., Fry, A. C., Weiss, L. W., Ireland, T. R., and McNight, M. M. Effect of rest interval length on repeated 1 repetition maximum back squats. *J. Strength Cond. Res.* 17: 634–637, 2003.

5. Weir, J. P., Wagner, L. L., and Housh, T. J. The effect of rest interval length on repeated maximal bench presses. *J. Strength Cond. Res.* 8: 58–60, 1994.

BACKGROUND

Surface electromyography (SEMG) involves the recording of muscle action potentials.

In SEMG, electrodes are placed over the muscle of interest on the surface of the skin (see photo 25.1). The amplitude of the SEMG signal reflects the amount of electrical current (expressed in microvolts; 1 µV = 1/1,000,000 of a volt) recorded from the muscle action potentials that are passing along the sarcolemmas of the active muscle fibers in the recording area (called the pick-up area) of the electrodes. The amplitude of the SEMG signal represents the level of muscle activation, including the number of muscle fibers recruited and their firing rates. The amplitude of the SEMG signal can be quantified by integration (resulting in a time-averaged, integrated SEMG amplitude value in µV) or as the root mean square (RMS) value (the standard deviation of the individually recorded voltages in µV).

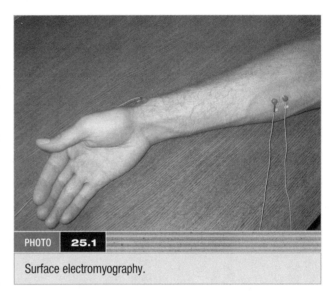

PHOTO 25.1

Surface electromyography.

Examination of the patterns of SEMG amplitude responses can provide information about various aspects of muscle function. In this laboratory, SEMG is used to examine the relationship between muscle activation and force production and also to examine the effect of fatigue on muscle activation.

The Muscle Activation Versus Force Production Relationship

The amplitude of the SEMG signal represents muscle activation. Thus, this section of the laboratory will determine the relationship between SEMG voltage and force. During isometric muscle actions, force production is modulated by motor unit recruitment and rate coding (changes in the firing rates of activated motor units). Increases in force are associated with the recruitment of additional motor units and increases in firing rates. Together, these factors result in increased muscle activation and, therefore, increased SEMG amplitude (see figure 25.1).

Under various conditions, the positive relationship between SEMG amplitude and force can be linear or curvilinear. In either case, however, increases in force are associated with greater muscle activation due to increases in motor unit recruitment and firing rates.

The Effect of Fatigue on Muscle Activation

During a submaximal fatiguing task, the amplitude of the SEMG signal increases with time, even though force remains stable. As fatigue progresses, the initial motor units recruited become fatigued and can no longer contribute to force

FIGURE 25.1 The positive relationship between SEMG amplitude and force can be linear or curvilinear.

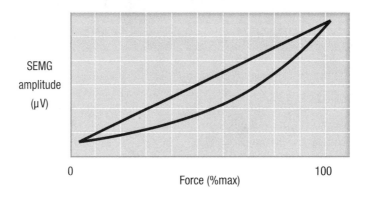

production. To maintain the force, additional motor units are recruited, and/ or there are increases in the firing rates of the initially activated motor units. The recruitment of additional motor units, added to those initially recruited (plus the increases in firing rates), leads to an increase in muscle activation and SEMG amplitude. Although the initially recruited motor units may not contribute to force production due to fatigue, their action potentials are still recorded by the surface electrodes and contribute to the amplitude of the SEMG signal. The change in muscle activation that accompanies fatigue can be described by comparing the SEMG amplitude with the time relationship during a continuous isometric muscle action.

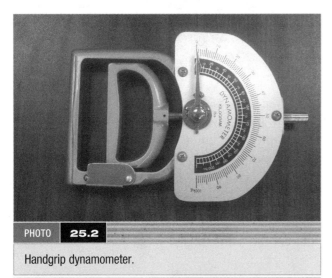

PHOTO **25.2**

Handgrip dynamometer.

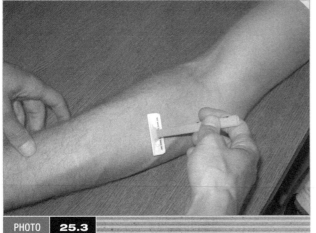

PHOTO **25.3**

Shaving the area to prepare for SEMG.

KNOW THESE TERMS & ABBREVIATIONS

○ MVIC = maximal, voluntary isometric contraction

○ SEMG = surface electromyography

PROCEDURES
For Determining the Relationship Between SEMG Amplitude and Force

The procedures in this laboratory will utilize a bipolar (two electrodes placed over the muscle and one reference electrode placed over a boney structure) SEMG electrode arrangement (see photo 25.1). Isometric force will be measured using a handgrip dynamometer (see photo 25.2). The SEMG amplitude and force data can be recorded on worksheet 25.1 (p. 199).

1. Before the electrodes are attached, the skin's surface must be prepared to remove hair and oils

that may affect the recording of the SEMG signal. This is accomplished by shaving the area and cleansing with an alcohol swab (see photos 25.3 and 25.4). In this laboratory, an area of the right forearm over the flexor digitorum superficialis muscle will be the site of placement for the active electrodes. The reference electrode will be placed over the lateral styloid process of the radius bone (see photo 25.1 and table 25.1, number 3 for specific instructions).

2. Because the voltages (μV) associated with the SEMG signal are so small, they are routinely amplified using a differential amplifier (see table 25.1, number 10). Conceptually, a differential amplifier subtracts the voltage recorded at one of the active electrodes from the voltage recorded at the other active electrode, compares this value to the voltage recorded at the reference electrode (theoretically zero μV), and then amplifies the difference scores.

3. Once the electrodes are in place, the subject's maximal, voluntary isometric contraction (MVIC) strength is measured. The subject will hold the handgrip dynamometer in the right hand with the palm up and the elbow at approximately 90° (see photo 25.5). MVIC will be determined by squeezing the handgrip dynamometer maximally for 3 seconds. The SEMG signal is recorded simultaneously with the 3-second MVIC. The MVIC is repeated, and the highest strength value (expressed in kg of force)

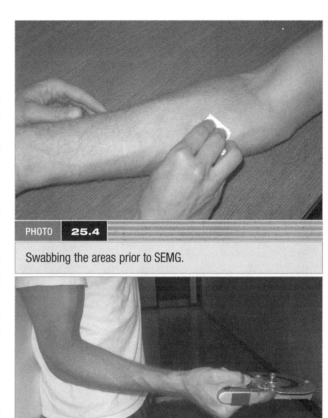

PHOTO **25.4**

Swabbing the areas prior to SEMG.

PHOTO **25.5**

Use of hand dynamometer.

Technical SEMG recommendations. TABLE 25.1

1. Electrodes: silver/silver chloride with conducting gel (see photo 25.6)

2. Electrode arrangement: bipolar, surface arrangement (see photo 25.1)

3. Electrode placement: a. active electrodes over the right flexor digitorum superficialis muscle, parallel to the long axis of the radius bone (see photo 25.1)

 b. reference electrode over the lateral styloid process of the radius bone (see photo 25.1)

4. Skin preparation: shave area and cleanse with alcohol swab

5. Interelectrode distance: 20 mm

6. Sampling frequency: 1,000 Hz

7. Bandpass filter: 10–500 Hz

8. Signal selection: middle 1 second of the 3-second signal

9. SEMG amplitude (μV): root mean square (RMS) or time averaged, integrated value

10. Signal amplification: differential amplification 1,000 times

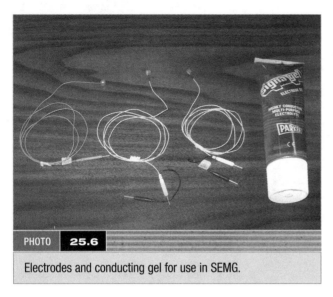

PHOTO **25.6**

Electrodes and conducting gel for use in SEMG.

is used as the subject's MVIC. The corresponding SEMG signal from the highest MVIC repetition is selected for analysis. Figure 25.2 includes an example of a raw SEMG signal recorded during a 3-second MVIC and the portion of the SEMG signal selected for analysis.

4. The middle 1 second of the SEMG signal is selected for determination of the amplitude (see figure 25.2). After filtering the signal, the amplitude will be expressed as RMS or time-averaged, integrated value in µV (see table 25.1, number 7 and number 9).

5. Calculate 25%, 50%, and 75% of MVIC force.

6. In random order, perform 3-second muscle actions at 25%, 50%, and 75% of MVIC. Collect the SEMG signal during each muscle action.

7. Select the middle 1 second of the 3-second signal at each level of force production, filter the signals with a bandpass filter (10–500 Hz), and determine the RMS or time-averaged, integrated amplitude values in µV.

FIGURE **25.2** Raw SEMG signal recorded during a 3-second MVIC. The portion of the SEMG signal between the dashed vertical lines was selected for analysis.

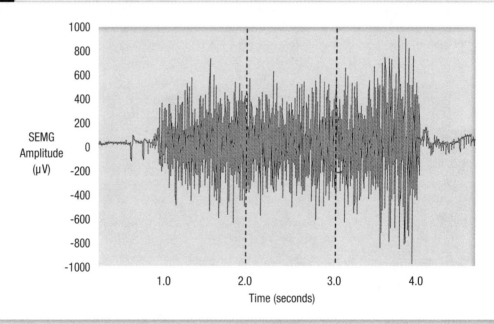

8. Record and plot the SEMG amplitude (µV) and isometric force (kg) data on worksheet 25.1 (p. 199). (See an example of a completed worksheet 25.1 on p. 198.)

For Determining the Relationship Between SEMG Amplitude and Time During a Submaximal, Fatiguing Isometric Muscle Action

This section of the laboratory will utilize the same SEMG signal acquisition and analysis procedures used in the earlier "Procedures" section (see table 25.1).

1. After skin preparation and electrode placement, the subject squeezes the handgrip dynamometer (palm up and elbow at 90°) continuously at 50% MVIC for 1 minute or as long as possible if 1 minute cannot be completed.

2. Samples of the SEMG signal are recorded every 5 seconds, and 1-second samples are selected for the amplitude analyses.

3. Each 1-second sample is bandpass filtered (10–500 Hz), and the amplitude (µV) is determined.

4. Record the SEMG amplitude (µV) data on worksheet 25.1. (See also an example of a completed worksheet 25.1 on the following page.) The isometric force values should be constant at 50% MVIC for each SEMG sample. If isometric force decreases across time, use only those SEMG samples that were recorded with the isometric force maintained at 50% MVIC.

5. Plot the SEMG amplitude–time relationship on worksheet 25.1.

Worksheet 25.1 EXAMPLE: SEMG RECORDING SHEET

Name Example   *Date* Today

1. SEMG amplitude–isometric force relationship

   MVIC trial 1 = _____55_____ kg   MVIC trial 2 = _____60_____ kg

   25% MVIC = _____15_____ kg   SEMG amplitude = _____55_____ µV

   50% MVIC = _____30_____ kg   SEMG amplitude = _____110_____ µV

   75% MVIC = _____45_____ kg   SEMG amplitude = _____145_____ µV

   100% MVIC = _____60_____ kg   SEMG amplitude = _____200_____ µV

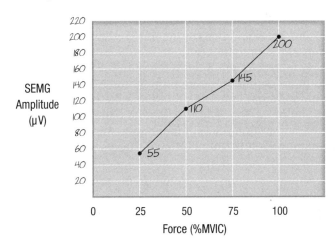

SEMG Amplitude (µV) vs Force (%MVIC)

2. SEMG amplitude–time relationship

   50% MVIC = _____30_____ kg

   SEMG amplitude (µV)

   Second 5 = _____112_____

   10 = _____118_____

   15 = _____121_____

   20 = _____125_____

   25 = _____130_____

   30 = _____133_____

   35 = _____138_____

   40 = _____141_____

   45 = _____144_____

   50 = _____149_____

   55 = _____152_____

   60 = _____157_____

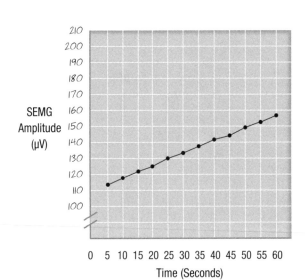

SEMG Amplitude (µV) vs Time (Seconds)

SEMG RECORDING SHEET   Worksheet **25.1**

Name _____   *Date* _____

1. SEMG amplitude–isometric force relationship

   MVIC trial 1 = _____ kg   MVIC trial 2 = _____ kg

   25% MVIC = _____ kg   SEMG amplitude = _____ μV

   50% MVIC = _____ kg   SEMG amplitude = _____ μV

   75% MVIC = _____ kg   SEMG amplitude = _____ μV

   100% MVIC = _____ kg   SEMG amplitude = _____ μV

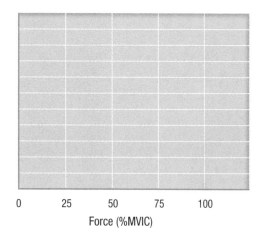

SEMG Amplitude (μV)

0   25   50   75   100

Force (%MVIC)

2. SEMG amplitude–time relationship

   50% MVIC = _____ kg

   SEMG amplitude (μV)

   Second 5 = _____

   10 = _____

   15 = _____

   20 = _____

   25 = _____

   30 = _____

   35 = _____

   40 = _____

   45 = _____

   50 = _____

   55 = _____

   60 = _____

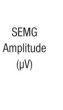
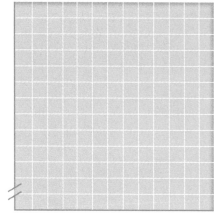

SEMG Amplitude (μV)

0 5 10 15 20 25 30 35 40 45 50 55 60

Time (Seconds)

Worksheet 25.2   EXTENSION ACTIVITIES

Name _____   *Date* _____

1. The following are randomly ordered SEMG amplitude values (μV) recorded during a fatiguing isometric muscle action. Given the typical pattern for the SEMG amplitude–time relationship, list the following values in the likely order associated with the appropriate time value:

   260, 140, 370, 180, 400, 60, 300, 220.

Time (seconds)	SEMG amplitude (μV)
5	_____
10	_____
15	_____
20	_____
25	_____
30	_____
35	_____
40	_____

2. Graph the relationship between SEMG amplitude and isometric force below.

   SEMG
   Amplitude
   (μV)

   0   100

   Force (%MVIC)

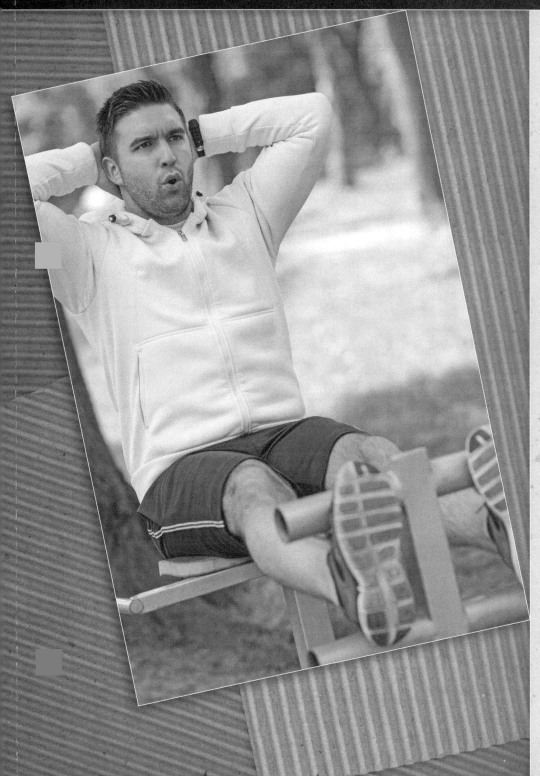

Unit 5

MUSCULAR ENDURANCE

1-Minute Sit-up Test of Muscular Endurance

BACKGROUND

Muscular endurance describes the ability to perform repeated muscle actions.[1,2,3,4] Muscular endurance is an important component of physical fitness, because most activities of daily living, as well as sporting activities, require multiple submaximal muscle actions. For example, household activities such as gardening, lawn mowing, shoveling snow, and vacuuming require repeated actions that often utilize the same muscles. Furthermore, although success in some sports, such as power lifting and Olympic lifting, is based on the ability to perform a single, maximal muscle action, most sports, such as rowing, swimming, cross-country skiing, bicycling, wrestling, boxing, sprinting, baseball pitching, and many others, involve repeated muscle actions. Thus, although muscular strength and muscular endurance are typically related, they involve the assessment of separate components of physical fitness.

The 1-Minute Sit-up Test is commonly used to assess the endurance of the abdominal muscles. Poor abdominal muscle endurance (as well as strength) is often thought to contribute to low back pain.[1] Thus, the 1-Minute Sit-up Test can provide valuable information about the potential risk of developing low back pain.

In this laboratory, you will learn to conduct the 1-Minute Sit-up Test of muscular endurance and to compare the results of the test to the norms in tables 26.1 and 26.2 to classify the subject based on age and gender.[2]

KNOW THESE TERMS & ABBREVIATIONS

○ muscular endurance = the ability to perform repeated muscle actions

---

TABLE	26.1	Male norms for the 1-Minute Sit-Up Test (number of correctly performed sit-ups).[2,3]

Classification	Age (years)					
	18–25	26–35	36–45	46–55	56–65	66+
Excellent	60–50	55–46	50–42	50–36	42–32	40–29
Good	48–45	45–41	40–36	33–29	29–26	26–22
Above average	42–40	38–36	34–30	28–25	24–21	21–20
Average	38–36	34–32	29–28	24–22	20–17	18–16
Below average	34–32	30–29	26–24	21–18	16–13	14–12
Poor	30–26	28–24	22–18	17–13	12–9	10–8
Very poor	24–12	21–6	16–4	12–4	8–2	6–2

	Age (years)					
Classification	18–25	26–35	36–45	46–55	56–65	66+
Excellent	55–44	54–40	50–34	42–28	38–25	36–24
Good	41–37	37–33	30–27	25–22	21–18	22–18
Above average	36–33	32–29	26–24	21–18	17–13	16–14
Average	32–29	28–25	22–20	17–14	12–10	13–11
Below average	28–25	24–21	18–16	13–10	9–7	10–6
Poor	24–20	20–16	14–10	9–6	6–4	4–2
Very poor	17–4	12–1	6–1	4–0	2–0	1–0

Female norms for the 1-Minute Sit-Up Test (number of correctly performed sit-ups).[2,3]   **TABLE**   **26.2**

○ muscular strength = the maximal force that can be exerted by a specific muscle or muscle group

PROCEDURES[2,3]

1. Have the subject lie on his or her back, with knees bent, feet flat on the floor, and fingers next to the ears. The subject's heels should be approximately 18 inches from the buttocks (photo 26.1). Have a partner hold the subject's feet firmly on the floor for stability.[2,3]

2. The subject should touch each elbow to the opposite knee, alternately, and perform as many sit-ups as possible in 1 minute (photo 26.2). The partner should count the number of sit-ups correctly performed during the test.[2,3]

3. Record the number of correctly performed sit-ups on worksheet 26.1.

Sample Classification

Gender: _Female_

Age: _37 years_

Number of sit-ups in 1 minute: _36_

Classification (see table 26.2): _excellent_

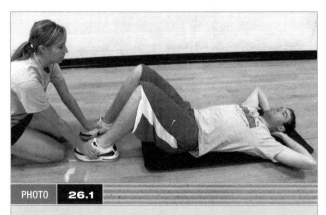

PHOTO **26.1**

Sit-up test. The subject's heels should be approximately 18 inches from the buttocks.

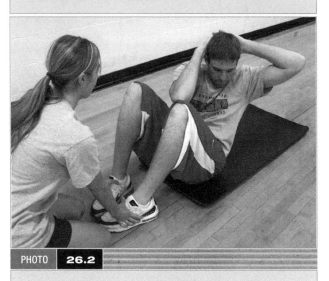

PHOTO **26.2**

Sit-up test. A partner holds the subject's feet firmly on the floor while the subject touches each elbow to the opposite knee.

Worksheet 26.1 THE 1-MINUTE SIT-UP TEST FORM

Name _____ Date _____

Gender: _____

Age: _____

1. Number of correctly performed sit-ups = _____

2. Classification = _____ (see tables 26.1 and 26.2)

Worksheet 26.2 EXTENSION ACTIVITIES

Name _____ Date _____

1. Given the following data, classify the results of a 1-Minute Sit-up Test.

   Gender: _____Female_____

   Age: ___26 years___

   Number of sit-ups in 1 minute: _____29_____

   Classification = _____ (see table 26.2).

2. Given the following data, classify the results of a 1-Minute Sit-up Test.

   Gender: _____Male_____

   Age: ___20 years___

   Number of sit-ups in 1 minute: _____33_____

   Classification = _____ (see table 26.1).

EXTENSION QUESTIONS

1. What are some common mistakes that may occur in administering this lab?

2. Identify possible sources of error in this lab.

3. Assess the practicality of using this lab in the field.

4. Research the reliability and/or validity of this lab using online resources, journal articles, and other credible sources.

REFERENCES

1. American College of Sports Medicine. *ACSM's Guidelines for Exercise Testing and Prescription,* 9th edition. Baltimore: Wolters Kluwer/Lippincott Williams & Wilkins, 2014.

2. Golding, L. A., Myers, C. R., and Sinning, W. E. *Y's Way to Physical Fitness,* 3rd edition. Champaign, IL: Human Kinetics, 1989, pp. 111–124.

3. Morrow, J. R., Jackson, A. W., Disch, J. G., and Mood, D. P. *Measurement and Evaluation in Human Performance,* 3rd edition. Champaign, IL: Human Kinetics, 2005, pp. 251–252.

4. Ryan, E. D., and Cramer, J. T. Fitness testing protocols and norms. In *NSCA's Essentials of Personal Training,* eds. R. W. Earle and T. K. Baechle, 2nd edition. Champaign, IL: Human Kinetics, 2004.

Lab 27

Push-up Test of Upper-Body Muscular Endurance

BACKGROUND

Muscular endurance, an important component of physical fitness, describes the ability to perform repeated muscle actions.[1,2,3] Muscular endurance contributes to our ability to accomplish many activities of daily living, such as gardening, lawn mowing, and shoveling snow. In addition, a number of sports, such as rowing, swimming, wrestling, and many others, require substantial muscular endurance to compete successfully.

The ability to perform repeated muscle actions is specific to the muscle group involved.[2] For example, depending on training status and/or the competitive sport, an individual may demonstrate considerable upper-body muscular endurance, but display less lower-body or abdominal muscular endurance. Thus, testing procedures are often designed to assess upper-body, lower-body, or abdominal muscular endurance.[1,2,3]

In this laboratory, you will learn to administer the Push-up Test of Upper-Body Muscular Endurance and to classify the subject based on age and gender.[1]

KNOW THESE TERMS & ABBREVIATIONS

- muscular endurance = the ability to perform repeated muscle actions

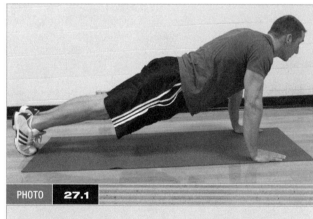

PHOTO **27.1**

Up position with arms fully extended and body straight. The hands should be pointed forward and approximately shoulder-width apart. Male subjects use the toes as the pivot point.

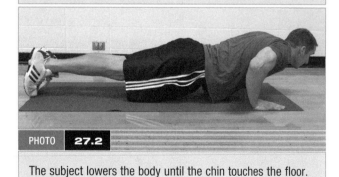

PHOTO **27.2**

The subject lowers the body until the chin touches the floor.

PROCEDURES[1,2] (see photos 27.1 to 27.4)

1. Have the subject begin in the up position with arms fully extended and body straight. The hands should be pointed forward and approximately shoulder-width apart (see photos 27.1 and 27.3). Male subjects use the toes as the pivot point. Female subjects should assume the "modified knee push-up" position with the knees bent and touching the floor (see photo 27.3).

2. The subject lowers his or her body until the chin touches the floor (see photos 27.2 and 27.4) and then returns to the up position by straightening the elbows.

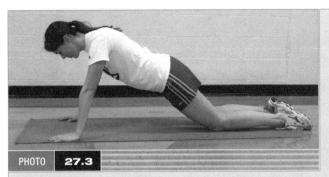

Up position with arms fully extended and body straight. The hands should be pointed forward and approximately shoulder-width apart. Female subjects should assume the "modified knee push-up" position with the knees bent and touching the floor.

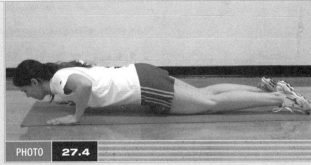

The subject lowers the body until the chin touches the floor.

3. A partner should count the number of push-ups performed correctly to exhaustion without stopping.
4. Record the number of correctly performed push-ups on worksheet 27.1.

Sample Classification

Gender: _____Male_____

Age: _23 years_

Number of consecutive push-ups to exhaustion: _____28_____

Classification (see table 27.1): _____good_____

Norms for the push-up test of upper body muscular endurance.[2] **TABLE** **27.1**

Category	Age (years)									
	20–29		30–39		40–49		50–59		60–69	
GENDER	MALE	FEMALE	MALE	FEMALE	MALE	FEMALE	MALE	FEMALE	MALE	FEMALE
Excellent	36	30	30	27	25	24	21	21	18	17
Very good	35	29	29	26	24	23	20	20	17	16
	29	21	22	20	17	15	13	11	11	12
Good	28	20	21	19	16	14	12	10	10	11
	22	15	17	13	13	11	10	7	8	5
Fair	21	14	16	12	12	10	9	6	7	4
	17	10	12	8	10	5	7	2	5	2
Needs improvement	16	9	11	7	9	4	6	1	4	1

Worksheet 27.1 | PUSH-UP TEST OF UPPER-BODY MUSCULAR ENDURANCE FORM

Name _____ Date _____

Gender: _____

Age: _____

1. Number of consecutive push-ups = _____

2. Classification = _____ (see table 27.1)

Worksheet 27.2 | EXTENSION ACTIVITIES

Name _____ Date _____

1. Given the following data, classify the results of a Push-up Test of Upper-Body Muscular Endurance.

   Gender: _____Male_____

   Age: __34 years__

   Number of consecutive push-ups: _____18_____

   Classification = _____ (see table 27.1)

2. Given the following data, classify the results of a Push-up Test of Upper-Body Muscular Endurance.

   Gender: ____Female____

   Age: __21 years__

   Number of consecutive push-ups: _____25_____

   Classification = _____ (see table 27.1)

EXTENSION QUESTIONS

1. What are some common mistakes that may occur in administering this lab?

2. Identify possible sources of error in this lab.

3. Assess the practicality of using this lab in the field.

4. Research the reliability and/or validity of this lab using online resources, journal articles, and other credible sources.

REFERENCES

1. American College of Sports Medicine. *ACSM's Guidelines for Exercise Testing and Prescription,* 9th edition. Baltimore: Wolters Kluwer/Lippincott Williams & Wilkins, 2014.

2. Hoffman, J. Norms for Fitness, Performance, and Health. Champaign, IL: Human Kinetics, 2006, pp. 41 and 196.

3. Ryan, E. D., and Cramer, J. T. Fitness testing protocols and norms. In *NSCA's Essentials of Personal Training,* eds. R. W. Earle and T. K. Baechle, 2nd edition. Champaign, IL: Human Kinetics, 2004.

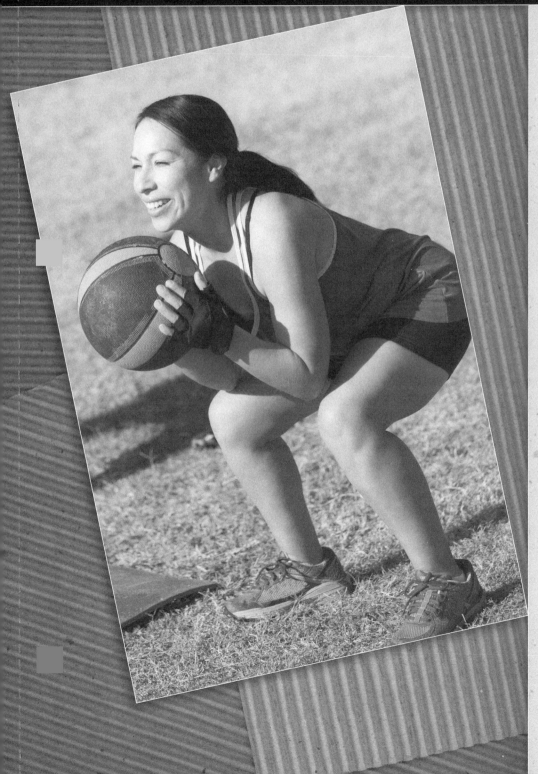

Unit 6

MUSCULAR POWER

BACKGROUND

Speed describes the ability to cover a specific distance as fast as possible. One of the most commonly used tests of speed is the 40-yard dash, and it is often included in a battery of tests for male and female athletes who compete in sports such as football, basketball, volleyball, and baseball.[1,2,3,4] Although it is likely that the original selection of 40 yards for this test was somewhat arbitrary, this distance has now become standard, and many coaches and athletes are familiar with the sprint times associated with this distance.[4]

In this laboratory, you will learn to perform and record the time for the 40-yard dash. You will also learn to estimate the approximate percentile rank associated with 40-yard dash times by gender and age, as well as compare 40-yard dash times with those of athletes in various sports.

KNOW THESE TERMS & ABBREVIATIONS

- ○ speed = the ability to cover a specific distance as fast as possible
- ○ percentile rank = in this lab, a score between 10% and 90% that shows how the subject performed relative to others in the age group. A percentile ranking of 70, for example, indicates that the subject can run the 40-yard dash faster than 70% of the others in the age group and slower than 30% of the others in the age group.

PROCEDURES[4] (see photos 28.1 and 28.2)

1. Typically, the 40-yard dash is performed on a track or football field, but any open area of sufficient size will work.

2. Mark off a distance of 40 yards using cones (on a field) or tape (on a track).

3. Have the subject warm up by jogging (and stretching if desired). After the initial warm-up, the subject should complete four to six intermittent sprints of approximately 10 to 20 yards at 80 to 100% of maximal speed.

4. Have the subject place one or two hands on the starting line of the 40-yard dash (for an example of a four-point stance, see photo 28.1). When ready, the subject starts running as fast as possible. The timer is located at the end line of the 40 yards and begins timing with a stopwatch when the subject's hands leave the starting line. The subject must run as fast as possible for the full 40 yards. The timer stops the stopwatch precisely when the subject crosses the end line (see photo 28.2).

5. The timer records the 40-yard dash time to the nearest 0.01 second on worksheet 28.1.

6. Repeat for a total of three trials and select the fastest time. The subject should rest for approximately 3 minutes (or more) between trials.

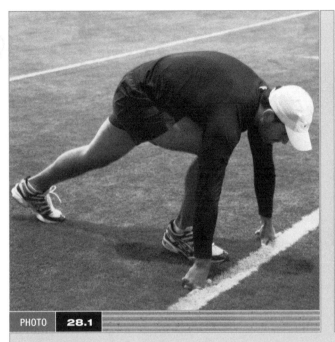

PHOTO **28.1**

Four-point stance at the starting line of the 40-yard dash.

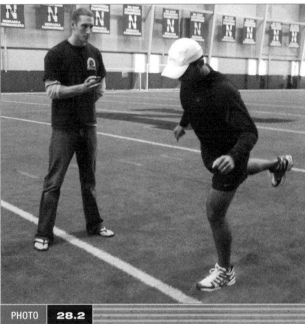

PHOTO **28.2**

Subject being timed as he crosses the finish line.

7. Table 28.1 provides the percentile ranks for 40-yard dash times in seconds for young males and females (12 to 18 years of age). For college-age subjects, use the percentile ranks in table 28.1 for 16- to 18-year-olds (even though the subject may be older than 18) for the appropriate gender. Table 28.2 provides mean 40-yard dash times in seconds for male and female athletes in selected sports.

Sample Calculation

Gender: *Male*

Age: *15 years*

40-yard dash time (to the nearest 0.01 second):

Trial 1	Trial 2	Trial 3
5.31	5.30	5.24

Fastest trial = _____ *5.24* _____ seconds

Approximate percentile rank = _____ *70* _____ (see table 28.1)

| TABLE | 28.1 | Percentile ranks for 40-yard dash times in seconds for young (age 12–18) males and females.[4] |

	Percentile rank					
	12–13 years		14–15 years		16–18 years	
	MALES	FEMALES	MALES	FEMALES	MALES	FEMALES
90	5.41	5.79	5.02	5.36	4.76	4.93
80	5.63	6.14	5.15	5.68	4.85	5.22
70	5.77	6.49	5.24	6.01	4.90	5.52
60	5.84	6.84	5.32	6.33	4.98	5.82
50	5.97	7.19	5.46	6.65	5.10	6.11
40	6.08	7.54	5.54	6.97	5.13	6.41
30	6.25	7.89	5.78	7.30	5.21	6.71
20	6.32	8.24	6.02	7.62	5.30	7.00
10	6.64	8.59	6.08	7.95	5.46	7.31

| TABLE | 28.2 | Mean (± SD) 40-yard dash times in seconds for male and female athletes in selected sports.[1,2,3,4] |

Sport	Gender	Age	$\bar{X} \pm SD$
American football	M	14–15 years	5.40 ± 0.53
American football	M	16–18 years	5.15 ± 0.45
American football	M	College (NCAA Division III)	4.99 ± 0.35
American football	M	College (NCAA Division II)	4.88 ± 0.30
American football	M	College (NCAA Division I)	4.74 ± 0.30
Basketball	M	College (NCAA Division I)	4.81 ± 0.26
Soccer	M	College (NCAA Division III)	4.73 ± 0.18
Ice hockey	F	8–16 years ($\bar{X} \pm SD$ = 12.2 ± 2.1 years)	7.19 ± 0.70
Soccer	F	College (NCAA Division III)	5.34 ± 0.17
Volleyball	F	College (NCAA Division I)	5.62 ± 0.24

Sample Calculations

Gender: _____Male_____

Body weight: ____70 kg____

Fat-free weight: ____63 kg____

Resistance = 0.075 × kg of body weight [BW] = 0.075 × 70 kg: ____5.25 kg____

Seconds	Resistance	×	6	×	Revolutions	=	Work (kgm • 5 sec⁻¹)
0–5	5.25	×	6	×	11	=	346.5
5–10	5.25	×	6	×	12	=	378.0
10–15	5.25	×	6	×	10	=	315.0
15–20	5.25	×	6	×	9	=	283.5
20–25	5.25	×	6	×	9	=	283.5
25–30	5.25	×	6	×	8	=	252.0
0–30	5.25	×	6	×	59	=	1858.5 kgm • 30 sec⁻¹

peak power (PP) = 5.25 kg of resistance × 6 m × 12 revolutions
= 378.0 kgm • 5 sec⁻¹ × 12 = 4536.0 kgm • min⁻¹ / 6.12 = 741.2 watts (W)

   Percentile rank (see table 29.1) = approximately 64th percentile

PP / BW (W • kgBW⁻¹) = 741.2 / 70 = 10.6 W • kgBW⁻¹

   Percentile rank (see table 29.1) = approximately 85th percentile

PP / FFW (W • kgFFW⁻¹) = 741.2 / 63 = 11.8 W • kgFFW⁻¹

   Percentile rank (see table 29.1) = approximately 88th percentile

mean power (MP) = 5.25 kg of resistance × 6 m × 59 revolutions
= 1858.5 kgm • 30 sec⁻¹ × 2 = 3717 kgm • min⁻¹ / 6.12 = 607.4 W

   Percentile rank (see table 29.2) = approximately 76th percentile

MP / BW (W • kgBW⁻¹) = 607.4 / 70 = 8.7 W • kgBW⁻¹

   Percentile rank (see table 29.2) = approximately 96th percentile

MP / FFW (W • kgFFW⁻¹) = 607.4 / 63 = 9.6 W • kgFFW⁻¹

   Percentile rank (see table 29.2) = approximately 99th percentile

$$\text{fatigue index} = \frac{378.0 \text{ kgm} \cdot 5 \text{ sec}^{-1} - 252.0 \text{ kgm} \cdot 5 \text{ sec}^{-1}}{378.0 \text{ kgm} \cdot 5 \text{ sec}^{-1}} \times 100 = 33.33$$

   Percentile rank (see table 29.3) = approximately 34th percentile

   % fast-twitch muscle fibers = 33.33 − 19 / 0.5 = 28.66%

See table 29.4 for approximate average percentage of fast-twitch muscle fibers in non-athletes and athletes.

TABLE	29.1	Percentile norms and descriptive statistics for peak power of the Wingate Anaerobic Test.

Percentile Rank	Watts (W)		$W \cdot kgBW^{-1}$		$W \cdot kgFFW^{-1}$	
	MALE	FEMALE	MALE	FEMALE	MALE	FEMALE
95	866.9	602.1	11.08	9.32	12.26	11.87
90	821.8	560.0	10.89	9.02	11.96	11.47
85	807.1	529.6	10.59	8.92	11.67	11.28
80	776.7	526.6	10.39	8.83	11.47	10.79
75	767.9	517.8	10.39	8.63	11.38	10.69
70	757.1	505.0	10.20	8.53	11.28	10.39
65	744.3	493.3	10.00	8.34	11.08	10.30
60	720.8	479.5	9.80	8.14	10.79	10.10
55	706.1	463.9	9.51	7.85	10.30	9.90
50	689.4	449.1	9.22	7.65	10.20	9.61
45	677.6	447.2	9.02	7.16	10.10	9.41
40	670.8	432.5	8.92	6.96	10.00	8.92
35	661.9	417.8	8.63	6.96	9.90	8.83
30	656.1	399.1	8.53	6.86	9.51	8.73
25	646.3	396.2	8.34	6.77	9.32	8.43
20	617.8	375.6	8.24	6.57	9.12	8.34
15	594.3	361.9	7.45	6.37	8.53	8.04
10	569.8	353.0	7.06	5.98	8.04	7.75
5	530.5	329.5	6.57	5.69	7.45	6.86
M	699.5	454.5	9.18	7.61	10.18	9.54
SD	94.7	81.3	1.43	1.24	1.46	1.51
Maximum	926.7	622.7	11.90	10.64	12.96	12.90
Minimum	500.1	239.3	5.31	4.58	6.55	5.20

Note: BW = body weight, FFW = fat-free weight

Reprinted with permission from *Research Quarterly for Exercise and Sport,* Vol. 60, No. 2, pp. 144–151. Reprinted by permission of the Society of Health and Physical Educators, www.shapeamerica.org.

Percentile norms and descriptive statistics for mean power of the Wingate Anaerobic Test.   **TABLE   29.2**

Percentile Rank	Watts (W)		$W \cdot kgBW^{-1}$		$W \cdot kgFFW^{-1}$	
	MALE	FEMALE	MALE	FEMALE	MALE	FEMALE
95	676.6	483.0	8.63	7.52	9.30	9.43
90	661.8	469.9	8.24	7.31	9.03	9.01
85	630.5	437.0	8.09	7.08	8.88	8.88
80	617.9	419.4	8.01	6.95	8.80	8.76
75	604.3	413.5	7.96	6.93	8.70	8.68
70	600.0	409.7	7.91	6.77	8.63	8.52
65	591.7	402.2	7.70	6.65	8.50	8.32
60	576.8	391.4	7.59	6.59	8.44	8.18
55	574.5	386.0	7.46	6.51	8.24	8.13
50	564.6	381.1	7.44	6.39	8.21	7.93
45	552.8	376.9	7.26	6.20	8.14	7.86
40	547.6	366.9	7.14	6.15	8.04	7.70
35	534.6	360.5	7.08	6.13	7.95	7.57
30	529.7	353.2	7.00	6.03	7.80	7.46
25	520.6	346.8	6.79	5.94	7.64	7.32
20	496.1	336.5	6.59	5.71	7.46	7.11
15	484.6	320.3	6.39	5.56	7.28	7.03
10	470.9	306.1	5.98	5.25	6.83	6.83
5	453.2	286.5	5.56	5.07	6.49	6.70
M	562.7	380.8	7.28	6.35	8.11	7.96
SD	66.5	56.4	0.88	0.73	0.82	0.88
Minimum	441.3	235.4	4.63	4.53	5.72	5.12
Maximum	711.0	528.6	9.07	8.11	9.66	9.66

Note: BW = body weight, FFW = fat-free weight

Reprinted with permission from *Research Quarterly for Exercise and Sport,* Vol. 60, No. 2, pp. 144–151. Reprinted by permission of the Society of Health and Physical Educators, www.shapeamerica.org.

TABLE	29.3	Percentile norms and descriptive statistics for fatigue index.

Percentile Rank	Fatigue Index	
	MALE	FEMALE
95	55.01	48.05
90	51.69	47.33
85	47.40	44.25
80	46.67	43.57
75	44.98	42.19
70	43.51	40.33
65	41.93	39.04
60	39.92	38.21
55	39.48	36.69
50	38.39	35.15
45	36.77	34.36
40	35.04	33.70
35	34.07	30.70
30	31.09	28.74
25	30.23	28.11
20	29.55	26.45
15	26.86	25.00
10	23.18	25.00
5	20.77	19.65
M	37.67	35.05
SD	9.89	8.32
Minimum	14.71	17.86
Maximum	57.51	48.94

Note: N = Males 52, Females 50

Reprinted with permission from *Research Quarterly for Exercise and Sport,* Vol. 60, No. 2, pp. 144–151. Reprinted by permission of the Society of Health and Physical Educators, www.shapeamerica.org.

Approximate average percentage of fast-twitch and slow-twitch fibers in the thigh muscles of male and female non-athletes and athletes in various sports.

TABLE 29.4

Females	% fast-twitch	% slow-twitch
1. Non-athletes	50	50
2. 800 meter runners	40	60
3. Cross-country skiers	40	60
4. Cyclists	49	51
5. Shot-putters and discus throwers	50	50
6. Long jumpers and high jumpers	52	48
7. Javelin throwers	60	40
8. Sprinters	73	27
Males	**% fast-twitch**	**% slow-twitch**
1. Non-athletes	50	50
2. Marathon runners	18	82
3. Swimmers	26	74
4. Distance runners	30	70
5. Speed skaters	30	70
6. Cross-country skiers	37	63
7. Ice hockey players	40	60
8. Cyclists	43	57
9. Shot-putters and discus throwers	63	37
10. Sprinters and jumpers	64	26
11. 800-meter runners	54	46
12. Weight lifters	53	47
13. Javelin throwers	52	48
14. Triathletes	37	63

Adapted from: Bowers, R.W., and Fox, E.L. *Sports Physiology,* 3rd ed. Dubuque: Wm. C. Brown Publishers, 1988, pp. 128–129. McArdle, W.D., Katch, F.I., and Katch, V.L. *Exercise Physiology,* 4th ed. Baltimore: Williams and Wilkins, 1996, p. 333. Wilmore, J.H., and Castill, D.C. *Physiology of Sport and Exercise,* 2nd ed. Champaign: Human Kinetics, 1999, p. 45.

Worksheet 29.1 WINGATE TEST FORM

Name _____ Date _____

Body weight: _____ kg

Seconds	Resistance	×	6	×	Revolutions	=	Work (kgm • 5 sec^{-1})
0–5	_____	×	6	×	_____	=	_____
5–10	_____	×	6	×	_____	=	_____
10–15	_____	×	6	×	_____	=	_____
15–20	_____	×	6	×	_____	=	_____
20–25	_____	×	6	×	_____	=	_____
25–30	_____	×	6	×	_____	=	_____
0–30	_____	×	6	×	_____	=	_____ kgm • 30 sec^{-1}

Resistance ($0.075 \times$ kg of body weight [BW]) = _____ kg

Peak power = _____ kgm • 5 sec^{-1} × 12 / 6.12 = _____ watts

Percentile rank (table 29.1) = _____

Peak power/body weight (W • kgBW^{-1}, table 29.1) = _____

Percentile rank = _____

Peak power/fat-free weight (W • kgFFW^{-1}, table 29.1) = _____

Percentile rank = _____

Mean power = _____ kgm • 30 sec^{-1} × 2 / 6.12 = _____ watts

Percentile rank (table 29.2) = _____

Mean power/body weight (W • kgBW^{-1}, table 29.2) = _____

Percentile rank = _____

Mean power/fat-free weight (W • kgFFW^{-1}, table 29.2) = _____

Percentile rank = _____

Fatigue index _____

Percentile rank (table 29.3) = _____

% fast-twitch muscle fibers = _____

See table 29.4 for approximate average percentage of fast-twitch muscle fibers in non-athletes and athletes.

EXTENSION ACTIVITIES

Worksheet **29.2**

Name _____   Date _____

1. Mary has a fatigue index of 28.5. What is her percentile rank for her fatigue index? Provide a brief interpretation of her fatigue index based on her percentile rank.

2. The 40-yard dash is frequently used to assess football players. Which of the three anaerobic work indices would be best correlated with the 40-yard dash time? Why?

3. Frank Fastwitch (who weighs 175 lbs) performed a Wingate Test, and his results are presented below. Use 0.075 x BW (kg) to determine resistance. Round off resistance to the nearest 0.25 kg.

Seconds	Revolutions
0–5	10
5–10	10
10–15	8
15–20	7
20–25	5
25–30	4

Determine:

A. Peak power _____

B. Mean power _____

C. Fatigue index _____

D. Percent fast-twitch
   muscle fibers _____

4. Use your own data to calculate the following:

   a. *Peak Power:* Calculate peak power in kgm • 5 sec^{-1} and watts. Report and briefly interpret the absolute (watts) and relative (W • kgBW^{-1}) percentile ranks (table 29.1).

   b. *Mean Power:* Calculate mean power in kgm • 30 sec^{-1} and watts. Report and briefly interpret the absolute (watts) and relative (W • kgBW^{-1}) percentile ranks (table 29.2).

   c. *Fatigue Index:* Calculate fatigue index and report your percentile rank (table 29.3). What does this imply in terms of how you fatigue in comparison to the rest of the population?

   d. *Percent Fast-Twitch Muscle Fibers:* Use the fatigue index to estimate your percent fast-twitch muscle fibers. What athletic group in table 29.4 are you most similar to?

EXTENSION QUESTIONS

1. What are some common mistakes that may occur in administering this lab?

2. Identify possible sources of error in this lab.

3. Assess the practicality of using this lab in the field.

4. Research the reliability and/or validity of this lab using online resources, journal articles, and other credible sources.

REFERENCES

1. Bar-Or, O. The Wingate Anaerobic Test: An update on methodology, reliability, and validity. *Sports Med.* 4: 381–394, 1987.

2. Maud, P. J., and Schultz, B. B. Norms for the Wingate Anaerobic Test with comparison to another similar test. *Res. Q. Exerc. Sport* 60: 144–151, 1989.

Vertical Jump Test for Measuring Muscular Power of the Legs

BACKGROUND

The vertical jump is a commonly used test to assess muscular power of the legs.[1,2,3,4,5,6] Power is defined as (*force × distance*) / *time*. Thus, performing the vertical jump and producing great muscular power depend on the ability to produce a high level of force very rapidly. There are two primary ways to test the vertical jump: the squat jump and the countermovement jump. During the squat jump, the subject lowers into the squat position, pauses for a moment, and then jumps vertically as high as possible. During the countermovement jump, the subject starts from a standing position, descends rapidly into a squat position, and then, without stopping at the bottom of the squat, performs a maximal vertical jump. The countermovement jump results in jump heights that are approximately 2 to 4 cm higher than the squat jump.[1] This occurs because there is a rapid transition from the descent (eccentric phase) to the ascent (concentric phase) of the movement. The squat jump, however, tends to result in more reliable scores, presumably due to the variability associated with the countermovement. In addition, muscular power of the legs is more accurately estimated using the squat jump than the countermovement jump.[5]

It is not necessary to use advanced equipment such as a force plate or Vertec device to determine vertical jump height. Vertical jump height can be measured simply by placing chalk on the fingertips of the subject, then having the subject jump next to a wall and touch the wall at the top of the jump. Vertical jump height is measured as the difference between the height of the chalk mark at the level of the highest jump and the height of a chalk mark made while standing with the arm fully extended overhead.

Power output cannot be measured directly from jump height alone, but for the squat jump technique, it can be estimated for both males and females from vertical jump height and body weight using the following regression equation of Sayers et al.:[5]

muscular power (watts) = (60.7 × vertical jump height (cm))
+ (45.3 × body weight (kg))
− 2055.

multiple correlation coefficient (R) = 0.94
standard error of estimate (SEE) = 372.9 watts

In addition, a nomogram has been developed[3] from the equation of Sayers et al.[5] to simplify the estimation of muscular power.

In this laboratory, you will learn to administer the vertical jump test using the squat jump technique and calculate muscular power of the legs from vertical jump height and body weight using the equation of Sayers et al.[5] You will also learn to use the nomogram of Keir et al.[3] to estimate muscular power. You will then compare the subject's vertical jump height in cm and muscular power in watts to percentile rank norms based on age and gender (tables 30.1–30.4).

FIGURE 30.1 Nomogram for estimating muscular power in watts from vertical jump height and body weight.[3,5]

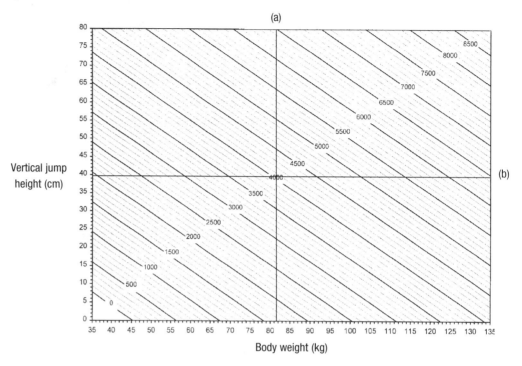

To estimate muscular power (watts) from the vertical jump height and body weight, first draw a vertical line (a) upward from the x-axis at a point equal to the subject's body weight (kg). Next, draw a horizontal line (b) to the right from the y-axis at a level equal to the subject's best vertical jump height (cm). Find the muscular power value (expressed in watts) that is closest to the intersection of the two lines.[3] For example, based on the data provided in the sample calculations (body weight = 81.6 kg and best vertical jump height = 40 cm), the estimated muscular power is approximately 4050 watts.

| Percentile ranks for vertical jump muscular power (watts) for males by age.[4] | | | | TABLE | 30.1 | |

Percentile rank	15–19	20–29	30–39	40–49	50–59	60–69
90	≥4978	≥5676	≥5602	≥5271	≥4841	≥4106
80	4643	5093	4859	4319	4018	3766
70	4506	4882	4685	3992	3703	3466
60	4184	4639	4388	3699	3566	3290
50	4049	4411	4222	3550	3342	3248
40	3857	4296	3966	3241	2937	2842
30	3678	4018	3750	3040	2747	2512
20	3322	3774	3484	2707	2511	2382
10	2908	3456	2764	2511	2080	1636
<10	<2908	<3456	<2764	<2511	<2080	<1636

Note: The percentile ranks in this table are for the squat jump technique.

| Percentile ranks for vertical jump muscular power (watts) for females by age.[4] | | | | TABLE | 30.2 | |

Percentile rank	15–19	20–29	30–39	40–49	50–59	60–69
90	≥3514	≥3667	≥3581	≥2989	≥2742	≥2604
80	3166	3249	3192	2674	2558	2474
70	2945	3007	2844	2503	2470	1779
60	2794	2803	2549	2287	2160	1717
50	2590	2628	2388	2157	1956	1465
40	2398	2477	2334	2100	1700	1316
30	2280	2374	2258	1824	1497	1262
20	2155	2270	2146	1687	1385	1197
10	1878	1971	1692	1330	1006	570
<10	<1878	<1971	<1692	<1330	<1006	<570

Note: The percentile ranks in this table are for the squat jump technique.

TABLE	30.3	Percentile ranks for vertical jump height (cm) for males by age.[4]

Percentile rank	15–19	20–29	30–39	40–49	50–59	60–69
90	≥57	≥60	≥54	≥51	≥47	≥34
80	55	57	51	42	40	32
70	53	55	48	38	36	30
60	50	53	45	35	34	28
50	47	50	42	33	30	26
40	45	47	39	31	27	24
30	43	44	36	29	24	22
20	41	41	30	25	17	17
10	38	38	23	21	10	12
<10	<38	<38	<23	<21	<10	<12

Note: The percentile ranks in this table are for the squat jump technique.

TABLE	30.4	Percentile ranks for vertical jump height (cm) for females by age.[4]

Percentile rank	15–19	20–29	30–39	40–49	50–59	60–69
90	≥41	≥40	≥37	≥32	≥26	≥20
80	39	37	35	30	24	18
70	37	35	33	28	22	16
60	35	33	31	26	20	14
50	33	30	29	24	18	12
40	31	28	27	22	15	10
30	29	26	25	20	12	8
20	27	24	23	17	9	6
10	25	19	19	14	5	3
<10	<25	<19	<19	<14	<5	<3

Note: The percentile ranks in this table are for the squat jump technique.

DETERMINATION OF VERTICAL JUMP HEIGHT AND MUSCULAR POWER

Name _____   Date _____

Gender: _____

Age: _____

Body weight: _____ kg

Height: _____ cm

Age: _____

standing reach height _____ cm

total jump height # 1 _____ cm

total jump height – standing reach height = vertical jump height

_____ cm – _____ cm = _____ cm

total jump height # 2 _____ cm

total jump height – standing reach height = vertical jump height

_____ cm – _____ cm = _____ cm

total jump height # 3 _____ cm

total jump height – standing reach height = vertical jump height

_____ cm – _____ cm = _____ cm

muscular power = (60.7 × _____ cm) + (45.3 × _____ kg) – 2055 = _____ watts

estimated muscular power from the nomogram (see figure 30.2) = _____ watts

percentile rank based on muscular power (see tables 30.1 and 30.2) _____ watts

percentile rank based on vertical jump height (see tables 30.3 and 30.4) _____ cm

FIGURE **30.2** Nomogram for estimating muscular power in watts from vertical jump height and body weight.[3,5]

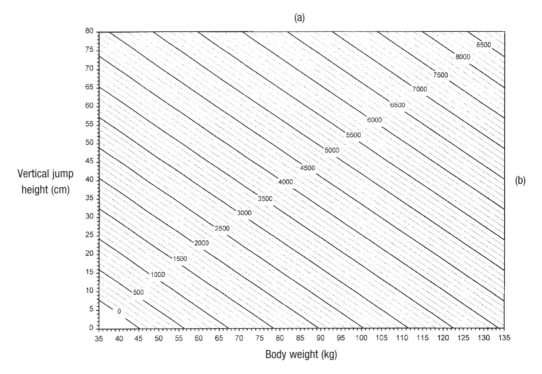

(a)

Vertical jump height (cm)

(b)

Body weight (kg)

To estimate muscular power (watts) from the vertical jump height and body weight, first draw a vertical line upward from the x-axis at a point equal to the subject's body weight (kg). Next, draw a horizontal line to the right from the y-axis at a level equal to the subject's best vertical jump height (cm). Find the muscular power value (expressed in watts) that is closest to the intersection of the two lines.[3]

Worksheet **30.2**

Name _____   Date _____

Gender: _Female_____

Age: _26 years_____

Body weight: _____54_____ kg

Vertical jump height: _____30_____ cm

muscular power = (60.7 × _____ cm) + (45.3 × _____ kg) – 2055 = _____ watts

estimated muscular power from the nomogram (see figure 21.2) = _____ watts

percentile rank based on muscular power (table 30.2) _____ watts

percentile rank based on vertical jump height (table 30.4) _____ cm

EXTENSION QUESTIONS

1. What are some common mistakes that may occur in administering this lab?

2. Identify possible sources of error in this lab.

3. Assess the practicality of using this lab in the field.

4. Research the reliability and/or validity of this lab using online resources, journal articles, and other credible sources.

REFERENCES

1. Bobbert, M. F., and Casius, J. R. Is the effect of a countermovement on jump height due to active state development? *Med. Sci. Sports Exerc.* 37: 440–446, 2005.

2. Burkett, L. N., Phillips, W. T., and Ziuraitis, J. The best warm up for the vertical jump in college-age athletic men. *J. Strength Cond. Res.* 19: 673–676, 2005.

3. Keir, P. J., Jamnik, V. K., and Gledhill, N. Technical-methodological report: A nomogram for peak leg power in the vertical jump. *J. Strength Cond. Res.* 17: 701–703, 2003.

4. Payne, N., Gledhill, N., Katzmarzyk, P. T., Jamnik, V. K., and Keir, J. P. Canadian musculoskeletal fitness norms. *Can. J. Appl. Physiol.* 25: 430–442, 2000.

5. Sayers, S. P., Harackiewicz, D. V., Harman, E. A., Frykman, P. N., and Rosenstein, M. T. Cross validation of three jump power equations. *Med. Sci. Sports Exerc.* 31: 572–577, 1999.

6. Stockbrugger, B. A., and Haennel, R. G. Contributing factors to performance of a medicine ball explosive power test: A comparison between jump and nonjump athletes. *J. Strength Cond. Res.* 17: 768–774, 2003.

Lab 31

BACKGROUND

The standing long jump is a test of muscular power (power = (force × distance) / time) of the legs and conceptually is similar to the vertical jump test. The standing long jump, however, involves jumping horizontally as far as possible, whereas the vertical jump test measures the height that the subject can jump. The standing long jump distance is highly correlated with other indices of muscular power, such as mean and peak power from the Wingate test (see Lab 29) and jumping height from the vertical jump test (see Lab 30).[2,6]

KNOW THESE TERMS & ABBREVIATIONS

- mean power = the total work performed (kgm • 30 sec^{-1}) during the 30-second Wingate test (see Lab 29)
- peak power = the greatest work performed (kgm • 5 sec^{-1}) during any 5-second period of the Wingate test (see Lab 29)
- power = (force × distance) / time

PROCEDURES

1. Have the subject perform a generalized warm-up.
2. Position the subject facing the starting line with feet parallel and shoulder-width apart (see photo 31.1).
3. Have the subject simultaneously drop into a squat position to a knee joint angle of about 90 degrees and thrust the arms backward behind the torso (see photo 31.2). A knee joint angle of 90 degrees allows force to be applied to the floor for a longer period of time than a knee joint angle of 45 degrees and, therefore, results in a jumping distance that is typically about 25 cm farther.[8] Many people appear to be less powerful than they really are in this test because they do not effectively coordinate the leg and arm motions. It is important for subjects to keep this in mind as they follow the procedures.
4. At the bottom of the squat (a knee joint angle of 90 degrees), have the subject rapidly transition to a jumping motion using both feet simultaneously. During the jumping motion, the subject should swing the arms and legs forward. Powerful arm swings can add 16–21% to the jumping distance.[1,7,8]
5. Have the subject land on both feet together simultaneously (see photo 31.3).

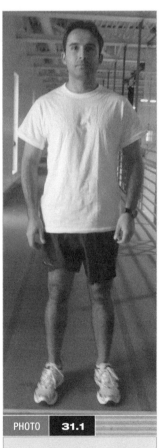

PHOTO **31.1**

Facing the starting line with feet parallel and shoulder-width apart.

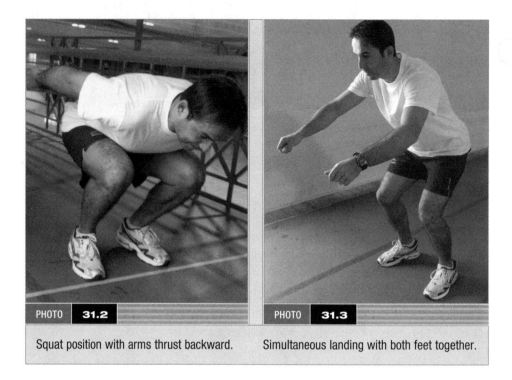

| PHOTO | 31.2 | | PHOTO | 31.3 |

Squat position with arms thrust backward. Simultaneous landing with both feet together.

6. Have the subject perform at least three practice standing long jumps and at least three recorded standing long jumps. The subject should continue the jumps as long as scores increase.

7. Record the jumping distance from the starting line to the more rearward of the two heels on worksheet 31.1.

8. Discard an attempt if the subject falls backward.

9. Compare the subject's best standing long jump distance in cm to the percentile rank norms in table 31.1 and the mean values for various samples in table 31.2.

| TABLE | 31.1 | Percentile ranks for the standing long jump distance (cm) for college age (17+ years of age) males and females.[3] |

Percentile rank	Males	Females
95	257	206
75	236	183
50	218	165
25	198	150
5	160	124

	TABLE 31.2
Age, height, body weight, and standing long jump distances (mean ± SD) for various athletic and non-athletic samples.	

Samples	Age (years)	Height (cm)	Body weight (kg)	Jump distance (cm)
Division 1 football players (all positions)[6]	21 ± 1	N/A	98.2 ± 16.4	268 ± 21
Division 1 football players (backs)[6]	21 ± 1	N/A	83.8 ± 6.1	284 ± 16
Division 1 football players (linebackers)[6]	21 ± 1	N/A	99.3 ± 3.9	271 ± 9
Division 1 football players (linemen)[6]	20 ± 1	N/A	117.0 ± 11.4	250 ± 19
Taiwanese college students (female)[8]	20 ± 1	160 ± 6	50.7 ± 10.8	93 ± 20
Untrained men[4]	31 ± 4	178 ± 6	75.0 ± 7.3	215 ± 23
Undergraduate kinesiology students (male)[5]	22 ± 3	179 ± 7	82.7 ± 15.5	227 ± 21

Sample Calculations

Gender: _Male_

Age: _21 years_

Standing Long Jump Distance #1 _191_ cm

Standing Long Jump Distance #2 _198_ cm

Standing Long Jump Distance #3 _202_ cm

Standing Long Jump Distance #4 _(204)_ cm

Standing Long Jump Distance #5 _200_ cm

Standing Long Jump Distance #6 _____ cm

Standing Long Jump Distance #7 _____ cm

Percentile rank = _32_ (see table 31.1)

Worksheet 31.1 STANDING LONG JUMP TEST

Name _____ *Date* _____

Gender: _____

Age: _____

Standing Long Jump Distance #1 _____ cm

Standing Long Jump Distance #2 _____ cm

Standing Long Jump Distance #3 _____ cm

Standing Long Jump Distance #4 _____ cm

Standing Long Jump Distance #5 _____ cm

Standing Long Jump Distance #6 _____ cm

Standing Long Jump Distance #7 _____ cm

Percentile rank = _____ (see table 31.1)

Worksheet 31.2 EXTENSION ACTIVITIES

Name _____ *Date* _____

1. On the blank graph below, draw the expected relationship between age and standing long jump distance.

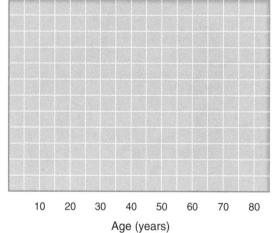

Standing long jump distance (cm)

Age (years)

2. Sally jumps 185 cm and John jumps 200 cm during the standing long jump test. Use table 31.1 to determine their approximate percentile ranks.

Sally: _____ percentile rank

John: _____ percentile rank

EXTENSION QUESTIONS

1. What are some common mistakes that may occur in administering this lab?

2. Identify possible sources of error in this lab.

3. Assess the practicality of using this lab in the field.

4. Research the reliability and/or validity of this lab using online resources, journal articles, and other credible sources.

REFERENCES

1. Ashby, B. M., and Heegaard, J. H. Role of arm motion in the standing long jump. *J. Biomech.* 35: 1631–1637, 2002.

2. Izquierdo, M., Aguado, X., Gonzalez, R., Lopez, J. L., and Hakkinen, K. Maximal and explosive force production capacity and balance performance in men of different ages. *Eur. J. Appl. Physiol.* 79: 260–267, 1999.

3. Johnson, B. L., and Nelson, J. K. *Practical Measurements for Evaluation in Physical Education.* Edina, MN: Burgess Publishing, 1986, p. 213.

4. Moriss, C. J., Tolfrey, K., and Coppack, R. J. Effects of short-term isokinetic training on standing long-jump performance in untrained men. *J. Strength Cond. Res.* 15: 498–502, 2001.

5. Murray, D. P., Brown, L. E., Zinder, S. M., Noffal, G. J., Bera, S. G., and Garrett, N. M. Effects of velocity-specific training on rate of velocity development, peak torque, and performance. *J. Strength Cond. Res.* 21: 870–874, 2007.

6. Seiler, S., Taylor, M., Diana, R., Layes, J., Newton, P., and Brown, B. Assessing anaerobic power in collegiate football players. *J. Appl. Sport Sci. Res.* 4: 9–15, 1990.

7. Wakai, M., and Linthorne, N. P. Optimum take-off angle in the standing long jump. *Human Move. Sci.* 24: 81–96, 2005.

8. Wu, W.-L., Wu, J.-H., Lin, H.-T., and Wang, G. J. Biomechanical analysis of the standing long jump. *Biomed. Eng.* 15: 186–192, 2003.

BACKGROUND

The backward, overhead medicine ball (BOMB) throw is a test of total body power. Both upper-body and lower-body power contribute to the distance the medicine ball can be thrown.[4] While the test is designed to assess total body power, to date there is no equation that can be used to estimate power output (expressed in watts) from the distance the medicine ball is thrown. Rather, it is assumed that longer distances are associated with greater muscular power output. Recent studies have shown that the distance the medicine ball is thrown is correlated with other indices of muscular power, such as the vertical jump.[2,3,4]

The BOMB throwing technique involves: (1) taking the medicine ball in both hands with the arms fully extended; (2) bending at the knees (squatting) until the ball reaches approximately the level of the knees; and (3) standing up quickly to throw the medicine ball backward over the top of the head as far as possible.[2] To maximize distance, the subject should perform the motion as fast as possible. The throwing motion is similar to a vertical jump and, in some cases, the subject may come off the ground when performing the test.

In this laboratory, you will learn to administer the BOMB throw test. You will then compare the distance the medicine ball is thrown to values for male and female athletes from various sports (table 32.1).

KNOW THESE TERMS & ABBREVIATIONS

- power = (force $\times$ distance) / time
- total body power = a combination of upper- and lower-body power ((force $\times$ distance) / time) output. Total body power is assessed using the distance that the medicine ball can be thrown.

TABLE 32.1	Data for the BOMB throw test for selected male and female athletes.

Athlete	Age (years)	Height (m)	Weight (kg)	Medicine ball weight (kg)	Throw distance (m)
Volleyball players (male and female)[3]	22.8 ± 3.7	N/A	75.7 ± 14.8	3	12.59 ± 3.31
Wrestlers (male)[4]	20.0 ± 2.9	1.74 ± 0.07	84.8 ± 25.3	3	14.2 ± 1.8
Volleyball players (male)[4]	18.9 ± 1.4	1.89 ± 0.07	82.3 ± 8.9	3	15.4 ± 1.1
Football players (male)[2]	20.6 ± 1.3	1.83 ± 5.6	102.8 ± 19.4	7	10.41 ± 1.45

Note: Values are mean ± standard deviation.

PROCEDURES[4]

1. Have the subject perform a generalized warm-up.

2. Position the subject facing away from the area where the medicine ball will be thrown (see photo 32.1).

3. Have the subject grasp the medicine ball with both hands, with arms extended and perpendicular to the ground (see photo 32.2).

4. Space the subject's heels slightly wider than the shoulders so the arms and medicine ball will have room to swing between the knees during the throw (see photo 32.2).

5. For each throw, have the subject rapidly descend into a squatting position. As the subject descends into the squatting position, the elbows should be kept extended. The ball should swing backward between the legs (see photo 32.3).

6. At the bottom of the squat, the subject should, without stopping, transition into the upward motion of the throw (photo 32.4). This upward motion is similar to that of a vertical jump, with the addition that the subject throws the medicine ball backward over the head. During the throw, the subject should try to keep the arms straight and use a "pendulum action" to maximize throwing distance.[3]

7. After each throw, measure the distance from between the subject's feet and the point where the medicine ball makes first contact with the ground or floor.

8. Repeat until three consecutive throws are within 0.50 meter of the best throw.[4] This will typically take up to six trials.[1] Provide at least 1 minute of rest between trials.[4] Record the distance of each throw on worksheet 32.1. The longest throw is selected as the subject's score.

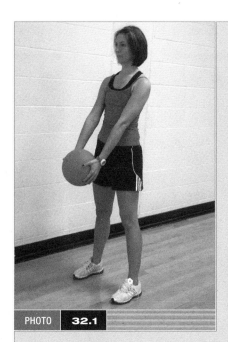

Starting position for the BOMB throw test.

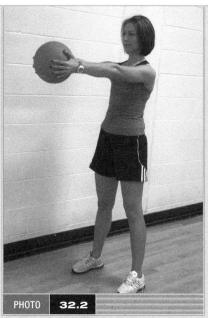

Grasping the medicine ball, with both hands extended and perpendicular to the ground.

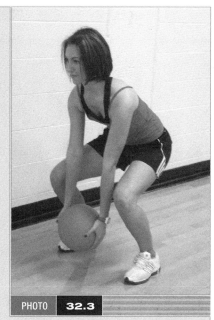

The subject in squatting position with the elbows extended.

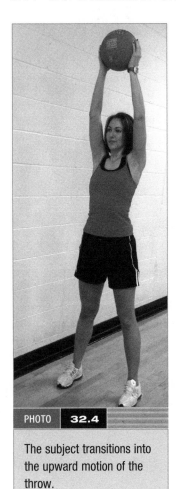

The subject transitions into the upward motion of the throw.

Sample Calculation

Gender: _____Male_____

Body weight: _____81.6_____ kg

Height: _____153_____ cm

Age: _____21 years_____

Throwing Distance #1 _____12.1_____ m

Throwing Distance #2 _____12.7_____ m

Throwing Distance #3 _____13.2_____ m

Throwing Distance #4 _____⟨13.4⟩_____ m

Throwing Distance #5 _____13.3_____ m

Throwing Distance #6 _____ m

BACKWARD OVERHEAD MEDICINE BALL THROW TEST

Worksheet **32.1**

Name _____   Date _____

Gender: _____

Body weight: _____ kg

Height: _____ cm

Age: _____ years

Throwing Distance #1 _____ m

Throwing Distance #2 _____ m

Throwing Distance #3 _____ m

Throwing Distance #4 _____ m

Throwing Distance #5 _____ m

Throwing Distance #6 _____ m

EXTENSION ACTIVITIES

Worksheet **32.2**

Name _____   Date _____

1. On the blank graph below, draw the expected relationship between the BOMB throw distance and vertical jump power in a sample of basketball players. Briefly explain your graph.

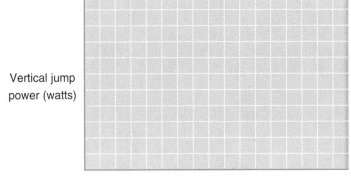

Vertical jump power (watts)

Throw distance (m)

2. Which of the following activities would most likely be correlated with the BOMB throw distance? Briefly explain your selection.

    a. maximal bench press strength

    b. 400-meter sprint time

    c. standing long jump

    d. pull-ups

EXTENSION QUESTIONS

1. What are some common mistakes that may occur in administering this lab?

2. Identify possible sources of error in this lab.

3. Assess the practicality of using this lab in the field.

4. Research the reliability and/or validity of this lab using online resources, journal articles, and other credible sources.

REFERENCES

1. Duncan, M. J., Al-Nakeeb, Y., and Nevill, A. M. Influence of familiarization on a backward, overhead medicine ball explosive power test. *Res. Sports Med.* 13: 345–352, 2005.

2. Mayhew, J. L., Bird, M., Cole, M. L., Koch, A. J., Jacques, J. A., Ware, J. S., Buford, B. N., and Fletcher, K. M. Comparison of the backward overhead medicine ball throw to power production in college football players. *J. Strength Cond. Res.* 19: 514–518, 2005.

3. Stockbrugger, B. A., and Haennel, R. G. Validity and reliability of a medicine ball explosive power test. *J. Strength Cond. Res.* 15: 431–438, 2001.

4. Stockbrugger, B. A., and Haennel, R. G. Contributing factors to performance of a medicine ball explosive power test: A comparison between jump and nonjump athletes. *J. Strength Cond. Res.* 17: 768–774, 2003.

Unit 7

BODY COMPOSITION AND BODY BUILD

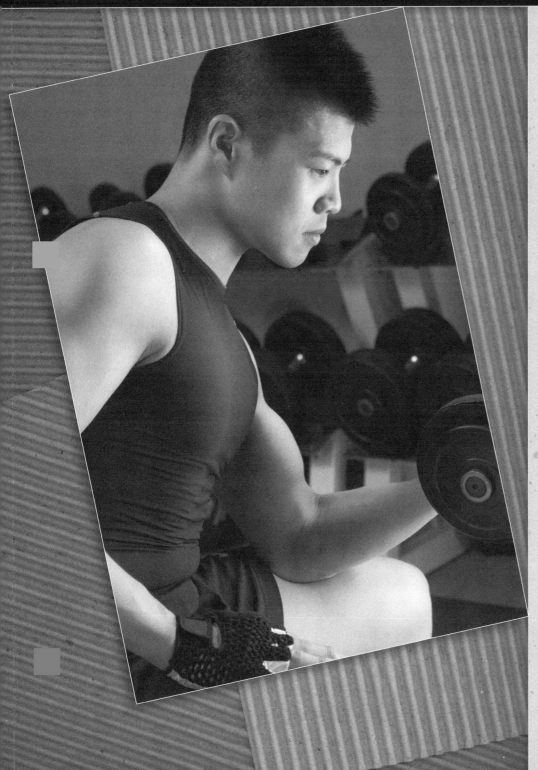

BACKGROUND

Underwater weighing is often considered the "gold standard" for determining the amounts of fat and fat-free tissues in a live human. Consequently, it serves as one of the principal means for assessment of body composition in many research studies, as well as a criterion technique in the development of field methods for estimating body composition such as skinfold equations.

Evaluation of body composition means determining the amount of fat and fat-free tissue comprising an individual's body. To facilitate procedures for this evaluation, the body is considered as a two-component system. The fat component of the body principally represents the lipid constituents of the body, chiefly found in adipose tissue and, to a much lesser extent, in neural tissue. Thus, the size of the fat component indicates the magnitude of adipose mass. The fat-free body component is made up of those tissues not represented by the fat component, such as muscle, bone, and internal organs. It is convenient to discriminate body tissues in this manner, since those comprising the fat component have a density of 0.90 kg $\bullet$ L^{-1}, while those tissues comprising the fat-free component have a density of 1.10 kg $\bullet$ L^{-1}. Muscle, bone, and organ tissue all have different densities. However, each normally represents a standard proportion of the fat-free component. Therefore, only one density value is used for this component.

Underwater weighing is an indirect method for determining body density and the amounts of the fat and fat-free components. Underwater, an individual weighs much less than on land. This is a reflection of Archimedes' Principle, which states that an object immersed in a fluid loses an amount of weight equivalent to the weight of the fluid displaced. Consequently, the difference between "dry" weight on land and underwater weight reflects the volume of water displaced, and this is equal to the individual's body volume. Therefore, underwater weighing actually allows us to determine body volume. Body density can then be determined by dividing "dry" weight (body weight) by body volume (density = weight / volume).

Since body density is the collective result of the amount of lower-density (fat component) and higher-density (fat-free component) tissues, theoretically we can determine the proportion to which each component contributes. Suppose we determine that an individual has a body density of 1.04 kg $\bullet$ L^{-1}. Mathematically we could determine that the fat component (density = 0.90 kg $\bullet$ L^{-1}) and the fat-free component (density = 1.10 kg $\bullet$ L^{-1}) account for 30% and 70% of the overall body density, respectively. The proportions to which the fat and fat-free components contribute to body volume would be the same as their respective contributions to body density. Given a body weight (dry) of 100 kg, the above body density (1.04 kg $\bullet$ L^{-1}) implies a body volume of 96.15 L. Therefore, 30% of this volume is fat (28.85 L) and 70% of it is fat-free (67.30 L). Based on the individual densities of these tissues, the resultant weight of fat would be 25.96 kg, and the fat-free weight would be 74.03 kg. This line of reasoning underlies the mathematical equations by which body density is converted to values of fat and fat-free weight.

Obesity indicates an excessive amount of body fat. The standard for obesity is 30% of body weight consisting of fat (% FAT) for males and females. Desirable levels are somewhat less than the above standards. For males it is desirable to be at 10 to 15 % FAT, while for females 15 to 20 % FAT may be desirable. For competitive athletes, even lower levels of body fatness may be consistent with optimal performance. Generally, the lowest healthy levels of body fatness are considered to be approximately 5 % FAT for adult males and 12 % FAT for adult females. Table 33.1 provides % FAT norms for adult athletes and non-athletes.

Overweightness indicates an excessive body weight compared with what is the standard body weight based on one's height, age, gender, and frame size. In many cases, overweightness may not indicate obesity and vice versa. Consequently, just knowing one's height and weight may not lend insight into the degree of obesity present. Frequently, we speak of weight reduction goals when what we really mean to refer to is fat reduction goals. After all, few people have a problem with excess amounts of fat-free tissue. Therefore, knowledge of one's fat weight can be most useful in evaluating the body structure and establishing any necessary goals for modifying levels of body fatness.

In this laboratory, we will further discuss and demonstrate the techniques of underwater weighing and determination of body composition. As a result, you should become familiar with the general procedures and the principles they are based on. Also, you should be able to interpret the results of body composition assessment and recommend any modification that may be indicated.

KNOW THESE TERMS & ABBREVIATIONS

- obesity = an excessive amount of body fat
- overweightness = an excessive body weight compared with the standard body weight based on an individual's height, weight, age, gender, and frame size
- RV = residual lung volume or the air left in the lungs following a maximal exhalation
- BW = body weight
- UWW = body weight while submerged under water or underwater weight
- % FAT = the percent body weight consisting of fat
- DBW = dry body weight
- VC = vital capacity
- BTPS = body temperature pressure saturated
- FW = fat weight (DBW × (% FAT / 100))
- FFW = fat-free weight (DBW – FW)
- DB = body density

PROCEDURES

To determine body composition, we must use three measures: RV, BW, and UWW. Record data on worksheet 33.1. RV must be determined so that its effects on body buoyancy can be accounted for when underwater weight is

TABLE	33.1	Percent body fat norms for adult athletes and non-athletes.

Non-Athletes[1]

FEMALES PERCENTILE	AGE					
	20–29	30–39	40–49	50–59	60–69	70–79
90	15.1	15.5	16.8	19.1	20.2	18.3
80	16.8	17.5	19.5	22.3	23.3	22.5
70	18.4	19.2	21.7	24.8	25.7	24.8
60	19.8	21.0	23.7	26.7	27.5	26.6
50	21.5	22.8	25.5	28.4	29.2	28.2
40	23.4	24.8	27.5	30.1	30.8	30.5
30	25.5	26.9	29.5	31.8	32.6	31.9
20	28.2	29.6	31.9	33.9	34.4	34.0
10	33.5	33.6	35.1	36.1	36.6	36.4

MALES PERCENTILE	AGE					
	20–29	30–39	40–49	50–59	60–69	70–79
90	7.9	12.4	15.0	17.0	18.1	17.5
80	10.5	14.9	17.5	19.4	20.2	20.1
70	12.6	16.8	19.3	21.0	21.7	21.6
60	14.8	18.4	20.8	22.3	23.0	22.9
50	16.6	20.0	22.1	23.6	24.2	24.1
40	18.6	21.6	23.5	24.9	25.6	25.3
30	20.7	23.2	24.9	26.3	27.0	26.5
20	23.3	25.1	26.6	28.1	28.8	28.4
10	26.6	27.8	29.2	30.6	31.2	30.7

Athletes[2]

SPORT	FEMALES	MALES
Basketball	20–27	7–11
Bicycling	15	8–10
Distance Running	10–19	6–13
Football	—	9–19
Gymnastics	10–17	5–10
Soccer	—	10
Softball	22	—
Sprinting	11–19	8–16
Swimming	14–24	9–12
Tennis	20	15–16
Volleyball	16–25	11–12

calculated. The air left in the lungs following a maximal exhalation (RV) will cause a person to float and incorrectly increase the estimated % FAT value.

I. Measurement of Vital Capacity
(see photos 33.1–33.3)

1. With the subject in a swimsuit, measure dry body weight (DBW) to the nearest 0.25 pound.

2. Apply a nose clip and have the subject sit, leaning slightly forward, in front of the spirometer.

3. Have the subject take several deep breaths and then, with the lungs filled maximally, seal the lips around the mouthpiece. From this position, have the subject blow as much air as possible into the spirometer with one long, forceful expiration (leaning forward to "squeeze out" as much air as possible), before removing the lips from the mouthpiece.

4. After a few moments to regain comfort, repeat the above step two more times, recording the volume expired each time (i.e., the vital capacity [VC]). Record the temperature of the air in the spirometer during the last trial.

II. Measurement of Underwater Weight
(see photos 33.4–33.7)

1. Strap the weight belt onto the subject and have the subject enter the tank and sit on the swing seat. Then have the subject remove any air that may be trapped in the swimsuit.

2. Have the subject grasp the swing, tuck the head underwater, empty the lungs (blow out all of the air), and then slowly count to 10 before raising the head back above the water. Repeat this 6 to 10 times, recording the weight each time after the subject has emptied the lungs and the scale reading has stabilized. Following six repetitions, further trials need be done only if weights from trial to trial continue to show large differences (>0.15 kg).

3. After the last trial, record water temperature. This will conclude the data collection.

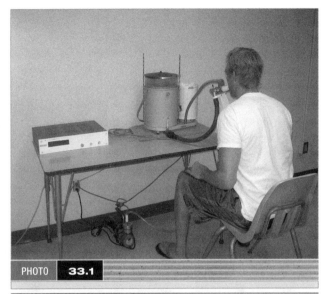

PHOTO **33.1**

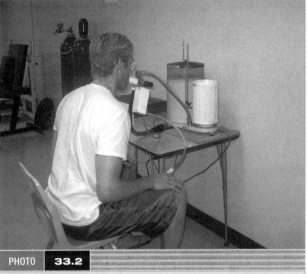

PHOTO **33.2**

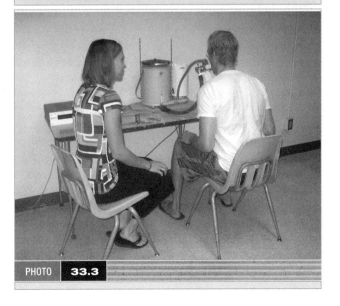

PHOTO **33.3**

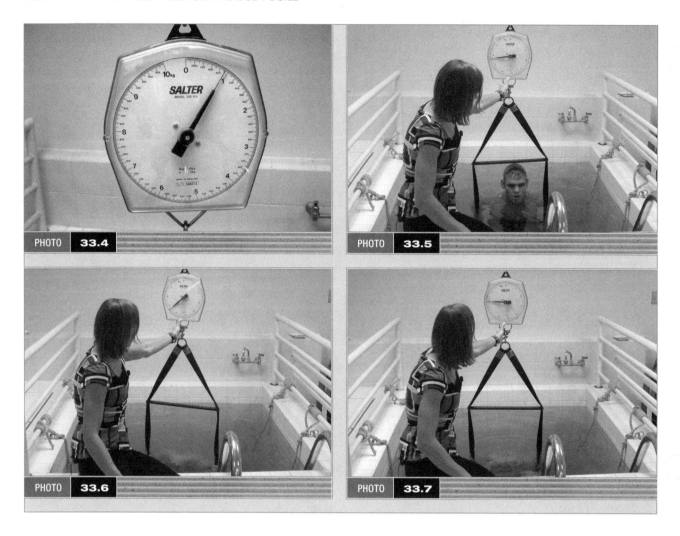

Sample Calculations

The following example demonstrates how data collected from the procedures described above can be used to calculate body composition characteristics. Follow the steps in the order shown:

1. Calculation of residual lung volume

a. Determine the BTPS (body temperature pressure saturated) correction factor from table 33.2, based on the recorded air temperature in the spirometer.

For instance, if air is 28° C, BTPS = 1.057

b. Select the highest of the three VC values and correct it for BTPS.

$$VC_{BTPS} = (VC \times BTPS)$$
Example: $VC_{BTPS} = (4.35\ L \times 1.057) = 4.598\ L$

c. Estimate RV based on:

$$RV = (VC_{BTPS} \times 0.24)\ \text{for males}$$
  or
$$RV = (VC_{BTPS} \times 0.28)\ \text{for females}$$
Example: (assume previous VC data was for a female)
$$RV = (4.598 \times 0.28) = 1.287\ L$$

VC Air Temp	BTPS
23° C	1.085
24° C	1.080
25° C	1.075
26° C	1.068
27° C	1.063
28° C	1.057
29° C	1.051
30° C	1.045

BTPS correction factors for air temperature.   **TABLE   33.2**

2. Calculation of body composition

a. Convert dry body weight (DBW) from pounds to kilograms by dividing by 2.2046.

   Example: (127.5 lbs / 2.2046) = 57.834 kg

b. Determine underwater weight (UWW) based on the average of the three "heaviest" trials.

c. Correct for the weight of the apparatus (swing seat, chains, and weight belt) to derive the true underwater weight (TUWW) of the subject. The weight of the apparatus is called tare weight.

   Example: If the average UWW of the best trials is 7.833 kg and the tare weighs 4.91 kg, TUWW = (7.833 − 4.91) = 2.923 kg

d. Determine water density (DH_2O) from water temperature using table 33.3.

   Example: If H_2O temp = 33° C, then DH_2O = 0.99471

e. Calculate body volume (BV) from DBW, TUWW, water density (DH_2O), and RV, as well as a constant of 0.1 L, which is an estimate of the air in the digestive tract based on:

   BV = (((((DBW − TUWW) / DH_2O) − RV) − 0.1)

   Example: BV = (((((57.834 − 2.923) / 0.99471) − 1.287) − 0.1) = 53.816L

f. Calculate body density (DB) from DBW and BV based on:

   DB = (DBW / BV)

   Example: DB = (57.834 / 53.816) = 1.0747 kg • L^{-1}

g. Convert body density to % FAT using the following standard formula:

   % FAT = (((4.57 / DB) − 4.142) × 100)

   Example: % FAT = (((4.57 / 1.0747) − 4.142) × 100) = 11.0%

TABLE	33.3	Density of water at various temperatures.

H$_2$O Temp	H$_2$O Density
25° C	0.99707
26° C	0.99681
27° C	0.99654
28° C	0.99626
29° C	0.99597
30° C	0.99567
31° C	0.99537
32° C	0.99505
33° C	0.99471
34° C	0.99438
35° C	0.99404
36° C	0.99369
37° C	0.99333

h. Calculate fat weight (FW) and fat-free weight (FFW) using the following calculations:

FW = (DBW × (% FAT / 100))

Example: FW = (57.834 × (11.0 / 100)) = 6.362 kg

FFW = (DBW − FW)

Example: FFW = (57.834 − 6.362) = 51.472 kg

3. Setting body weight goal

If current body composition is to be used as the basis for setting a body weight goal corresponding to a target value for a new % FAT level, base this on the following:

a. Select a target value for the % FAT level you want to achieve.

Example: Currently at 11 % FAT, and the goal is 10 % FAT.

b. Using the target value for % FAT and the current value for FFW, calculate the BW goal as follows:

BW goal = FFW / (1 − (TARGET % FAT / 100))

Example: BW goal = 51.472 / (1 − (10 / 100)) = 57.191 kg

Thus, at 10 % FAT, this subject would weigh 57.191 kg and would need to lose 0.643 kg of body weight to reach this goal (assuming all of the weight lost was from FW).

UNDERWATER WEIGHING LABORATORY DATA

Worksheet **33.1**

Age _____   *Gender* _____

I. Residual Volume Determination

Dry body weight, DBW = _____

Vital Capacity (L):   1. _____

2. _____

3. _____

Air Temperature (°C) _____   BTPS Correction Factor (table 33.2) _____

$VC_{BTPS} = VC \times BTPS =$ _____ $\times$ _____ = _____ L

Male RV = $0.24 \times VC_{BTPS}$ _____ = _____ L

Female RV = $0.28 \times VC_{BTPS}$ _____ = _____ L

II. Underwater Weighing

Underwater Weighing Trials (kg)

1. _____   6. _____

2. _____   7. _____

3. _____   8. _____

4. _____   9. _____

5. _____   10. _____

Average of 3 heaviest trials (UWW) _____ kg

DBW _____ kg

Tare Weight _____ kg

TUWW = UWW − Tare Weight = _____ − _____ = _____ kg

III. Body Density Calculation

H_2O Temp _____ °C

DH_2O (see table 33.3) _____

BV = $((((DBW − TUWW) / DH_2O) − RV) − 0.1) =$ _____ L

DB = DBW/BV = _____ / _____ = _____ $kg \cdot L^{-1}$

IV. Body Fat Calculation

% FAT = $((4.57 / DB) − 4.142) \times 100 =$ _____ %

FW = DBW $\times$ (% FAT / 100) = _____ 3 _____ (_____ / 100) = _____ kg

FFW = DBW − FW = _____ − _____ = _____ kg

Worksheet 33.2 | EXTENSION ACTIVITIES

Name   Date

1. Graph the following relationships:

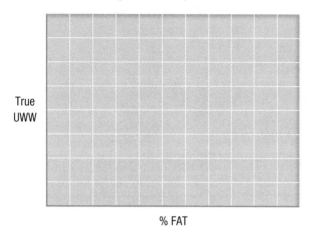

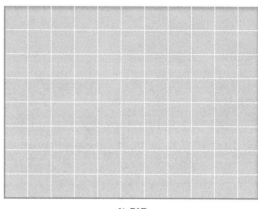

2. Given the following information, calculate:

   a. This male athlete's % FAT

   b. How much weight would this athlete need to lose if he desired a % FAT level of 6.5%?

   Dry Body Weight = 153.5 lbs H_2O Temp = 32° C
   Underwater Weight = 7.65 kg   Air Temp = 23° C
   Tare Weight = 3.75 kg   Vital Capacity = 5.5 L

3. Use your own data to calculate:

   a. % FAT

   b. Fat weight

   c. Fat-free weight

   d. Body weight goal at a more desirable level of % FAT (if you already have a desirable level of % FAT, use a target % FAT that is 1% below your current level).

REFERENCES

1. American College of Sports Medicine, *ACSM's Guidelines for Exercise Testing and Prescription*, 9th edition. Baltimore: Wolters Kluwer/Lippincott Williams & Wilkins, pp. 73–74, 2014.

2. Heyward, V. H., and Stolarozyk, L. M. *Applied Body Composition Assessment*. Champaign, IL: Human Kinetics, p. 151, 1996.

BACKGROUND

Laboratory methods for body composition assessment represent the most accurate means available for determining the amount of fat and fat-free tissue in live subjects. Generally, underwater weighing is considered the "gold standard" for determining body composition characteristics. Often, however, underwater weighing is not practical for assessing large groups of subjects in field situations.

Assessment of body composition by skinfold measurements is a simple and relatively accurate method that requires minimal equipment and can be used with large numbers of subjects in a field setting. Skinfold measurements can be used in multiple regression "prediction" equations to estimate body composition (body density [DB], percent fat [% FAT], fat-free weight [FFW], fat weight [FW]). The results of skinfold methods to determine body composition are usually within 3% to 5% of underwater weighing.

The ability to predict body composition from skinfolds is simply based on the fact that fat or fat-free tissues accumulate in relatively predictable patterns in similarly aged individuals of the same gender. Therefore, if specific sites are measured, the measurements will be influenced by the amount of the individual's adipose or fat-free tissue.

In this laboratory the technique for skinfold measurement will be outlined, and you will use the measurements to predict various aspects of body composition.

KNOW THESE TERMS & ABBREVIATIONS

- DB = body density
- FFW = fat-free weight
- FW = fat weight
- % FAT = percent fat

PROCEDURES[2]

1. Measure and mark the anatomical sites with a marker (see sites below in photos 34.1 through 34.15). Three sites are to be measured for each gender. Both males and females are measured at the thigh site. Males are also measured at the chest and abdomen, females at the triceps and suprailium.

2. Take all measurements on the right side of the body.

3. Grasp the skinfold of the subject firmly with the thumb and forefinger and pull away from the body.

4. Hold the caliper perpendicular to the skinfold. The caliper should be approximately 1 cm away from the thumb and forefinger so that the pressure of the caliper will not be affected.

5. Read the skinfold size approximately 1 to 2 seconds after the caliper thumb grip has been released.

6. Take three measurements per site at least 15 seconds apart to allow the skinfold site to return to normal. If the repeated measurements vary by more than 1 mm, more measurements should be taken. Use the mean of the recorded measurements that are within 1 mm as the representative skinfold value in the equation.

7. Calculate body composition characteristics using worksheet 34.1.

Equations

Males (ages 18–61 years)[3]

$DB = 1.1093800 - (0.0008267 (X_2)) + (0.0000016 (X_2)^2) - (0.0002574 (X_4))$

$R = 0.91$

$SEE = 0.008$ kg $\cdot$ L^{-1}

X_2 = sum of chest, abdomen, and thigh skinfolds in mm

X_4 = age in years

Females (ages 18–55 years)[3]

$DB = 1.099421 - (0.0009929 (X_3)) + (0.0000023 (X_3)^2) - (0.0001392 (X_4))$

$R = 0.84$

$SEE = 0.009$ kg $\cdot$ L^{-1}

X_3 = sum of triceps, thigh, and suprailium skinfolds in mm

X_4 = age in years

SEE = standard error of estimate, R = multiple correlation coefficient

% FAT $= (((4.57 / DB) - 4.142) \times 100)$[1]

FW = body weight $\times$ (% FAT / 100)

FFW = body weight $-$ FW

body weight goal = FFW / (1 $-$ (target % FAT / 100))

Sample Calculations

Gender: _____Male_____

Body weight: _____80.0 kg_____

Age: _____25 years_____

Sum of chest, abdomen, and thigh skinfolds: _____40 mm_____

$DB = 1.1093800 - (0.0008267 (40)) + (0.0000016 (40)^2) - (0.0002574 (25))$

$DB = 1.1093800 - 0.03307 + 0.00256 - 0.006435 = 1.0724$ kg $\cdot$ L^{-1}

% FAT $= ((4.57 / 1.0724) - 4.142) \times 100 = 11.9$ % FAT

FW $= 80.0 \times (11.9 / 100) = 9.5$ kg

FFW = 80.0 − 9.5 = 70.5 kg

body weight goal of 8.0 % FAT = 70.5 / (1 − (8.0 / 100)) = 76.6 kg

Gender: _____Female_____

Body weight: _____65 kg_____

Age: ___30 years___

Sum of triceps, thigh, and suprailium skinfolds: _____55 mm_____

DB = 1.099421 − (0.0009929 (55)) + (0.0000023 (55)^2) − 0.0001392 (30)

DB = 1.099421 − 0.05461 + 0.00696 − 0.004176 = 1.0476

% FAT = ((4.57 / 1.0476) − 4.142) × 100 = 22.0 % FAT

FW = 65 × (22.0 / 100) = 14.3 kg

FFW = 65 − 14.3 = 50.7 kg

body weight goal of 15.0 % FAT = 50.7 / (1 − (15.0 / 100)) = 59.6 kg

Skinfold Sites[3]

CHEST (see photos 34.1–34.3): a diagonal fold taken one half of the distance between the anterior axillary line and the nipple (males).

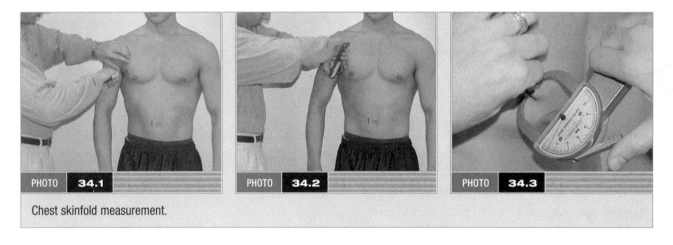

| PHOTO **34.1** | PHOTO **34.2** | PHOTO **34.3** |

Chest skinfold measurement.

ABDOMEN (see photos 34.4–34.6): a vertical fold taken at a lateral distance of approximately 2 cm from the umbilicus (males).

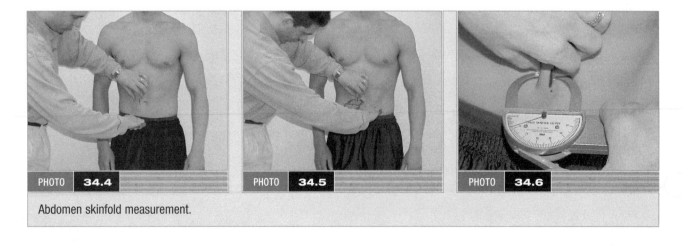

| PHOTO **34.4** | PHOTO **34.5** | PHOTO **34.6** |

Abdomen skinfold measurement.

THIGH (see photos 34.7–34.9): a vertical fold on the anterior aspect of the thigh, midway between hip and knee joints (males and females).

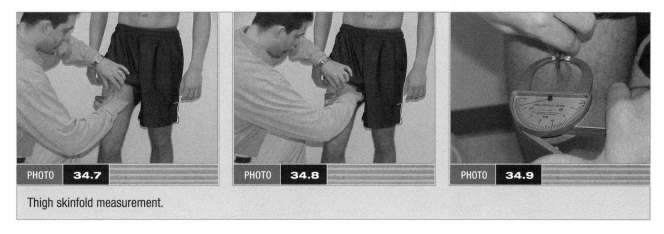

Thigh skinfold measurement.

TRICEPS (see photos 34.10–34.12): a vertical fold on the posterior midline of the upper arm, halfway between the acromion and olecranon processes; the elbow should be extended and relaxed (females).

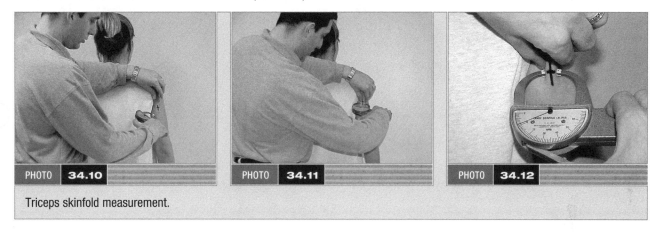

Triceps skinfold measurement.

SUPRAILIUM (see photos 34.13–34.15): a diagonal fold above the crest of the ilium at the spot where an imaginary line would come down from the anterior axillary line (females).

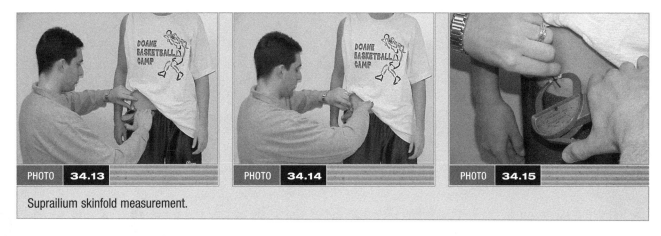

Suprailium skinfold measurement.

Note: For accurate measures, do not take measurements when the skin is wet, immediately after exercise, or when the subject is overheated.

Worksheet 34.1 — SKINFOLD ESTIMATIONS OF BODY COMPOSITION

Name _____ Date _____

Gender: _____

Age: _____ years

Body weight: _____ kg

Skinfold Measurements (mm)

	Trial 1	Trial 2	Trial 3	Mean
Triceps	_____	_____	_____	_____
Suprailium	_____	_____	_____	_____
Abdomen	_____	_____	_____	_____
Thigh	_____	_____	_____	_____
Chest	_____	_____	_____	_____

Sum of chest, abdomen, and thigh skinfolds = _____

Sum of triceps, thigh, and suprailium skinfolds = _____

Use the gender-specific equations on p. 259 to calculate DB.

DB = _____ $kg \cdot L^{-1}$

Use the equations on p. 259 to calculate % FAT, FW, and FFW.

% FAT = _____ %   FW = _____ kg   FFW = _____ kg

Worksheet 34.2 — EXTENSION ACTIVITIES

Name _____ Date _____

1. A subject's % FAT, determined by skinfolds, was estimated to be 16.9% (DB = 1.0600 $kg \cdot L^{-1}$). If the SEE of the predicted body density value is equal to 0.0050 $kg \cdot L^{-1}$, then this subject's % FAT is likely to fall between what two values?

2. List potential sources of error when estimating body composition from skinfold equations.

3. Using the skinfold prediction equations on p. 259, calculate your body density and convert this value to % FAT.

EXTENSION QUESTIONS

1. What are some common mistakes that may occur in administering this lab?

2. Assess the practicality of using this lab in the field.

3. Research the reliability and/or validity of this lab using online resources, journal articles, and other credible sources.

REFERENCES

1. Brozek, J., Grande, F., Anderson, J. T., and Keys, A. Densitometric analysis of body composition: Revision of some quantitative assumptions. *Ann. N.Y. Acad. Sci.* 110: 113–140, 1963.

2. Harrison, G. G., Buskirk, E. R., Carter, J. E. L., Johnston, F. E., Lohman, T. G., Pollock, M. L., Roche, A. F., and Wilmore, J. Skinfold thicknesses and measurement techniques. In *Anthropometric Standardization Reference Manual*, eds. T. G. Lohman, A. F. Roche, and R. Martorell. Champaign, IL: Human Kinetics, pp. 55–70, 1988.

3. Jackson, A. S., and Pollock, M. L. Practical assessment of body composition. *Phys. Sportsmed.* 13: 76–90, 1985.

BACKGROUND

Three primary anthropometric-based parameters that can provide information regarding the risk of developing cardiovascular disease, type 2 diabetes, dyslipidemia, obesity, and/or hypertension are body mass index (BMI), waist-to-hip ratio, and waist circumference.[1,3,4,5,8] Each of these parameters can be used to classify individuals with regard to their health risk. In addition, they are commonly used in epidemiological studies because they are associated with various diseases and risk factors, require few measurements, and are simple to calculate.

In this laboratory, the techniques and landmarks for measuring height and body weight, as well as waist 1, waist 2, and hips circumferences, will be described, and you will use them to determine the BMI, waist-to-hip ratio, and waist 2 circumference. You will also learn to classify an individual's health risk based on these parameters.

KNOW THESE TERMS & ABBREVIATIONS

- anthropometric = relating to the measurement of the size and proportions of the human body
- BMI = body mass index: body weight in kg/height in meters squared $(kg \cdot m^{-2})$
- epidemiological studies = studies performed on human populations that attempt to link health effects to a cause; e.g., waist circumference and type 2 diabetes

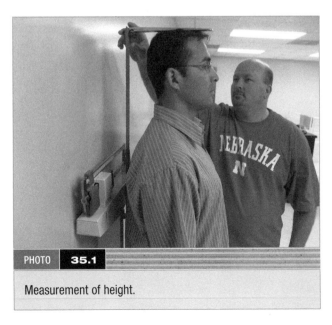

PHOTO **35.1**

Measurement of height.

PROCEDURES[1,5,6]

1. Measure the subject's height in meters (cm/100) and body weight in kg with the shoes removed (see photos 35.1 and 35.2). Record the values on worksheet 35.1.

2. Identify the landmarks for the waist 1, waist 2, and hips circumferences (see photos 35.3, 35.4, and 35.5).

3. Place the tape parallel to the floor (horizontal).

4. Hold the tape firmly around the circumference site, but do not compress the underlying tissue.

5. Take three measurements per site and use the mean of repeated recordings that agree within 0.5 cm. Record measurements on worksheet 35.1.

Circumference Sites in cm[1,2,6,8]

Waist 1 (see photo 35.3): at the level of the "natural waist," midway between the xyphoid process and umbilicus

Waist 2 (see photo 35.4): at the level of the umbilicus and iliac crests

Hips (see photo 35.5): at the level of the pubis symphysis and the maximal protrusion of the gluteal muscles

Sample Calculations

Gender: _____*Male*_____

Body weight: _____*80 kg*_____

Height: _____*1.85 m*_____

Waist 1 (also called abdomen 1 in Lab 38) circumference: ___*84.0 cm*___

Waist 2 (also called abdomen 2 in Lab 38) circumference: ___*87.0 cm*___

Hips circumference: _____*96 cm*_____

body mass index (BMI) = body weight in kg / height in meters squared (kg • m^{-2})

BMI = 80/1.85^2 = 80/3.42 = 23.4

waist-to-hip ratio   = waist 1 circumference in cm / hips circumference in cm

waist-to-hip ratio   = 84.0/96.0 = 0.875

waist 2 circumference   = 87.0 cm

Tables 35.1, 35.2, and 35.3 provide mean height, body weight, and BMI values by age categories.[8]

Tables 35.4, 35.5, and 35.6 provide health risk classifications for BMI, waist-to-hip ratio, and waist 2 circumference.[3,4,5,6,7]

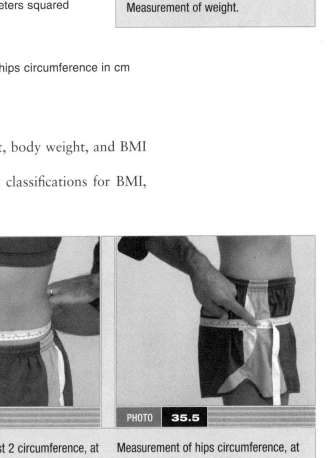

PHOTO **35.2**

Measurement of weight.

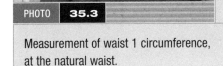

PHOTO **35.3**	PHOTO **35.4**	PHOTO **35.5**
Measurement of waist 1 circumference, at the natural waist.	Measurement of waist 2 circumference, at the level of the umbilicus and iliac crests.	Measurement of hips circumference, at the level of the symphysis pubis and maximal gluteal protrusion.

TABLE 35.1 Mean (± SEM) height (cm) values by age categories.[8]

Age (years)	Males	Females
17	175.3 ± 0.57	163.1 ± 0.56
18	176.4 ± 0.65	163.1 ± 0.44
19	176.7 ± 0.64	162.9 ± 0.64
20–29	176.7 ± 0.29	162.8 ± 0.31
30–39	176.4 ± 0.26	163.1 ± 0.28
40–49	177.2 ± 0.33	163.4 ± 0.24
50–59	175.8 ± 0.32	162.3 ± 0.35
60–69	174.8 ± 0.33	160.6 ± 0.27
70–79	172.7 ± 0.44	159.0 ± 0.31
80 and over	170.7 ± 0.44	155.8 ± 0.34

TABLE 35.2 Mean (± SEM) body weight (kg) values by age categories.[8]

Age (years)	Males	Females
17	75.6 ± 1.38	61.7 ± 1.21
18	75.6 ± 1.12	65.2 ± 1.52
19	78.2 ± 1.29	67.9 ± 1.21
20–29	83.4 ± 0.70	71.1 ± 0.90
30–39	86.0 ± 0.90	74.1 ± 0.91
40–49	89.1 ± 0.73	76.5 ± 1.09
50–59	88.8 ± 0.94	76.9 ± 1.15
60–69	88.2 ± 0.73	76.3 ± 0.76
70–79	82.7 ± 0.71	71.0 ± 0.76
80 and over	76.0 ± 0.66	63.7 ± 1.31

Mean (± SEM) BMI values by age categories.[8]   TABLE   35.3

Age (years)	Males	Females
17	24.5 ± 0.41	23.1 ± 0.41
18	24.2 ± 0.34	24.4 ± 0.48
19	24.9 ± 0.36	25.5 ± 0.43
20–29	26.6 ± 0.19	26.8 ± 0.29
30–39	27.5 ± 0.26	27.9 ± 0.33
40–49	28.4 ± 0.25	28.6 ± 0.40
50–59	28.7 ± 0.31	29.2 ± 0.40
60–69	28.9 ± 0.20	29.6 ± 0.30
70–79	27.7 ± 0.18	28.0 ± 0.29
80 and over	26.1 ± 0.23	26.1 ± 0.48

Health risk classifications for BMI.[5]   TABLE   35.4

BMI (kg · m^{-2})	Weight classification	Health risk
<18.5	Underweight	Increased
18.5–24.9	Normal weight	Average
25.0–29.9	Overweight	Increased
≥30	Obese	High

Note: Underweight, overweight, and obese classifications are associated with various diseases such as hypertension, dyslipidemia, and cardiovascular disease.[1]

TABLE	35.5	Health risk classifications for cardiovascular disease associated with waist-to-hip ratio by age categories.[4,6,7]

Males

AGE (YEARS)	LOW	MODERATE	HIGH	VERY HIGH
20–29	<0.83	0.83–0.88	0.89–0.94	>0.94
30–39	<0.84	0.84–0.91	0.92–0.96	>0.96
40–49	<0.88	0.88–0.95	0.96–1.00	>1.00
50–59	<0.90	0.90–0.96	0.97–1.02	>1.02
60–69	<0.91	0.91–0.98	0.99–1.03	>1.03

Females

AGE (YEARS)	LOW	MODERATE	HIGH	VERY HIGH
20–29	<0.71	0.71–0.77	0.78–0.82	>0.82
30–39	<0.72	0.72–0.78	0.79–0.84	>0.84
40–49	<0.73	0.73–0.79	0.80–0.87	>0.87
50–59	<0.74	0.74–0.81	0.82–0.88	>0.88
60–69	<0.76	0.76–0.83	0.84–0.90	>0.90

Note: Waist-to-hip ratio uses waist 1 circumference.

TABLE	35.6	Chronic disease classifications for waist 2 circumference.[3]

CHRONIC DISEASE RISK	FEMALES	MALES
Very low	<70	<80
Low	70–89	80–99
High	90–110	100–120
Very high	>110	>120

Note: Chronic diseases include type 2 diabetes, hypertension, and cardiovascular disease.[1]

ANTHROPOMETRIC MEASURES OF HEALTH RISK FORM   Worksheet 35.1

Name _____   *Date* _____

Gender: _____

Age: _____ years

Body Weight: _____ kg

Height: _____ cm / 100 = _____ meters

	Trial 1	Trial 2	Trial 3	Mean
Waist 1 circumference (cm)	_____	_____	_____	_____
Waist 2 circumference (cm)	_____	_____	_____	_____
Hips circumference (cm)	_____	_____	_____	_____

BMI = body weight in kg / height in m^2 = _____ kg / _____ m^2 = _____

    Classification = _____ (table 35.4)

Waist-to-hip ratio = waist 1 circumference in cm / hips circumference in cm =

    _____ cm / _____ cm = _____

    Classification = _____ (table 35.5)

Waist 2 circumference = _____ cm

    Classification = _____ (table 35.6)

Worksheet 35.2 — EXTENSION ACTIVITIES

Name _____ Date _____

Use the following data and tables 35.4, 35.5, and 35.6 to answer the questions below.

Gender: _____Female_____

Age: _____20_____ years

Body weight: _____78_____ kg

Height: _____1.75_____ m

Waist 1 circumference = _____82.0_____ cm

Waist 2 circumference = _____89.0_____ cm

Hips circumference = _____98.0_____ cm

1. Calculate the subject's BMI and classify her health risk (see table 35.4).

   BMI = _____

   Classification = _____

2. Calculate the subject's waist-to-hip ratio and classify her health risk for cardiovascular disease (see table 35.5).

   Waist-to-hip ratio = _____

   Classification = _____

3. Based on the subject's waist 2 circumference, classify her health risk for chronic diseases (see table 35.6).

   Classification = _____

EXTENSION QUESTIONS

1. What are some common mistakes that may occur in administering this lab?

2. Identify possible sources of error in this lab.

3. Assess the practicality of using this lab in the field.

4. Research the reliability and/or validity of this lab using online resources, journal articles, and other credible sources.

REFERENCES

1. American College of Sports Medicine. *ACSM's Resource Manual for Guidelines for Exercise Testing and Prescription*, 9th edition. Baltimore: Wolters Kluwer/Lippincott Williams & Wilkins, 2014.

2. Behnke, A. R., and Wilmore, J. H. *Evaluation and Regulation of Body Build and Composition.* Englewood Cliffs, NJ: Prentice-Hall, 1974.

3. Bray, G. A. Don't throw the baby out with the bath water. *Am. J. Clin. Nutr.* 79: 347–349, 2004.

4. Bray, G. A., and Gray, D. S. Obesity Part 1—Pathogenesis. *West. J. Med.* 149: 429–441, 1988.

5. Expert Panel on the Identification, Evaluation, and Treatment of Overweight in Adults. Clinical guidelines on the identification, evaluation, and treatment of overweight and obesity in adults: Executive summary. *Am. J. Clin. Nutr.* 68: 899–917, 1998.

6. Heyward, V. H., and Stolarczyk, L. M. *Applied Body Composition Assessment.* Champaign, IL: Human Kinetics, 1996, pp. 81–82.

7. Hoffman, J. *Norms for Fitness, Performance, and Health.* Champaign, IL: Human Kinetics, 2006, p. 87.

8. McDowell, M. A., Fryar, C. D., Hirsch, R., and Ogden, C. L. *Anthropometric Reference Data for Children and Adults: U.S. Population, 1999–2002.* Hyattsville, MD: Centers for Disease Control and Prevention, 2005.

BACKGROUND

The quantification of muscle cross-sectional area (CSA) has been used clinically to evaluate the nutritional status of children, the elderly, and individuals with muscle-wasting diseases or injuries.[3] In nonclinical settings, the quantification of muscle CSA has been used to describe and compare athletic and non-athletic populations, predict muscular strength and strength per unit of muscle CSA, and examine the effects of various interventions on hypertrophy and atrophy.[3]

The most common laboratory techniques used to determine muscle CSA are computed tomography (CT scan) and magnetic resonance imaging (MRI), which are valid and reliable but also expensive (see figures 36.1 and 36.2). Many laboratories do not have access to this technology and, therefore, must rely on more practical methods, such as anthropometry, for assessing muscle CSA. Recently, multiple regression equations for estimating thigh muscle CSA have been developed based on the measurement of the anterior thigh skinfold and mid-thigh circumference.[3] The accuracy (validated against MRI) of these equations is comparable to that of skinfold estimates of percent body fat as well as field tests such as the Astrand–Rhyming test (see Lab 8) for estimating maximal oxygen consumption rate ($\dot{V}O_2$ max).[3] The equations are applicable to both males and females. The mid-thigh circumference reflects all tissues of the thigh, including muscle, skin, subcutaneous fat, bone, connective tissue, and vessels. Theoretically, the skinfold accounts for the amount of subcutaneous fat (and skin) that covers the muscle.

In this laboratory, the mid-thigh circumference and anterior thigh skinfold will be measured and used in multiple regression equations to estimate the quadriceps CSA, hamstring CSA, and total thigh muscle CSA. The quadriceps CSA includes the vastus intermedius, vastus lateralis, vastus medialis, and rectus femoris muscles. The hamstring CSA includes the semimembranosus, semitendinosus, and biceps femoris muscles. The total thigh muscle CSA includes the quadriceps, hamstrings, adductor longus, adductor magnus, gracilis, and sartorius muscles.

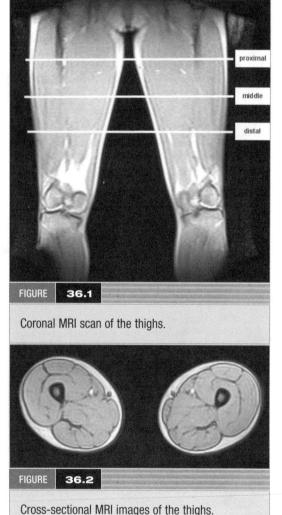

proximal

middle

distal

FIGURE **36.1**

Coronal MRI scan of the thighs.

FIGURE **36.2**

Cross-sectional MRI images of the thighs.

KNOW THESE TERMS & ABBREVIATIONS

- anthropometry = the measurement of the size and proportions of the human body

- CSA = cross-sectional area. Muscle CSA in this lab is determined using circumferences, skinfolds, and multiple regression equations.

- ⊙ CT scan = computed tomography scan
- ⊙ MRI = magnetic resonance imaging
- ⊙ multiple regression equation = a combination of a number of measurements (independent variables) that best predict a common variable (the dependent variable, in this case muscle CSA)
- ⊙ R = multiple correlation coefficient, a numerical measure of how well a dependent variable can be predicted from a combination of independent variables (a number between –1 and 1)
- ⊙ SEE = standard error of estimate, a measure of the accuracy of predictions made using a regression equation

PROCEDURES

1. Measure and mark the anatomical sites with a marker (see sites below). The mid-thigh circumference and anterior thigh skinfold measurements are taken on the dominant limb. To determine the dominant limb, ask the subject, "Which leg do you prefer to kick with?"

2. Calculate quadriceps CSA, hamstrings CSA, and total thigh muscle CSA using worksheet 36.1. The CSA values from the equations are expressed in cm^2.

Skinfold Site[2]

Anterior thigh (see photos 36.1–36.3): a vertical fold (measured in mm) on the anterior aspect of the thigh, midway between the hip (inguinal fold) and knee joints (superior border of the patella).

a. Grasp the skinfold firmly with the thumb and forefinger and pull away from the body (photo 36.2).

b. Hold the caliper perpendicular to the skinfold (photo 36.3). The caliper should be approximately 1 cm away from the thumb and forefinger so that the pressure of the caliper will not be affected.

c. Read the skinfold size approximately 1 to 2 seconds after the caliper thumb grip has been released.

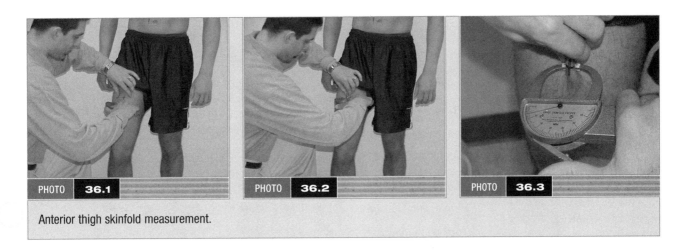

PHOTO **36.1**   PHOTO **36.2**   PHOTO **36.3**

Anterior thigh skinfold measurement.

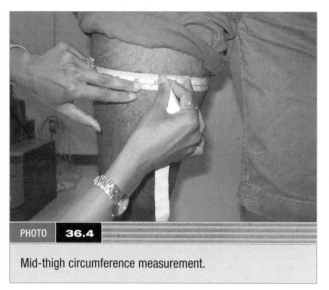

PHOTO **36.4**

Mid-thigh circumference measurement.

d. Take three measurements (record the measurements on worksheet 36.1) at least 15 seconds apart to allow the skinfold site to return to normal. If the repeated measurements vary by more than 1 mm, more measurements should be taken. Use the mean of the recorded measurements that are within 1 mm as the representative skinfold value in the equations.

Circumference Site[1]

Mid-thigh (see photo 36.4): the distance (expressed in cm) around the thigh, midway between the hip (inguinal fold) and knee joints (superior border of the patella), with the subject standing and feet slightly apart.

a. Place the tape perpendicular to the long axis of the limb.

b. Hold the tape tightly around the limb, but do not compress the underlying tissue.

c. Take three measurements (record the measurements on worksheet 36.1) and use the mean of repeated recordings that agree within 0.5 cm.

Equations[3]

Quadriceps CSA (cm²) = (2.52 × mid-thigh circumference in cm) − (1.25 × anterior thigh skinfold in mm) − 45.13

  R = 0.86

  SEE = 5.2 cm²

Hamstrings CSA (cm²) = (1.08 × mid-thigh circumference in cm) − (0.64 × anterior thigh skinfold in mm) − 22.69

  R = 0.75

  SEE = 3.5 cm²

Total thigh muscle CSA (cm²) = (4.68 × mid-thigh circumference in cm) − (2.09 × anterior thigh skinfold in mm) − 80.99

  R = 0.86

  SEE = 9.5 cm²

Sample Calculations

TRIAL	1	2	3	MEAN
Anterior thigh skinfold (mm)	19.5	20.5	20.0	20
Mid-thigh circumference (cm)	55.0	54.8	55.2	55

Quadriceps CSA (cm²) = (2.52 × 55) − (1.25 × 20) − 45.13 = 68.5 cm²

Hamstrings CSA (cm²) = (1.08 × 55) − (0.64 × 20) − 22.69 = 23.9 cm²

Total thigh muscle CSA (cm²) = (4.68 × 55) − (2.09 × 20) − 80.99 = 134.6 cm²

Table 36.1 includes typical quadriceps, hamstrings, and total thigh muscle CSA values.

	TABLE 36.1
Typical mean (± SD) values for quadriceps, hamstrings, and total thigh muscle cross-sectional area.[3]	

Muscle group	Mean ± SD
Quadriceps CSA	75.5 ± 9.9 cm^2
Hamstrings CSA	27.5 ± 5.1 cm^2
Total thigh muscle CSA	145.9 ± 18.3 cm^2

Note: The values listed on this table are for untrained adults (age range = 19–36 years). Training status and age will likely affect the subject's estimated CSA values.

Worksheet 36.1 — ANTHROPOMETRIC ESTIMATION OF THIGH MUSCLE CROSS-SECTIONAL AREA

Name _____   Date _____

Measurements

	Trial 1	Trial 2	Trial 3	Mean
Anterior thigh skinfold (mm)	_____	_____	_____	_____
Mid-thigh circumference (cm)	_____	_____	_____	_____

Use the equations on page 274 to calculate:

Quadriceps CSA = _____ cm²

Hamstrings CSA = _____ cm²

Total thigh muscle CSA = _____ cm²

Worksheet 36.2 — EXTENSION ACTIVITIES

Name _____   Date _____

1. A subject's quadriceps CSA estimated from the anthropometric equation in the present laboratory is 70.5 cm². Given that the SEE for this equation is 5.2 cm², the subject's true quadriceps CSA is likely to fall between what two values?

2. Have your anterior thigh skinfold and mid-thigh circumference measured, and use the anthropometric equations on page 274 to calculate your:

Quadriceps CSA = _____ cm²

Hamstrings CSA = _____ cm²

Total thigh muscle CSA = _____ cm²

EXTENSION QUESTIONS

1. What are some common mistakes that may occur in administering this lab?

2. Identify possible sources of error in this lab.

3. Assess the practicality of using this lab in the field.

4. Research the reliability and/or validity of this lab using online resources, journal articles, and other credible sources.

REFERENCES

1. Callaway, C. W., Chumlea, W. C., Bouchard, C., Himes, J. H., Lohman, T. G., Martin, A. D., Mitchell, C. D., Mueller, W. H., Roche, A. F., and Seefeldt, V. D. Circumferences. In *Anthropometric Standardization Reference Manual*, eds. T. G. Lohman, A. F. Roche, and R. Martorell. Champaign, IL: Human Kinetics, 1988, pp. 39–54.

2. Harrison, G. G., Buskirk, E. R., Carter, J. E. L., Johnston, F. E., Lohman, T. G., Pollock, M. L., Roche, A. F., and Wilmore, J. Skinfold thicknesses and measurement technique. In *Anthropometric Standardization Reference Manual*, eds. T. G. Lohman, A. F. Roche, and R. Martorell. Champaign, IL: Human Kinetics, 1988, pp. 55–70.

3. Housh, D. J., Housh, T. J., Weir, J. P., Weir, L. L., Johnson, G. O., and Stout, J. R. Anthropometric estimation of thigh muscle cross-sectional area. *Med. Sci. Sports Exerc.* 27: 784–791, 1995.

Lab 37

BACKGROUND

The calculation of an individual's reference weight utilizes diameter measurements (the distance between two bony landmarks) to estimate an appropriate (or normal) body weight based on skeletal size.[1] The reference weight is based on the assumption that diameters and height reflect frame size. In adulthood, frame size provides a stable characteristic from which to estimate how much an individual should weigh with respect to the size of his or her skeleton. The reference weight is the average weight for an adult with a given frame size. Thus, the reference weight can serve as the basis for determining whether an individual is underweight or overweight based on his or her frame size.

The reference weight may also be used in combination with known body composition characteristics (body weight, % FAT, fat weight, and fat-free weight) to estimate the changes in fat weight and fat-free weight that are needed to meet a % FAT goal at the subject's reference weight. This lab will describe the procedures used to: (1) measure the diameters for the determination of reference weight, (2) calculate the reference weight, and (3) use known body composition characteristics, in conjunction with reference weight, to estimate the changes in fat weight and fat-free weight that are needed to meet a % FAT goal at the subject's reference weight.

KNOW THESE TERMS & ABBREVIATIONS

- % FAT = percent body fat, the proportion of the body that is composed of adipose (fat) tissue
- anthropometer = an instrument used to measure the human trunk and limbs, consisting of two horizontal arms (one movable and one fixed) attached to a vertical rod
- fat weight (FW) = weight of adipose tissue (subcutaneous and intermuscular and/or intravisceral) and neural tissue
- fat-free weight (FFW) = weight of bone, muscle, tendons, viscera, and connective tissue
- reference weight = the average weight for an adult with a given frame size

PROCEDURES[1,2]

1. Measure the subject's height in cm and body weight in kg with the shoes removed (see photos 37.1 and 37.2).

2. Palpate for bony landmarks at the diameter sites (see photos 37.4 through 37.11).

3. Hold the anthropometer (see photo 37.3) so that the tips of the index fingers are adjacent to the tips of the blades of the anthropometer.

4. Position the blades of the anthropometer with sufficient pressure to assure that they are measuring bony landmarks.

5. Take three measurements per site (record on worksheet 37.1) and use the mean of repeated recordings that agree within 0.5 cm.

6. The wrist, elbow, knee, and ankle diameters should be measured on both limbs.

7. Reference weight may be calculated using worksheet 37.1.

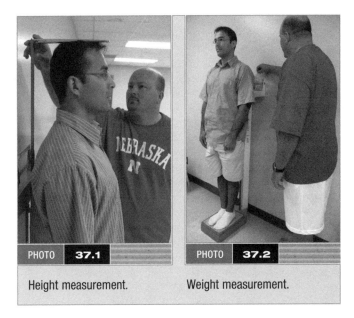

PHOTO **37.1**

PHOTO **37.2**

Height measurement.   Weight measurement.

Diameter Sites (cm)

Wrist: the distance between the styloid processes of the radius and ulna (see photo 37.4).

Elbow: the distance between the medial and lateral epicondyles of the humerus (see photo 37.5).

Knee: the distance between the medial and lateral epicondyles of the femur (see photo 37.6).

Ankle: the distance between the malleoli (see photo 37.7).

Biacromial: the distance between the most lateral projections of the acromial processes (see photo 37.8).

Chest: the distance across the chest at the level of the fifth and sixth ribs (approximately the nipple line; see photo 37.9).

Bi-iliac: the distance between the most lateral projections of the iliac crests (see photo 37.10).

Bitrochanteric: the distance between the most lateral projections of the greater trochanters (see photo 37.11).

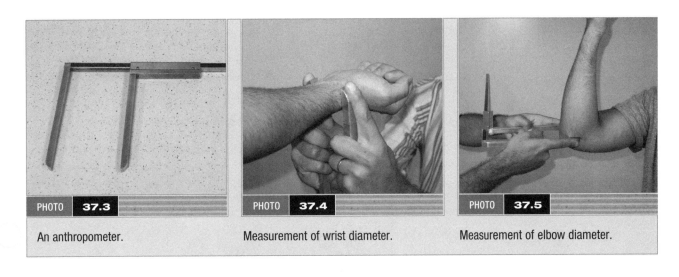

PHOTO **37.3**

PHOTO **37.4**

PHOTO **37.5**

An anthropometer.   Measurement of wrist diameter.   Measurement of elbow diameter.

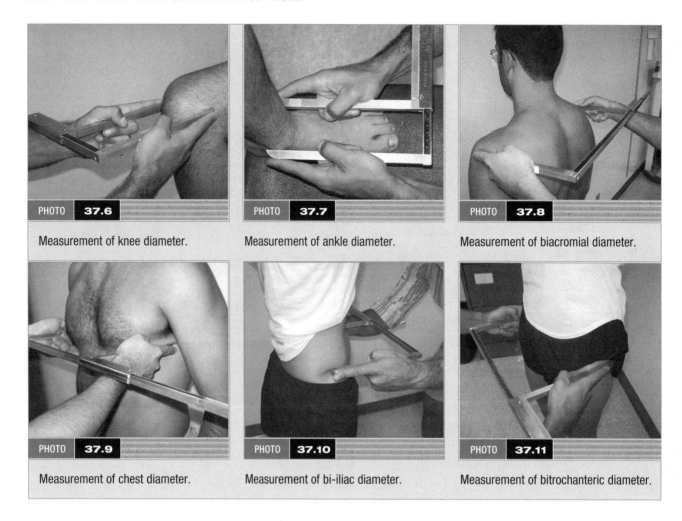

PHOTO 37.6

Measurement of knee diameter.

PHOTO 37.7

Measurement of ankle diameter.

PHOTO 37.8

Measurement of biacromial diameter.

PHOTO 37.9

Measurement of chest diameter.

PHOTO 37.10

Measurement of bi-iliac diameter.

PHOTO 37.11

Measurement of bitrochanteric diameter.

Equation

Sum of diameters = _____ cm

divided by   body constants (31.10 for females, 31.58 for males) = _____

squared   = _____

times   height (cm)   = _____

times   0.0111 = reference weight   = _____ kg

Body weight (kg) – reference weight (kg) = _____ kg

Classification = _____

Underweight: body weight is at least 5 kg less than reference weight

Normal weight: body weight is within 5 kg of reference weight

Overweight: body weight is at least 5 kg greater than reference weight

Sample Calculations

Height: _176.1 cm_

Body weight: _67.0 kg_

Gender: _Female_

Diameters:

wrist (sum of right and left) = _10.9 cm_

elbow (sum of right and left) = _13.1 cm_

knee (sum of right and left) = _18.0 cm_

ankle (sum of right and left) = _13.3 cm_

biacromial   = _34.7 cm_

chest   = _24.5 cm_

bi-iliac   = _26.9 cm_

bitrochanteric   = _31.6 cm_

sum of diameters   = _173.0 cm_

	Sum of diameters (cm)	= _173.0 cm_
divided by	31.10 (body constant for female)	= _5.563_
squared	5.563 × 5.563	= _30.94_
times	height (cm) = 30.94 × 176.1	= _5449.2_
times	0.0111 × 5449.2 = reference weight	= _60.5 kg_

Body weight minus reference weight = _6.5_ kg of change

Classification = _overweight_

Current body composition characteristics and reference weight may be combined to estimate the change in fat-free weight and fat weight needed to meet a body composition goal at the reference weight.

EXAMPLE:

Current	Goal	Change (goal – current)
Body weight = 67.0 kg	Reference weight = 60.5 kg	60.5 kg – 67.0 kg = –6.5 kg (loss)
% FAT = 30%	Target % FAT = 20%	20 % FAT – 30 % FAT = –10 % FAT (loss)
Fat weight = 20.1 kg	FW goal (20% of 60.5 kg) = 12.1 kg	12.1 kg – 20.1 kg = –8.0 kg of FW (loss)
Fat-free weight = 46.9 kg	FFW goal (60.5 kg – 12.1 kg) = 48.4 kg	48.4 kg – 46.9 kg = +1.5 kg of FFW (gain)

Note: A positive (+) change means to increase the variable and a negative (–) change means to decrease the variable. Under some circumstances, the combination of body composition and reference weight can result in a recommendation to lose fat-free weight.

Worksheet 37.1 DETERMINATION OF REFERENCE WEIGHT

Name _____   *Date* _____

Height: _____ cm

Body weight: _____ kg

Gender: _____

DIAMETER (cm)

	Right		Mean		Left		Mean		Sum of means
Wrist	____	____	____	____	____	____	____	____	____
Elbow	____	____	____	____	____	____	____	____	____
Knee	____	____	____	____	____	____	____	____	____
Ankle	____	____	____	____	____	____	____	____	____
Biacromial	____	____	____	____					
Chest	____	____	____	____					
Bi-iliac	____	____	____	____					
Bitrochanteric	____	____	____	____					

Equation

Sum of diameters = _____ cm

divided by body constants (31.10 for females, 31.58 for males)   = _____

squared   = _____

times   height (cm)   = _____

times   0.0111 = reference weight   = _____ kg

Body weight (kg) – reference weight (kg) = _____ kg

Classification = _____

Underweight: body weight is at least 5 kg less than reference weight

Normal weight: body weight is within 5 kg of reference weight

Overweight: body weight is at least 5 kg greater than reference weight

Name _____   Date _____

1. Given the following data, calculate the subject's reference weight.

    Height: ___180.0 cm___

    Body weight: ___75.0 kg___

    Gender: ___Male___

    Diameters:

    Wrist (sum of right and left)   ___11.5 cm___

    Elbow (sum of right and left)   ___15.0 cm___

    Knee (sum of right and left)   ___22.0 cm___

    Ankle (sum of right and left)   ___14.5 cm___

    Biacromial   ___37.0 cm___

    Chest   ___27.5 cm___

    Bi-iliac   ___28.0 cm___

    Bitrochanteric   ___32.5 cm___

    Sum of diameters   _____

    Reference weight (see equation on p. 280) = _____ kg

2. Given the data and reference weight from question 1, calculate the required changes in body weight, fat weight, and fat-free weight if the subject currently has 20 % FAT and has a goal of 15 % FAT.

Current	Goal	Change (goal – current)
Body weight = 75.0 kg	Reference weight = _____ kg	_____ kg
% FAT = 20%	Target % FAT = 15%	_____ %
FW = _____ kg	FW = _____ kg	_____ kg
FFW = _____ kg	FFW = _____ kg	_____ kg

3. Have your diameters measured and calculate your reference weight. Based on your reference weight, classify yourself as underweight, normal weight, or overweight.

    Reference weight = _____ kg

    Classification = _____

EXTENSION QUESTIONS

1. What are some common mistakes that may occur in administering this lab?

2. Identify possible sources of error in this lab.

3. Assess the practicality of using this lab in the field.

4. Research the reliability and/or validity of this lab using online resources, journal articles, and other credible sources.

REFERENCES

1. Behnke, A. R., and Wilmore, J. H. *Evaluation and Regulation of Body Build and Composition.* Englewood Cliffs, NJ: Prentice-Hall, 1974.

2. Wilmore, J. H., Frisancho, R. A., Gordon, C. C., Himes, J. H., Martin, A. D., Martorell, R., and Seefeldt, V. D. Body breadth equipment and measurement techniques. In *Anthropometric Standardization Reference Manual,* eds. T. G. Lohman, A. F. Roche, and R. Martorell. Champaign, IL: Human Kinetics, 1988, pp. 27–38.

BACKGROUND

The Somatogram describes an individual's body build or physique. Specifically, the Somatogram uses circumference measures (the distance around a landmark on the body) to determine the distribution of tissues on the body when compared to that of the average (or "normal") adult male or female.[1] For example, it is likely that a weightlifter would have proportionally larger biceps, forearms, shoulders, calves, and chest than the average person. An obese individual, however, may deviate from average by having larger than normal abdominal, hips, and thigh circumferences, while a person who is chronically underweight would likely have a proportionally small abdomen circumference, but large wrist, knee, and ankle circumferences relative to total body measurements.[1] Thus, the Somatogram characterizes the various segments (limbs and torso) of the body based on what is considered proportional for adults. This is accomplished by dividing circumference measures by "segmental constant" values that represent what is average for each site. Segmental constants differ for males and females, because of their differing body build characteristics.

In this laboratory, you will learn the techniques and landmarks for measuring circumferences and use the circumference measurements to develop a Somatogram. See figure 38.1 for an example.

KNOW THESE TERMS & ABBREVIATIONS

- ⊙ circumference = the distance around a landmark on the body
- ⊙ segmental constant = a value that represents what is average for each circumference site measured
- ⊙ Somatogram = a graphic description of body proportions based on circumference measurements (figure 38.1)

PROCEDURES[1,2]

1. Identify the anatomical landmarks for each circumference (see photos 38.1 through 38.12).

2. Place the tape perpendicular to the long axis of the limb for the extremity sites or parallel to the floor (horizontal) for the torso sites: shoulder, chest, abdomen 1, abdomen 2, and hips.

3. Record all extremity circumferences (wrist, forearm, flexed arm, thigh, knee, calf, and ankle) for both the left and right limbs.

4. Hold the tape tightly around the circumference site, but do not compress the underlying tissue.

5. Take three measurements per site and use the mean of repeated recordings that agree within 0.5 cm.

FIGURE 38.1 Example Somatogram.

Name   I. M. Sample

Gender   Female

MEASURE	CIRCUMFERENCES (cm)	FEMALE SEGMENTAL CONSTANT	MALE SEGMENTAL CONSTANT	CIRCUMFERENCE/ SEGMENTAL CONSTANT	PROPORTIONAL SCORE	SOMATOGRAM GRID
Wrist	15.20	2.73	2.88	5.568	99	
Forearm	23.70	4.15	4.47	5.711	102	
Flexed Arm	27.85	4.80	5.29	5.802	103	
Shoulder	97.60	17.51	18.47	5.574	99	
Chest	83.60	14.85	15.30	5.630	100	
Abdomen $\bar{X}$	70.15	12.90	13.07	5.438	97	
Hips	94.10	16.93	15.57	5.558	99	
Thigh	55.00	10.03	9.13	5.484	98	
Knee	36.30	6.27	6.10	5.789	103	
Calf	35.75	6.13	5.97	5.832	104	
Ankle	21.45	3.70	3.75	5.797	103	
Total Body Circumferences	560.70	100.00	100.00	5.607		

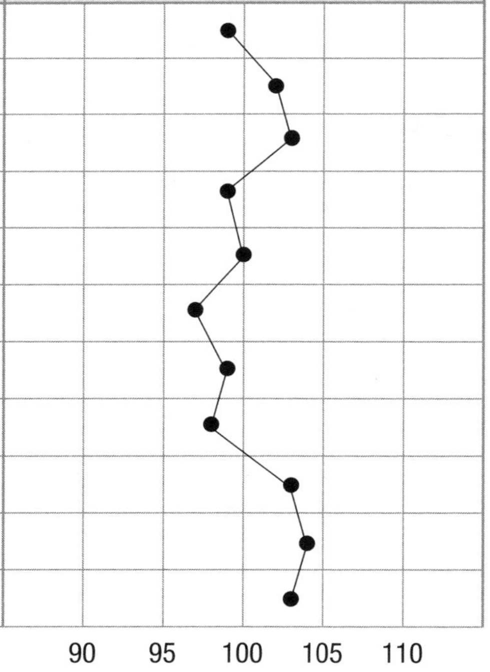

6. Record on worksheet 38.1 the circumference values for each site. For the extremity sites (wrist, forearm, flexed arm, thigh, knee, calf, and ankle), the circumference value used in the Somatogram is the average of the right and left limbs.

7. Calculate the sum of all circumferences and record it in the bottom row, in the box labeled "Total body circumferences." Divide this value by 100 (Total body circumferences/100) and record it in the box directly to the right, under the column "Circumference/segmental constant."

8. Divide each circumference value by the appropriate gender-specific segmental constant and record the values in the boxes to the right under "Circumference/segmental constant."

9. For each circumference, divide the value listed under "Circumference/ segmental constant" by the value listed for "Total body circumferences/ 100," then multiply by 100, and record the value in the appropriate box under "Proportional score."

> Proportional score = [(Circumference/segmental constant) divided by (Total body circumferences/100)] × 100

10. Plot each proportional score on the adjacent Somatogram grid and connect the points to determine the pattern of the Somatogram.

11. Interpret the Somatogram patterns as follows:

    a. An average body build is indicated when all proportional scores are between 95 and 105. See figure 38.1 for an example.

    b. Body weight versus frame size relationships are reflected in the wrist, knee, and ankle proportional scores. If two or more of these proportional scores are less than 95, overweightness is indicated. If two or more are greater than 105, underweightness is indicated.

    c. Excessive body fat distribution is often reflected in a large proportional score (greater than 105) for the abdomen $\bar{X}$ circumference. Large proportional scores (greater than 105) for the chest, hips, and thigh circumferences may also reflect excessive body fat distributions. The chest and thigh, however, may also be large due to extreme muscularity in some males.

    d. Pronounced muscular development is reflected in large proportional scores (greater than 105) for the forearm, flexed arm, shoulders, and calf circumferences.

Circumference Sites (cm)

Wrist: the maximal girth (distance around) distal to the styloid processes of the radius and ulna (see photo 38.1).

Forearm: the maximal girth with the arm extended and hand supinated (see photo 38.2).

Flexed arm: the maximal girth over the biceps muscle with the elbow flexed and muscle contracted (see photo 38.3).

Shoulder: across the maximal protrusion of the deltoids (see photo 38.4).

Chest: at the nipple line in males and just above the breast tissue in females (see photos 38.5a and 38.5b).

Abdomen 1 (also called waist 1 in Lab 35): at the level of the "natural waist," midway between the xyphoid process and umbilicus (see photo 38.6).

Abdomen 2 (also called waist 2 in Lab 35): at the level of the umbilicus and iliac crests (see photo 38.7).

Abdomen x̄: Average of Abdomen 1 and Abdomen 2 circumferences.

Hips: at the level of the pubis symphysis and the maximal protrusion of the gluteal muscles (see photo 38.8).

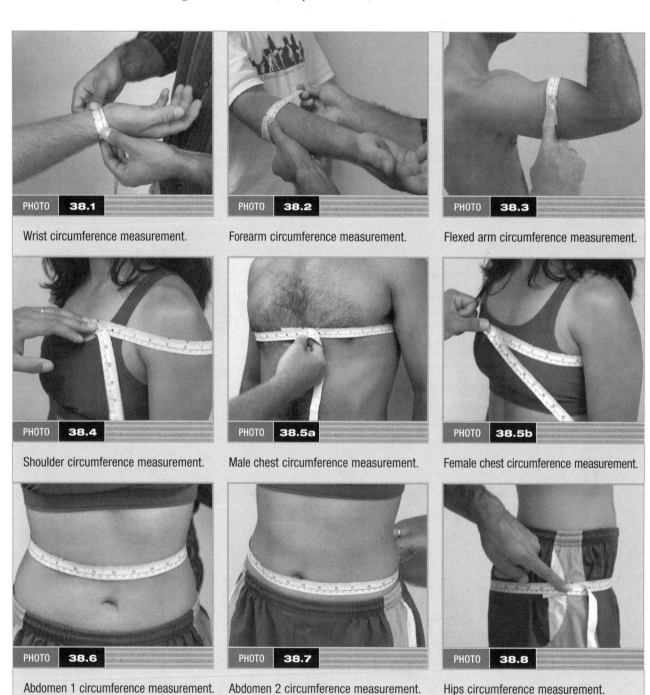

PHOTO **38.1**

Wrist circumference measurement.

PHOTO **38.2**

Forearm circumference measurement.

PHOTO **38.3**

Flexed arm circumference measurement.

PHOTO **38.4**

Shoulder circumference measurement.

PHOTO **38.5a**

Male chest circumference measurement.

PHOTO **38.5b**

Female chest circumference measurement.

PHOTO **38.6**

Abdomen 1 circumference measurement.

PHOTO **38.7**

Abdomen 2 circumference measurement.

PHOTO **38.8**

Hips circumference measurement.

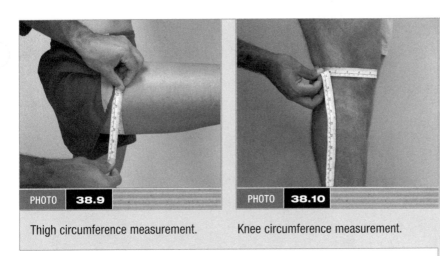

PHOTO **38.9**

Thigh circumference measurement.

PHOTO **38.10**

Knee circumference measurement.

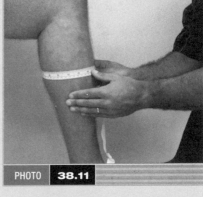

PHOTO **38.11**

Calf circumference measurement.

Thigh: the maximal girth inferior to the gluteal fold (see photo 38.9).

Knee: at the level of mid-patella (see photo 38.10).

Calf: the maximal girth (see photo 38.11).

Ankle: the minimal girth superior to the malleoli (see photo 38.12).

Sample Calculations

Figure 38.1 provides a completed sample Somatogram.

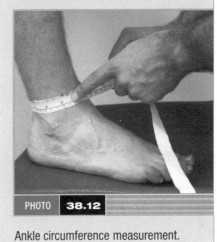

PHOTO **38.12**

Ankle circumference measurement.

Worksheet 38.1 SOMATOGRAM

Name _____

Gender _____

MEASURE	CIRCUMFERENCES (cm)	FEMALE SEGMENTAL CONSTANT	MALE SEGMENTAL CONSTANT	CIRCUMFERENCE/ SEGMENTAL CONSTANT	PROPORTIONAL SCORE	SOMATOGRAM GRID
Wrist		2.73	2.88			
Forearm		4.15	4.47			
Flexed Arm		4.80	5.29			
Shoulder		17.51	18.47			
Chest		14.85	15.30			
Abdomen $\bar{X}$		12.90	13.07			
Hips		16.93	15.57			
Thigh		10.03	9.13			
Knee		6.27	6.10			
Calf		6.13	5.97			
Ankle		3.70	3.75			
Total Body Circumferences		100.00	100.00			

90 95 100 105 110

Name   Date

1. An individual who had proportional scores on the Somatogram of wrist = 90, knee = 93, and ankle = 94 would be classified as (circle one answer below):

   a. Underweight

   b. Overweight

   c. Normal weight

2. An individual with pronounced muscular development would likely exhibit which of the following proportional scores on the Somatogram (circle all correct answers)?

   a. Abdomen $\bar{X}$ = 103

   b. Knee = 92

   c. Flexed arm = 107

   d. Shoulders = 98

   e. Hips = 105

   f. Ankle = 97

   g. Calf = 108

3. Have your circumferences measured, record them on worksheet 38.1, and plot your proportional scores on the Somatogram grid. Based on your Somatogram, classify yourself as underweight, normal weight, or overweight.

   Classification = _____

   What did you base this classification on?

EXTENSION QUESTIONS

1. What are some common mistakes that may occur in administering this lab?

2. Identify possible sources of error in this lab.

3. Assess the practicality of using this lab in the field.

4. Research the reliability and/or validity of this lab using online resources, journal articles, and other credible sources.

REFERENCES

1. Behnke, A. R., and Wilmore, J. H. *Evaluation and Regulation of Body Build and Composition.* Englewood Cliffs, NJ: Prentice-Hall, 1974.
2. Callaway, C. W., Chumlea, W. C., Bouchard, C., Himes, J. H., Lohman, T. G., Martin, A. D., Mitchell, C. D., Mueller, W. H., Roche, A. F., and Seefeldt, V. D. Circumferences. In *Anthropometric Standardization Reference Manual,* eds. T. G. Lohman, A. F. Roche, and R. Martorell. Champaign, IL: Human Kinetics, 1988, pp. 39–54.

BACKGROUND

Body build characteristics describe an individual's physique.[1,4,5,6] Unlike body composition measurements that determine the relative proportions of fat and fat-free tissue (see Labs 33 and 34 on underwater weighing and on skinfold estimations), body build assessments describe the distribution of body weight on the skeleton.

Athletes in various sports, as well as non-athletes, have unique body build characteristics. For example, basketball players tend to be tall and thin, while football linemen are usually much heavier with a lower center of gravity. Wrestlers and gymnasts, however, tend to be lean and muscular.

In addition to contributing to successful sports performance, body build characteristics can also have health-related implications.[6] For example, the endomorphic rating from the somatotyping procedures in this laboratory has been associated with the risk of developing a number of diseases including coronary heart disease, obesity, and diabetes.[6] Thus, there are both performance and health-related reasons for assessing body build characteristics.

Somatotyping

Somatotyping characterizes body build in terms of the predominance of each of three components: endomorphy, mesomorphy, and ectomorphy. There are a number of ways to perform somatotyping, including the use of photographs (photoscopic method), anthropometry (using height, weight, skinfolds, circumferences, and diameters), or a combination of the two. In this laboratory, the anthropometric method is used to determine the "decimalized anthropometric somatotype."[5,6]

Endomorphy. *Endomorphy*, the first component of the somatotyping classification, rates the individual in terms of fatness or roundness characteristics.

Mesomorphy. *Mesomorphy*, the second somatotype component, describes the individual's muscularity or musculoskeletal development.

Ectomorphy. The third component of the somatotyping classification, *ectomorphy*, rates the individual in terms of linearity of body build based on the relationship between height and weight.

After the separate endomorphy, mesomorphy, and ectomorphy components are calculated, the individual's somatotype characteristics are defined by a three-number combination of the components. That is, an individual who has an endomorphic rating of 2, mesomorphic rating of 3.5, and ectomorphic rating of 5.5 has a somatotype rating of 2-3.5-5.5 (read as 2, 3.5, 5.5). The first (endomorphy), second (mesomorphy), and third (ectomorphy) components are always listed in the same order. There is no upper limit to the rating scale for each component, but values of 2 to 2.5 are considered low, 3 to 5 moderate, 5.5 to 7 high, and greater than 7.5 very high.[5] Thus, an individual with a somatotype rating of 2-3.5-5.5 has a body build characterized by a low level of fatness (endomorphic rating of 2), moderate muscularity (meso-morphic rating of 3.5), and a high degree of linearity (ectomorphic rating of 5.5). This somatotype rating is typical of a basketball player at the center or forward position.[6] On the other hand, a male body builder may have a somatotype rating of 2-8-1, which reflects a low level of fatness (endomor-phic rating of 2), extreme muscularity (mesomorphic rating of 8), and a very low linearity of build (ectomorphic rating of 1).[6] Table 39.1 lists examples of somatotype ratings for non-athletes and athletes in various sports.

| TABLE | 39.1 | Examples of somatotype ratings for non-athletes and athletes in various sports. |

Females	Endomorphy	Mesomorphy	Ectomorphy
1. College students[6]	4.2	3.7	2.6
2. Non-athletes[3]	3.57	3.35	2.9
3. Junior Olympic swimmers[14]	3.6	3.4	3.3
4. Professional soccer players[4]	3.07	3.55	2.43
5. Olympic canoers[9]	2.8	4.0	2.9
6. Olympic gymnasts[9]	2.2	3.9	3.4
7. Olympic rowers[9]	3.0	3.9	2.8
8. Olympic swimmers[9]	3.2	3.8	3.1
9. Olympic track & field athletes[9]	2.3	3.4	3.5
10. College basketball players[6]	3.3	3.5	2.8
11. College volleyball players[6]	3.1	3.4	3.2
12. South Australian athletes[17]	3.8	4.2	2.6
13. Body builders[6]	2.5	5.1	2.5

Males	Endomorphy	Mesomorphy	Ectomorphy
1. College students[6]	3.1	5.1	2.7
2. Physical Education majors[7]	2.9	5.4	2.4
3. Young adults 18–29 years[6]	4.1	4.4	2.7
4. Junior Olympic swimmers[14]	2.8	4.5	3.3
5. High school wrestlers[8]	2.77	4.49	3.15
6. South Australian track & field athletes[16]	2.0	4.7	3.4
7. International soccer players[6]	2.5	5.0	2.5
8. Olympic canoers[6]	1.8	5.4	2.6
9. Olympic gymnasts[6]	1.4	5.8	2.5
10. Olympic rowers[6]	2.3	5.0	2.7
11. Olympic swimmers[6]	2.1	5.1	2.8
12. Olympic marathoners[6]	1.4	4.4	3.4
13. Olympic sprinters[6]	1.7	5.2	2.8
14. Olympic basketball players[6]	2.0	4.2	3.5
15. Olympic volleyball players[6]	2.3	4.4	3.4
16. Body builders[6]	1.6	8.7	1.2
17. College football players[6]	4.6	6.3	1.4

KNOW THESE TERMS & ABBREVIATIONS

○ ectomorphy = the third component of the somatotyping classification, a rating of the individual in terms of linearity of body build based on the relationship between height and weight

○ endomorphy = the first component of the somatotyping classification, a rating of the individual in terms of fatness or roundness characteristics

○ mesomorphy = the second somatotype component, a rating of the individual in terms of the individual's muscularity or musculoskeletal development

○ ponderal index = height in cm / cube root of body weight in kg—a height/weight ratio, estimated either from a nomogram or by use of a calculator

○ somatochart = a two-dimensional graph on which the X and Y coordinates are calculated from the three somatotype components (endomorphy, mesomorphy, and ectomorphy)

PROCEDURES

To calculate the three components of the somatotype rating, 10 anthropometric measurements need to be taken: height, body weight, four skinfolds, two diameters, and two circumferences. The following list includes all of the measurements needed to determine an individual's somatotype rating.

1. Height in centimeters without shoes (inches × 2.54 = cm; see photo 39.1)

2. Body weight in kilograms without shoes (pounds / 2.2046 = kg; see photo 39.2)

3. Skinfolds in millimeters (inches × 25.4 = mm)

   Procedures to measure skinfolds:

   a. Measure and mark the anatomical site with a marker (see sites below).

   b. Take all measurements on the right side of the body.

   c. Grasp the skinfold firmly with the thumb and finger and pull away from the body.

   d. Hold the caliper perpendicular to the skinfold. The caliper should be approximately 1 cm away from the thumb and forefinger so that the pressure of the caliper will not be affected.

   e. Read the skinfold size approximately 1 to 2 seconds after the caliper thumb grip has been released.

   f. Take three measurements per site at least 15 seconds apart to allow the skinfold site to return to normal. Record the skinfold values on worksheet 39.1. If the repeated measurements vary by more than 1 mm, more measurements should be taken. Use the mean of the recorded measurements that agree within 1 mm.

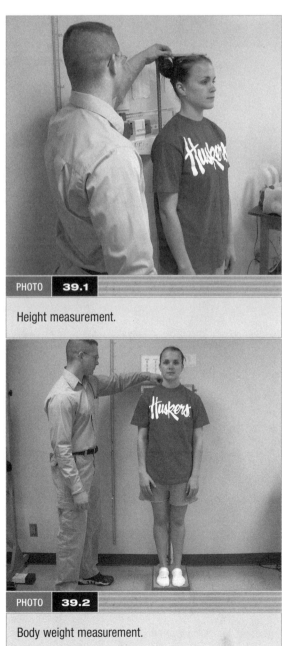

PHOTO **39.1**

Height measurement.

PHOTO **39.2**

Body weight measurement.

Skinfold Sites[6,10,12]

Triceps: a vertical fold on the posterior midline of the upper arm, halfway between the acromion and olecranon processes; the elbow should be extended and relaxed (see photo 39.3).

Suprailium: a diagonal fold above the crest of the ilium at the spot where an imaginary line would come down from the anterior axillary line (see photo 39.4).

Subscapular: a diagonal fold adjacent to the inferior angle of the scapula (see photo 39.5).

Medial calf: a vertical fold on the medial side of the leg, at the level of maximum circumference of the calf (see photo 39.6).

4. *Procedures to measure diameters:*
   a. Palpate for bony landmarks of the right limbs (see sites below).
   b. Hold anthropometer so that the tips of the index fingers are adjacent to the tips of the blades of the anthropometer.
   c. Position the blades of the anthropometer with sufficient pressure to assure they are measuring bony landmarks.
   d. Take three measurements per site and use the mean of repeated recordings that agree within 0.5 cm. Record the diameter values on worksheet 39.1.

Diameter Sites[6,15]

Elbow: the distance between the medial and lateral epicondyles of the humerus (see photo 39.7).

Knee: the distance between the medial and lateral epicondyles of the femur (see photo 39.8).

5. *Procedures to measure circumferences (see photos 39.9–39.10):*
   a. Identify the landmarks of the right limbs (see sites below).
   b. Place the tape perpendicular to the long axis of the limb.
   c. Hold the tape tightly around the limb, but do not compress the underlying tissue.

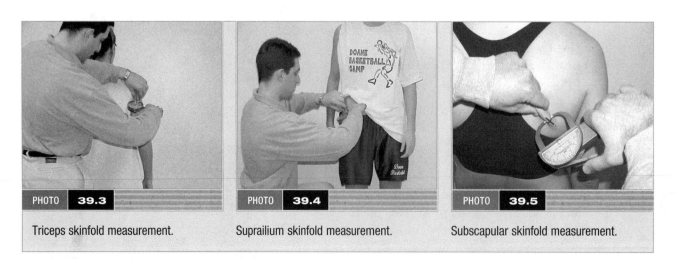

PHOTO **39.3**
Triceps skinfold measurement.

PHOTO **39.4**
Suprailium skinfold measurement.

PHOTO **39.5**
Subscapular skinfold measurement.

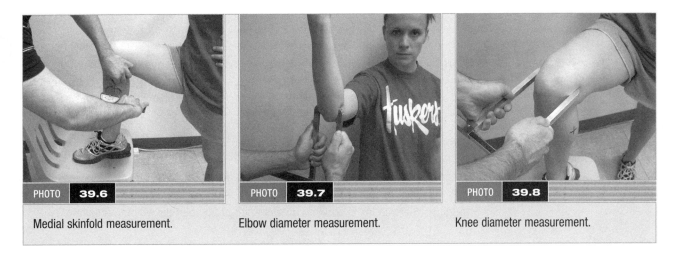

| PHOTO **39.6** | PHOTO **39.7** | PHOTO **39.8** |
| Medial skinfold measurement. | Elbow diameter measurement. | Knee diameter measurement. |

d. Take three measurements per site and use the mean of repeated recordings that agree within 0.5 cm. Record the circumference values on worksheet 39.1.

Circumference Sites[2,6]

Flexed arm: the maximal distance around the flexed biceps and triceps (see photo 39.9).

Calf: the maximal distance around the calf with the subject standing and feet slightly apart (see photo 39.10).

Equations

The following equations are used to calculate the endomorphic, mesomorphic, and ectomorphic ratings.[5,6]

Endomorphy

Height-corrected endomorphic rating

$= -0.7182 + 0.1451$ ((sum of triceps, suprailium, and subscapular skinfolds) $\times$ (170.18/height in cm))

$- 0.00068$ (sum of 3 skinfolds $\times$ (170.18/height in cm))^2

$+ 0.0000014$ (sum of 3 skinfolds $\times$ (170.18/height in cm))^3

Mesomorphy

Mesomorphic rating

$= [(0.858 \times$ elbow diameter) $+ (0.601 \times$ knee diameter) $+ (0.188 \times$ (flexed arm circumference $-$ triceps skinfold/10))

$+ (0.161 \times$ (calf circumference $-$ calf medial skinfold/10))]

$- (0.131 \times$ height) $+ 4.50$

Ectomorphy

The ectomorphic rating is based on the height–body weight ratio or ponderal index.[3,11]

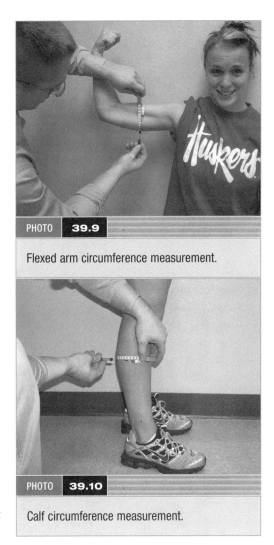

PHOTO **39.9**

Flexed arm circumference measurement.

PHOTO **39.10**

Calf circumference measurement.

ponderal index = height in cm/cube root of body weight in kg

The ponderal index can be estimated from the nomogram in figure 39.1. The cube root of body weight can be determined by use of a calculator with a y^x key. To get the cube root, enter body weight, press y^x, enter 0.333, and press "equals."[5]

Based on the ponderal index, the ectomorphic rating is determined as follows:

If the ponderal index is greater than or equal to 40.75, then the ectomorphic rating = 0.732 × ponderal index − 28.58.

If the ponderal index is less than 40.75 and greater than 38.25, then the ecto-morphic rating = 0.463 × ponderal index − 17.63.

If the ponderal index is equal to or less than 38.25, then the ectomorphic rating = 0.1.

Sample Calculations

Height: __176.0 cm__

Body weight: __62.8 kg__

Triceps skinfold: __11.0 mm__

Suprailium skinfold: __14.0 mm__

Subscapular skinfold: __9.0 mm__

Medial calf skinfold: __15.0 mm__

Elbow diameter: __6.5 cm__

Knee diameter: __9.0 cm__

Flexed arm circumference: __27.85 cm__

Calf circumference: __35.75 cm__

Height-corrected endomorphic rating = −0.7182 + 0.1451 ((11+14+9) × (170.18/176)) − 0.00068 $(32.9)^2$ + 0.0000014 $(32.9)^3$ = 3.36

Mesomorphic rating = [(0.858 × 6.5) + (0.601 × 9.0) + (0.188 × (27.85 − 1.1)) + (0.161 × (35.75 − 1.5))] − (0.131 × 176) + 4.50 = 3.03

Ectomorphic rating

ponderal index = $176.0/\sqrt[3]{62.8}$ = 176.0/3.97 = 44.33

Thus, ectomorphic rating = 0.732 × 44.33 − 28.58 = 3.87

Somatotyping rating = 3.36 − 3.03 − 3.87

Somatochart

Somatotype ratings can be visualized and compared to characteristics of various populations by plotting them on a somatochart (figures 39.2–39.4). While the somatotype includes three components (endomorphy, mesomor-phy, and ectomorphy), the somatochart plots the somatotype on a two-dimensional graph. To do so, X and Y coordinates are calculated from the three components as shown on p. 300.[5,13]

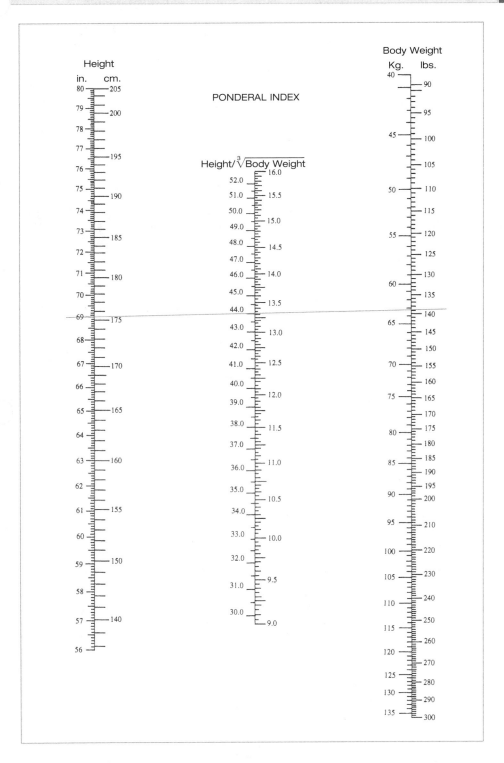

To estimate the ponderal index, lay a ruler between the height on the left column and body weight on the right column. Read the ponderal index value where the ruler crosses the center column. For example, the subject in the sample calculation had a height of 176.0 cm, body weight of 62.8 kg, and a ponderal index of 44.33.

X = ectomorphic rating – endomorphic rating

Y = 2 × mesomorphic rating – (endomorphic + ectomorphic ratings)

The X and Y coordinates can then be plotted on the somatochart. For example, figure 39.2 is the somatochart for the individual with a somatotype of 3.36 (endomorphy)-3.03 (mesomorphy)-3.87 (ectomorphy).

X = 3.87 – 3.36 = 0.51

Y = 2 × 3.03 – (3.36 + 3.87) = –1.17

Figures 39.3 and 39.4 include the somatotypes of various male and female athletes as well as non-athletes (see table 39.1) on somatocharts. Figures 39.5 and 39.6 are blank somatocharts.

FIGURE **39.2** Somatochart for somatotype ratings of 3.36-3.03-3.87 (X coordinate = 0.51 and Y coordinate = –1.17).

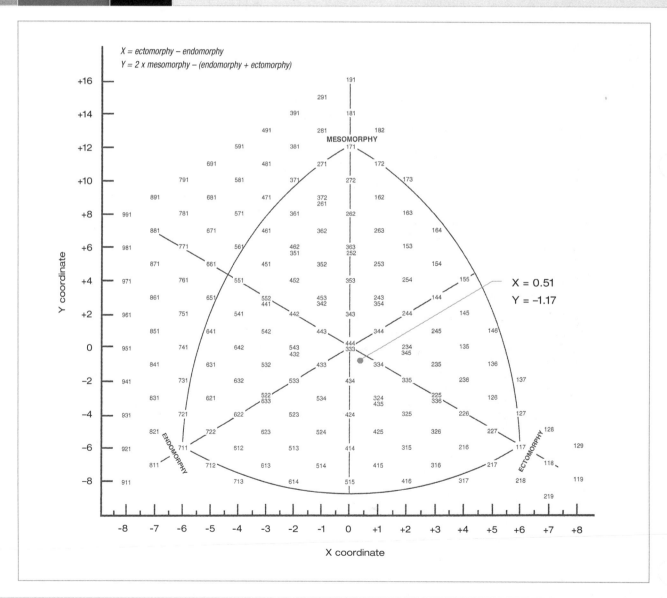

Somatochart examples of male athletes and non-athletes (see table 39.1).   FIGURE   39.3

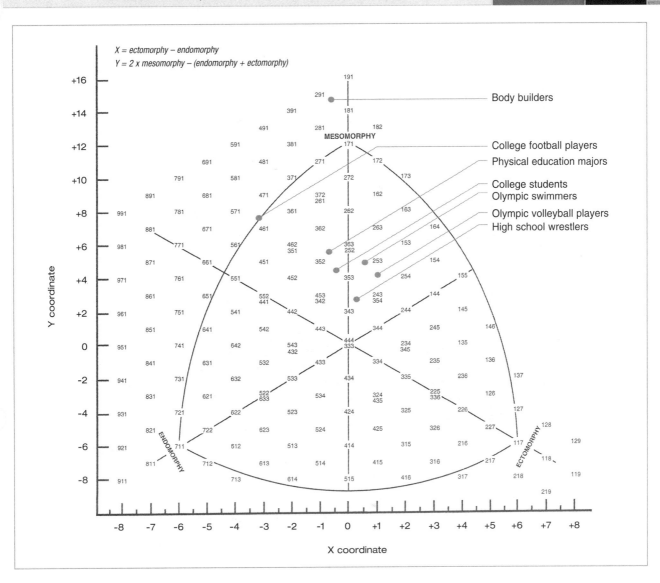

FIGURE   39.4   Somatochart examples of female athletes and non-athletes (see table 39.1).

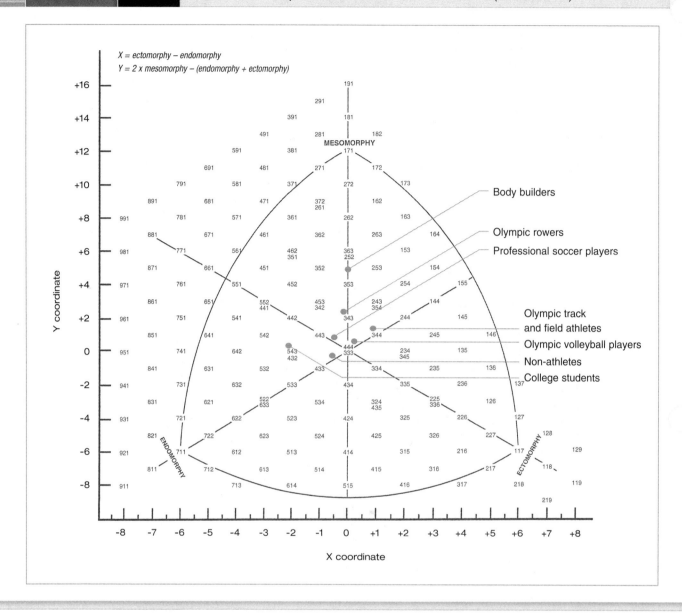

ANTHROPOMETRIC SOMATOTYPING

Name _____   Date _____

Height: _____ cm

Height-correction = 170.18 / height in cm: _____

Body weight: _____ kg

	Trial 1	Trial 2	Trial 3	Mean
Triceps skinfold (mm)	_____	_____	_____	_____
Suprailium skinfold (mm)	_____	_____	_____	_____
Subscapular skinfold (mm)	_____	_____	_____	_____
Sum of triceps, suprailium, and subscapular skinfolds (mm) =				_____
Medial calf skinfold (mm)	_____	_____	_____	_____
Elbow diameter (cm)	_____	_____	_____	_____
Knee diameter (cm)	_____	_____	_____	_____
Flexed arm circumference (cm)	_____	_____	_____	_____
Flexed arm circumference (cm) minus triceps skinfold (mm) / 10 =				_____
Calf circumference	_____	_____	_____	_____
Calf circumference (cm) minus calf skinfold (mm) / 10 =				_____

Endomorphic rating: _____

Mesomorphic rating: _____

Ectomorphic rating: _____

Somatotype rating: _____ – _____ – _____

X coordinate: _____

Y coordinate: _____

Somatochart: Use figure 39.5.

FIGURE **39.5** Blank somatochart.

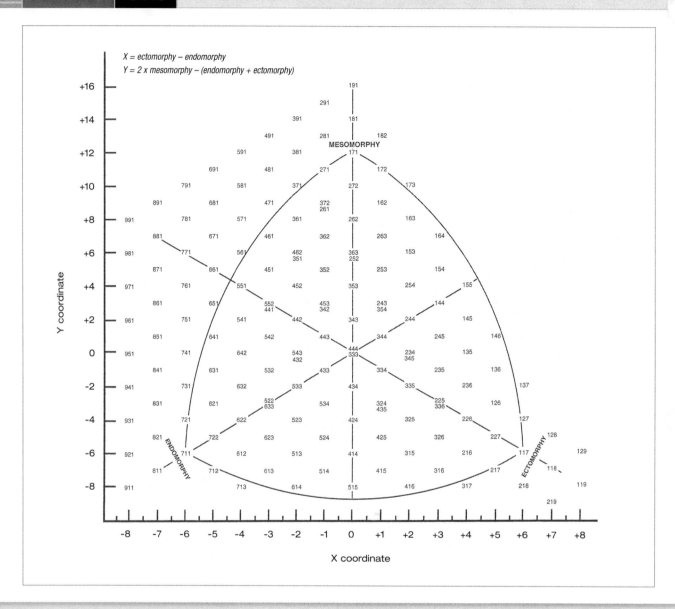

Worksheet **39.2**

Name _____ *Date* _____

1. Given the following data, calculate: (a) endomorphic rating, (b) mesomorphic rating, (c) ectomorphic rating, (d) X coordinate, and (e) Y coordinate.

   Data:

   Height: _172.0 cm_

   Body weight: _68.5 kg_

   Triceps skinfold: _17.0 mm_

   Suprailium skinfold: _16.0 mm_

   Subscapular skinfold: _13.0 mm_

   Medial calf skinfold: _14.0 mm_

   Elbow diameter: _7.5 cm_

   Knee diameter: _9.0 cm_

   Flexed arm circumference: _29.6 cm_

   Calf circumference: _37.9 cm_

   a. Endomorphic rating: _____

   b. Mesomorphic rating: _____

   c. Ectomorphic rating: _____

   d. X coordinate: _____

   e. Y coordinate: _____

2. Using the somatotype ratings in table 39.1: (a) calculate the X and Y coordinates for female Junior Olympic swimmers; female Olympic canoers; and male Olympic marathoners, and (b) plot these three sets of X and Y coordinates on the blank somatochart in figure 39.6.

	X	Y
Female Junior Olympic swimmers	_____	_____
Female Olympic canoers	_____	_____
Male Olympic marathoners	_____	_____

FIGURE **39.6** Blank somatochart.

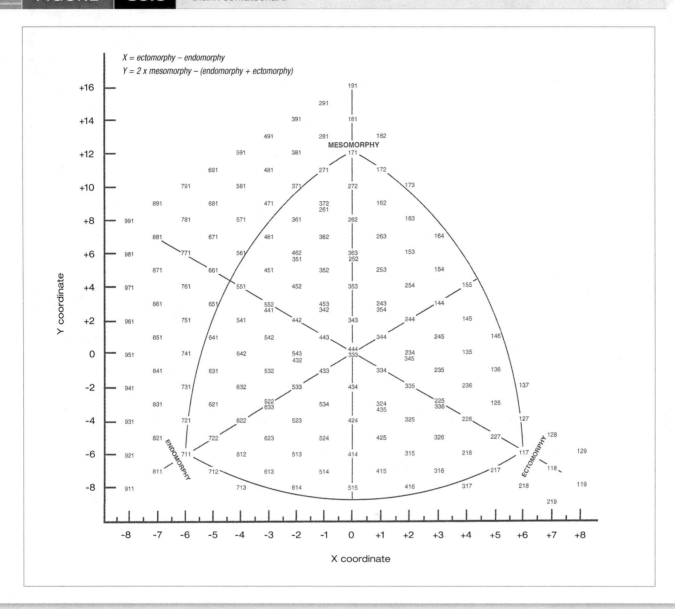

EXTENSION QUESTIONS

1. What are some common mistakes that may occur in administering this lab?

2. Identify possible sources of error in this lab.

3. Assess the practicality of using this lab in the field.

4. Research the reliability and/or validity of this lab using online resources, journal articles, and other credible sources.

REFERENCES

1. Behnke, A. R., and Wilmore, J. H. *Evaluation and Regulation of Body Build and Composition.* Englewood Cliffs, NJ: Prentice-Hall, 1974.

2. Callaway, C. W., Chumlea, W. C., Bouchard, C., Himes, J. H., Lohman, T. G., Martin, A. D., Mitchell, C. D., Mueller, W. H., Roche, A. F., and Seefeldt, V. D. Circumferences. In *Anthropometric Standardization Reference Manual,* eds. T. G. Lohman, A. F. Roche, and R. Martorell. Champaign, IL: Human Kinetics, 1988, pp. 39–54.

3. Can, F., Yilmaz, I., and Erden, Z. Morphological characteristics and performance variables of women soccer players. *J. Strength Cond. Res.* 18: 480–485, 2004.

4. Carter, J. E. L. *The Heath–Carter Somatotype Method.* San Diego, CA: San Diego University Press, 1980.

5. Carter, J. E. L. Somatotyping. In *Anthropometrica,* eds. K. Norton and T. Olds. Sidney, Australia: University of New South Wales Press, 1996, pp. 147–170.

6. Carter, J. E. L., and Heath, B. H. *Somatotyping—Development and Applications.* Cambridge, MA: Cambridge University Press, 1990.

7. Carter, J. E. L., Stepnicka, J., and Clarys, J. P. Somatotypes of male physical education majors in four countries. *Res. Q. Exerc. Sport* 44: 361–371, 1973.

8. Cisar, C. J., Johnson, G. O., Fry, A. C., Housh, T. J., Hughes, R. A., Ryan, A. J., and Thorland, W. G. Preseason body composition, build, and strength as predictors of high school wrestling success. *J. Appl. Sport Sci. Res.* 1: 66–70, 1987.

9. Cressie, N. A. C., Withers, R. T., and Craig, N. P. The statistical analysis of somatotype data. *Yearbook of Physical Anthropology* 29: 197–208, 1986.

10. Harrison, G. G., Buskirk, E. R., Carter, J. E. L., Johnston, F. E., Lohman, T. G., Pollock, M. L., Roche, A. F., and Wilmore, J. Skinfold thicknesses and measurement techniques. In *Anthropometric Standardization Reference Manual,* eds. T. G. Lohman, A. F. Roche, and R. Martorell. Champaign, IL: Human Kinetics, 1988, pp. 55–70.

11. Housh, T. J., Thorland, W. G., Johnson, G. O., Tharp, G. D., and Cisar, C. J. Anthropometic and body build variables as discriminators of event participation in elite adolescent male track and field athletes. *J. Sports Sci.* 2: 3–11, 1984.

12. Jackson, A. S., and Pollock, M. L. Practical assessment of body composition. *Phys. Sportsmed.* 13: 76–90, 1985.

13. Ross, W. D., and Wilson, B. D. A somatotype dispersion index. *Res. Q. Exerc. Sport* 44: 372–374, 1973.

14. Thorland, W. G., Johnson, G. O., Housh, T. J., and Refsell, M. J. Anthropometric characteristics of elite adolescent competitive swimmers. *Human Biol.* 55: 735–748, 1983.

15. Wilmore, J. H., Frisancho, R. A., Gordon, C. G., Himes, J. H., Martin, A. D., Martorell, R., and Seefeldt, V. D. Body breadth equipment and measurement techniques. In *Anthropometric Standardization Reference Manual,* eds. T. G. Lohman, A. F. Roche, and R. Martorell. Champaign, IL: Human Kinetics, 1988, pp. 27–38.

16. Withers, R. T., Craig, N. P., and Norton, K. I. Somatotypes of South Australian male athletes. *Human Biol.* 58: 337–356, 1986.

17. Withers, R. T., Whittingham, N. O., Norton, K. I., and Dutton, M. Somatotypes of South Australian female games players. *Human Biol.* 59: 575–584, 1987.

Unit 8

FLEXIBILITY

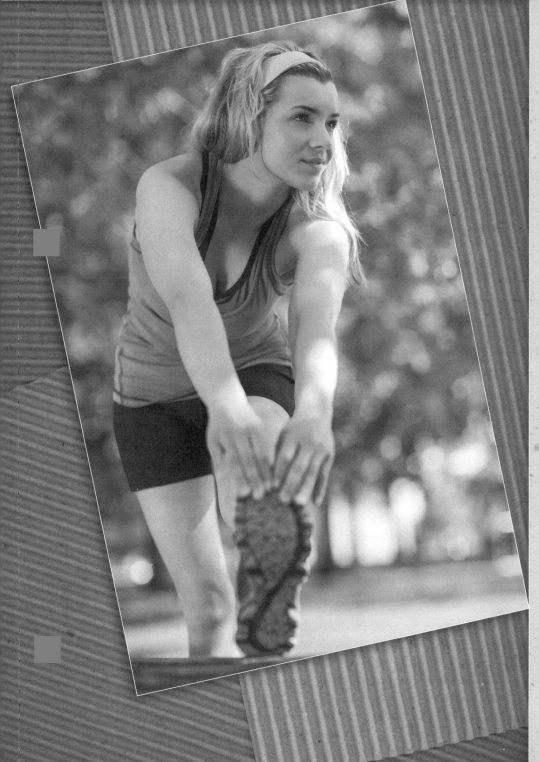

Lab 40

BACKGROUND

Flexibility is a measure of the range of motion at a specific joint. Just because an individual has a large range of motion at the shoulder joint does not mean the person is also "flexible" at the hip joint. Therefore, no single test can adequately represent overall body flexibility. However, many people experience low back pain, which is often related to poor flexibility in the low back and hamstring muscles. Therefore, the sit-and-reach test is the most commonly used measure of flexibility. The sit-and-reach test requires the subject to reach forward, stretching the muscles of the low back and hamstrings. In this laboratory experience, you will learn how to use the sit-and-reach test to evaluate an individual's flexibility, and you will compare the results to norms for individuals of the same age and gender (see tables 40.1 and 40.2).

KNOW THESE TERMS & ABBREVIATIONS

- flexibility = a measure of the range of motion at a specific joint
- percentile rank = in this lab, a score between 1% and 99% that shows how the subject performed relative to others in the age and gender group. A percentile ranking of 70, for example, indicates that the subject's low back and hamstring muscles are equal to or more flexible than 70% of the others in the age and gender group and less flexible than 30% of the others in the age and gender group.

PROCEDURES

1. Have the subject warm up by walking or riding a stationary cycle ergometer and by doing static stretching exercises.

2. Leg position: Have the subject sit down with shoes off with full extension at the knee and with the feet no more than 8 inches apart. The heels should be at the 15-inch mark on the measuring scale (see note below).

3. Arm position: The arms should be extended straight forward with one hand over the top of the other, fingertips even, and palms down (see photo 40.1).

4. For the test, have the subject reach forward along the measuring scale and hold the position for 1 or 2 seconds. Record the point reached on worksheet 40.1, and repeat for a total of three trials.

5. Record on worksheet 40.1 the most distant point reached to the nearest 0.25 inch. If the fingertips are uneven or if flexion at the knee occurs, the test should be repeated (see photo 40.2).

Note: A sit-and-reach box can easily be constructed. The box should be 12 inches high with an overlap toward the subject so that readings can be obtained if the subject is unable to reach the feet. The foot line is set at 15 inches. A bench (or a floor) with a ruler taped onto it can also be used (see photo 40.3).

Sample Calculations

Gender: _Female_

Age: _20 years_

Trial	1	2	3
Score (inches)	20	22	21

High Score = _22_ inches

Approximate percentile rank = _75_ (table 40.1)

Classification = _good_ (table 40.1)

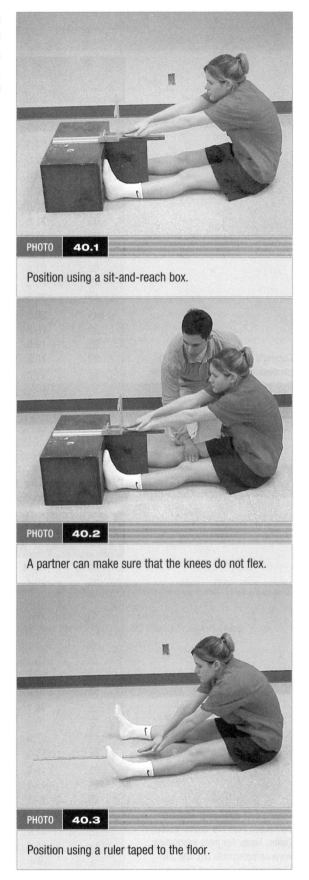

PHOTO **40.1**

Position using a sit-and-reach box.

PHOTO **40.2**

A partner can make sure that the knees do not flex.

PHOTO **40.3**

Position using a ruler taped to the floor.

EXTENSION QUESTIONS

1. What are some common mistakes that may occur in administering this lab?

2. Identify possible sources of error in this lab.

3. Assess the practicality of using this lab in the field.

4. Research the reliability and/or validity of this lab using online resources, journal articles, and other credible sources.

REFERENCES

1. *Physical Fitness Assessments and Norms for Adults and Law Enforcement,* 2007. Cooper Institute, Dallas, TX. Available online at www.cooperinstitute.org.

BACKGROUND

Flexibility is a measure of the range of motion at a specific joint. Just because an individual has a large range of motion at the hip joint does not mean the person is also "flexible" at the shoulder joint. Furthermore, the need for flexibility at a specific joint depends on the sports or activities in which the individual participates. For example, baseball pitchers, gymnasts, swimmers, and wrestlers require great flexibility at the shoulder joint, while swimmers, dancers, divers, and jumpers (long jump, high jump, triple jump, etc.) need substantial ankle flexibility. Therefore, flexibility assessments should be selected based on the demands of the sport or activity.

In this laboratory, you will learn to use the shoulder elevation and trunk extension tests to evaluate an individual's flexibility, and you will compare the results to gender-specific norms for young adults.

KNOW THESE TERMS & ABBREVIATIONS

- flexibility = a measure of the range of motion at a specific joint

- percentile rank = in this lab, a score between 10% and 90% that shows how the subject performed relative to others in the gender group. A percentile ranking of 70, for example, indicates that the subject's flexibility rating and scores are higher than 70% of the others in the gender group and lower than 30% of the others in the gender group.

- static stretching = a stretching method where specified joints are locked into a position that places the muscles and connective tissues passively at their greatest possible length, and held for 10 to 60 seconds

PROCEDURES

Shoulder Elevation Test[1,2]

1. The shoulder elevation test requires measuring the subject's arm length, which is defined as the distance between the acromion process (top of the shoulder) and the palm of the hand. To do so, have the subject stand and grasp a yardstick with the arms fully extended and hands pronated (see photo 41.1). Measure the distance (in inches) between the acromion process and the top of the yardstick. Record the arm length on worksheet 41.1.

2. Have the subject warm up by walking or riding a stationary cycle ergometer and doing static stretching exercises of the trunk, shoulders, and arms.

3. Have the subject lie face-down on the floor with the arms fully extended above the head and grasp a yardstick (see photo 41.2). The chin should be touching the floor. Have the subject slowly raise the yardstick from

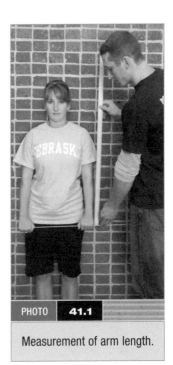

PHOTO **41.1**

Measurement of arm length.

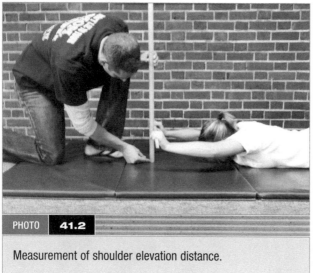

PHOTO **41.2**

Measurement of shoulder elevation distance.

the floor as high as possible. It is important that the subject keep the chin on the floor and arms fully extended while raising the yardstick. Record the distance (in inches) between the yardstick and floor on worksheet 41.1. Repeat for a total of four trials. Use the greatest distance from the four trials in all calculations.

4. Calculate the shoulder elevation score as:

    greatest shoulder elevation distance in inches
    × 100 / arm length in inches

5. Determine the subject's approximate percentile rank and flexibility rating from table 41.1.

Sample Calculations

Gender: _____Male_____

Arm length: _____29 inches_____

Greatest shoulder elevation distance: _____20 inches_____

shoulder elevation score = _20_ (inches) × 100 / _29_

= _____2000 / 29_____ = _____69 inches_____

approximate percentile rank: _49_ (see table 41.1)

flexibility rating: _____below average_____ (see table 41.1)

Trunk Extension Test[1,2]

1. The trunk extension test requires measuring the subject's trunk length, which is defined as the distance between the tip of the nose and the seat of the chair in which the subject is sitting (see photo 41.3). To do so, have the subject sit in a chair, with the back straight and chin level. Place the zero end of a yardstick on the seat of the chair between the subject's legs, and measure the distance between the seat of the chair and the tip of the subject's nose. Record the trunk length on worksheet 41.2.

TABLE	41.1	Percentile ranks, flexibility ratings, and shoulder elevation scores.[1]

Percentile rank	Rating	Shoulder elevation score (inches)	
		MALES	FEMALES
90	Well above average	106–123	105–123
70	Above average	88–105	86–104
50	Average	70–87	68–85
30	Below average	53–69	50–67
10	Well below average	35–52	31–49

2. Have the subject warm up by walking or riding a stationary cycle ergometer and doing upper-body static stretching exercises.

3. Have the subject lie face-down on the floor and place the hands on the lower back (see photo 41.4). Have a second person hold down the legs to stabilize the subject. The subject then slowly raises the trunk (hyperextending the back) from the floor as high and as far back as possible. Record the distance (in inches) between the floor and the tip of the subject's nose on worksheet 41.2. Repeat for a total of four trials. Use the greatest distance from the four trials in all calculations.

4. Calculate the trunk extension score as:

    greatest trunk extension distance in inches × 100 / trunk length in inches

5. Determine the subject's approximate percentile rank and flexibility rating from table 41.2.

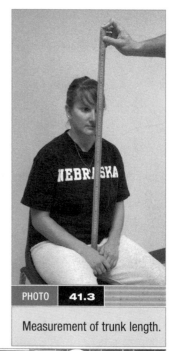

PHOTO   **41.3**

Measurement of trunk length.

Sample Calculations

Gender: ___Female___

Trunk length: ___34 inches___

Greatest trunk extension distance: ___13 inches___

trunk extension score = ___13___ inches × 100 / ___34___

= ___1300 / 34___ = ___38 inches___

approximate percentile rank: ___60___ (see table 41.2)

flexibility rating: ___average___ (see table 41.2)

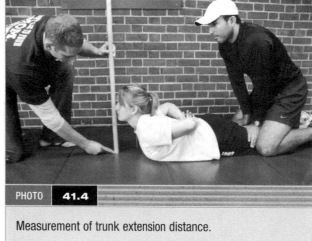

PHOTO   **41.4**

Measurement of trunk extension distance.

| | Percentile ranks, flexibility ratings, and trunk extension scores.[1] | TABLE | 41.2 |

Percentile rank	Rating	Shoulder elevation score (inches)	
		MALES	FEMALES
90	Well above average	50–64	48–63
70	Above average	43–49	42–47
50	Average	37–42	35–41
30	Below average	31–36	29–34
10	Well below average	28–30	23–28

Worksheet 41.1 — SHOULDER ELEVATION TEST FORM

Name _____   Date _____

Gender: _____

Arm length: _____ inches

Shoulder elevation distance (inches)

1	2	3	4
_____	_____	_____	_____

Shoulder elevation score = _____

Greatest shoulder elevation distance in inches × 100 / arm length in inches

_____ (inches) × 100 / _____ (inches) = _____ (inches)

Approximate percentile rank: _____ (see table 41.1)

Flexibility rating: _____ (see table 41.1)

Worksheet 41.2 — TRUNK EXTENSION TEST FORM

Name _____   Date _____

Gender: _____

Trunk length: _____ inches

Trunk extension distance (inches)

1	2	3	4
_____	_____	_____	_____

Trunk extension score = _____

Greatest trunk extension distance in inches × 100 / trunk length in inches

_____ (inches) × 100 / _____ (inches) = _____ (inches)

Approximate percentile rank: _____ (see table 41.2)

Flexibility rating: _____ (see table 41.2)

Name _____   Date _____

1. Use your own data from the shoulder elevation test to determine your approximate percentile rank and flexibility rating (see table 41.1).

   Approximate percentile rank: _____

   Flexibility rating: _____

2. Use your own data from the trunk extension test to determine your approximate percentile rank and flexibility rating (see table 41.2).

   Approximate percentile rank: _____

   Flexibility rating: _____

3. Briefly interpret the meaning of a percentile rank of 50.

4. Identify athletes who might benefit from high shoulder extension and/or trunk extension flexibility.

EXTENSION QUESTIONS

1. What are some common mistakes that may occur in administering this lab?

2. Identify possible sources of error in this lab.

3. Assess the practicality of using this lab in the field.

4. Research the reliability and/or validity of this lab using online resources, journal articles, and other credible sources.

REFERENCES

1. Acevedo, E. O., and Starks, M. A. *Exercise Testing and Prescription Lab Manual.* Champaign, IL: Human Kinetics, 2003, pp. 76–79.

2. Johnson, B. L., and Nelson, J. K. *Practical Measurements for Evaluation in Physical Education.* Edina, MN: Burgess Publishing, 1986, pp. 91–95.

Units and Conversions

Distance

1 inch (in) = 2.54 centimeters (cm)

1 foot (ft) = 12 in = 30.48 cm

= 0.3048 meters (m)

1 yard (yd) = 3 ft = 0.9144 m

1 mile (mi) = 5,280 ft

= 1,760 yd

= 1,609.35 m

= 1.61 kilometers (km)

1 m = 39.37 in = 3.28 ft = 1.09 yd

1 km = 0.62 mi

1 m = 100 cm

1 cm = 10 millimeters (mm)

Weights

1 ounce (oz) = 0.0625 pounds (lb)

= 28.35 grams (g)

= 0.029 kilogram (kg)

1 lb = 16 oz = 454 g = 0.454 (kg)

1 g = 0.035 oz = 0.002205 lb

1 kg = 35.27 oz = 2.205 lb

1 kg = 1,000 g

Volume

1 oz = 29.57 milliliters (mL)

1 pint (pt) = 16 oz = 473.1 mL

1 quart (qt) = 32 oz = 2 pt

= 0.9463 liters (L)

= 946.3 mL

1 gallon (gal) = 128 oz = 8 pt = 4 qt

= 3.785 L = 3785.2 mL

1 L = 1,000 mL = 1.057 qt

Energy

1 kilocalorie (kcal) = 1,000 calories (cal)

= 4,184 joules (J)

= 4.184 kilojoules (kJ)

1 L of oxygen (O_2) = 4.9 kcal = 21.139 kJ

1 kilogram meter (kgm) = energy required to move 1 kg 1 m

Power

power = work/time

1 watt (W) = 0.0134 kcal $\cdot$ min^{-1}

= 6.118 kgm $\cdot$ min^{-1}

1 kgm $\cdot$ min^{-1} = 0.1635 W

1 kcal $\cdot$ min^{-1} = 69.78 W

1 MET = 3.5 mL O_2 $\cdot$ kg^{-1} $\cdot$ min^{-1}

= 0.01768 kcal $\cdot$ kg^{-1} $\cdot$ min^{-1}

Velocity

1 mile per hour (mph) = 88 ft $\cdot$ min^{-1}

= 1.47 ft $\cdot$ s^{-1}

= 0.45 m $\cdot$ s^{-1}

= 26.8 m $\cdot$ min^{-1}

= 1.61 kilometers per hour (kph)

1 kph = 16.7 m $\cdot$ min^{-1}

= 0.28 m $\cdot$ s^{-1}

= 0.91 ft $\cdot$ s^{-1}

= 0.62 mph

Temperature

°F (Fahrenheit) = (1.8 × °C) + 32

°C (Celcius, centigrade) = 0.555 × (°F − 32)

°Kelvin = °C + 273

Pressure

1 atmosphere (atm) = 760 mmHg

% FAT percent fat, the proportion of the body composed of adipose (fat) tissue

1 mile 1.6 km

1-RM one repetition maximum, a standard index to quantify muscle strength, referring to the maximum amount of weight that can be lifted one time

ACSM American College of Sports Medicine

anthropometer an instrument used to measure the diameters of the human trunk and limbs; consisting of two horizontal arms (one movable and one fixed) attached to a vertical rod.

anthropometric relating to the measurement of the size and proportions of the human body

anthropometry the measurement of the size and proportions of the human body

ARC anaerobic running capacity (km), the y-intercept of the total distance (TD) versus time limit (TL) relationship (see figure 19.3b)

ATP adenosine triphosphate

auscultation listening to sounds arising from organs to aid in diagnosis and treatment

AWC anaerobic work capacity (kgm), the y-intercept of the work limit (WL) versus time limit (TL) relationship (see figure 16.2b)

BMI body mass index; body weight in kg/height in meters squared ($kg \cdot m^{-2}$)

BP blood pressure, a measurement of the forces of the blood acting against the vessel walls during and between heartbeats, measured in millimeters of mercury (mmHg)

bradycardia slow resting heart rate <60 bpm

BTPS body temperature pressure saturated

BW body weight

CER caloric expenditure rate ($\dot{V}O_2$ × kilocalories expended per liter of O_2 consumed)

circumference the distance around a landmark on the body

correlation coefficient a numerical measure of the degree to which two variables are linearly related (a number between −1 and 1)

CP critical power (kgm · min^{-1}), the slope coefficient of the work limit (WL) versus time limit (TL) relationship (see figure 16.2b)

CSA cross-sectional area

CT scan computed tomography scan

CV critical velocity (km · hr^{-1}), the slope coefficient of the total distance (TD) versus time limit (TL) relationship (see figure 19.3b)

DB body density

DBW dry body weight

DCER dynamic constant external resistance

diastolic blood pressure the pressure recorded between heartbeats (diastole)

ectomorphy the third component of the somatotyping classification, a rating of the individual in terms of linearity of body build based on the relationship between height and weight

EKG electrocardiogram

endomorphy the first component of the somatotyping classification, a rating of the individual in terms of fatness or roundness characteristics

epidemiological studies studies performed on human populations that attempt to link health effects to a cause, e.g., waist circumference and type 2 diabetes

expiratory reserve volume (ERV) (approximately 800–1200 mL) the maximum volume of gas that can be expired from the end-tidal expiratory level. It is also known as the volume of air present in the resting lungs after a passive exhalation, or resting lung volume (RLV).

fatigue index a number that reflects the anaerobic fatigue capabilities of the muscles that are active during cycling

FFW (fat-free weight) bone, muscle, tendons, viscera, and connective tissue; calculated DBW − FW.

flexibility a measure of the range of motion at a specific joint

FW (fat weight) adipose tissue (subcutaneous and intermuscular and/or intravisceral) and neural tissue; calculated DBW × (% FAT / 100).

hand grip dynamometer an instrument that measures isometric hand grip strength, providing a simple method for characterizing overall body strength

hip extensors the gluteal muscles (gluteus maximus and gluteus medius) and the hamstrings (biceps femoris, semitendinosus, and semimembranosus)

HR heart rate, measured in beats per minute (bpm)

HR monitor equipment used to measure and monitor heart rate, usually including a chest strap (which identifies the heartbeats and transmits the signal telemetrically) and a digital display (which displays the signal as a real-time HR value)

hyperextend to extend a joint beyond the normal range of motion

hypertension an abnormally high BP reading ($\geq$140/90)

inspiratory reserve volume (IRV) (approximately 1900–3100 mL) the maximum amount of gas that can be inspired from the end-tidal (the end of a breath) inspiratory level.

isometric strength tension production by a muscle without movement at the joint or shortening of the muscle fibers

J joule

kgm • min⁻¹ kilogram meters per minute

Korotkoff sounds sounds emitted as a result of pressure exerted against blood vessel walls, providing the basis of traditional BP assessments

leg extensors the quadriceps, made up of the rectus femoris, vastus lateralis, vastus intermedius, and vastus medialis

maximal effort vertical jump total jump height

mean power the total work performed during the 30-second Wingate test (measured in kgm • 30 sec⁻¹) (see Lab 29)

mesomorphy the second somatotype component, a rating of the individual in terms of muscularity or musculoskeletal development

MET metabolic equivalent of task; a measure of the energy cost of exercise defined as the ratio of the metabolic cost of the exercise (mL • kg⁻¹ • min⁻¹) to a reference metabolic cost (resting = 3.5 mL • kg⁻¹ • min⁻¹)

MRI magnetic resonance imaging

multiple regression equation a combination of a number of measurements (independent variables) that best predict a common variable (the dependent variable)

muscular endurance the ability to perform repeated muscle actions that often utilize the same muscles

muscular strength the maximal force that can be exerted by a specific muscle or muscle group

MVIC maximal, voluntary isometric contraction

nomogram a graph that shows the relationship between variables

obesity an excessive amount of body fat

overweightness an excessive body weight compared with the standard body weight based on an individual's height, weight, age, gender, and frame size

P power output (measured in kgm • min⁻¹ or watts)

palpation the act of examining by touch

PAR-Q Physical Activity Readiness Questionnaire, a medical screening assessment that determines who may be at risk during exercise

peak power the greatest work performed during any five-second period (measured in kgm • 5 sec⁻¹) of the Wingate test (see Lab 29)

percentile rank a score, expressed as a percentage, that shows how the subject performed relative to others in a specified group. A percentile ranking of 70, for example, indicates that the subject's score is higher than 70% of the others in the group and lower than 30% of the others in the group.

ponderal index a height/weight ratio, estimated either from a nomogram or the use of a calculator, equal to height in cm / cube root of body weight in kg

power (force $\times$ distance) / time

P wave portion of an EKG that reflects atrial depolarization

PR segment isoelectric point; flat baseline between the P wave and QRS complex in an EKG

Purkinje fibers large-diameter cardiomyocytes that conduct electrical impulses

PVC premature ventricular contraction

PWC$_{HRT}$ physical working capacity at the heart rate threshold (measured in watts), defined as the y-intercept of the power output versus HR slope coefficient relationship (see figure 20.1b)

PWC$_{RPE}$ physical working capacity at the rating of perceived exertion threshold (measured in watts), defined as the y-intercept of the power output versus RPE slope coefficient relationship (see figure 21.2b)

QRS complex portion of an EKG that reflects ventricular depolarization

R multiple correlation coefficient, a numerical measure of how well a dependent variable can be predicted from a combination of independent variables (a number between –1 and 1)

recovery heart rate the HR taken after the end of exercise

reference weight the average weight for an adult with a given frame size

regression equation a statistical method developed and used to relate two or more variables

residual volume (RV) (approximately 1000–1200 mL) the volume of air that remains in the lungs even after a maximal exhalation. After a maximal exhalation, approximately one quarter of total lung capacity (24% for males and 28% for females) will remain as residual volume.

RFWT Rockport Fitness Walking Test

risk stratification categorization of the likelihood of untoward events based on the screening and evaluation of patient health characteristics

RPE rating of perceived exertion

R value respiratory exchange ratio ($\dot{V}CO_2 / \dot{V}O_2$)

RV residual lung volume or the air left in the lungs following a maximal exhalation

SEE standard error of estimate, a measure of the accuracy of predictions made using a regression equation

segmental constant a value that represents what is average for each circumference site measured

SEMG surface electromyography

Somatochart a two-dimensional graph on which the X and Y coordinates are calculated from the three somatotype components (endomorphy, mesomorphy, and ectomorphy)

Somatogram a graphic description of body proportions based on circumference measurements

speed the ability to cover a specific distance as fast as possible

sphygmomanometer the instrument used to measure blood pressure in an artery, consisting of a pressure gauge and a rubber cuff and used with a stethoscope. Mercury and aneroid sphygmomanometers are available.

static stretching a stretching method where specified joints are locked into a position that places the muscles and connective tissues passively at their greatest possible length and held for 10 to 60 seconds

STPD standard temperature pressure dry correction factor

ST segment flat baseline between the QRS complex and T wave in an EKG

systolic blood pressure the pressure exerted against the vessels during a heartbeat (systole)

tachycardia fast resting heart rate >100 bpm

tidal volume (TV) (approximately 500 mL at rest) reflects the depth of breathing; it is the volume of gas inspired or expired during each respiratory cycle.

TL time limit or time to exhaustion (min)

total body power a combination of upper- and lower-body power [(force $\times$ distance) / time] output

T wave portion of an EKG during repolarization of the ventricles

UWW body weight while submerged under water or underwater weight

V velocity (km $\cdot$ hr^{-1})

VC vital capacity

$\dot{V}CO_2$ the volume of CO_2 produced

$\dot{V}CO_2$ L $\cdot$ min^{-1} volume of CO_2 produced

$\dot{V}CO_{2E}$ L $\cdot$ min^{-1} volume of CO_2 expired

$\dot{V}CO_{2I}$ L $\cdot$ min^{-1} volume of CO_2 inspired

V_E volume of gas expired or minute ventilation

$\dot{V}_E$ L $\cdot$ min^{-1} volume of expired gas

$\dot{V}_I$ L $\cdot$ min^{-1} volume of inspired gas (room air)

$\dot{V}O_2$ oxygen consumption rate, an indirect measure of aerobic energy production

$\dot{V}O_2$ L $\cdot$ min^{-1} O_2 consumed per minute

$\dot{V}O_2$ max maximal oxygen consumption rate

$\dot{V}O_{2E}$ L $\cdot$ min^{-1} volume of O_2 expired

$\dot{V}O_{2I}$ L $\cdot$ min^{-1} volume of O_2 inspired

VT ventilatory threshold, an estimation of the exercise intensity above which anaerobic ATP production must supplement aerobic metabolism

W watts

WanT Wingate Anaerobic Test

WL work limit or total work performed (kgm)